Genital Cutting: Protecting Children from Medical, Cultural, and Religious Infringements

George C. Denniston · Frederick M. Hodges
Marilyn Fayre Milos
Editors

Genital Cutting: Protecting Children from Medical, Cultural, and Religious Infringements

Proceedings of the 11th International Symposium on Circumcision, Genital Integrity, and Human Rights, 29–31 July 2010, University of California–Berkeley

Springer

Editors
George C. Denniston
Department of Family Medicine
University of Washington
Nordland, WA
USA

Marilyn Fayre Milos
National Organization of Circumcision
Information Resource Centers
San Anselmo, CA
USA

Frederick M. Hodges
University of Berkeley
Berkeley, CA
USA

ISBN 978-94-007-6406-4 ISBN 978-94-007-6407-1 (eBook)
DOI 10.1007/978-94-007-6407-1
Springer Dordrecht Heidelberg New York London

Library of Congress Control Number: 2013938177

Printed on acid-free paper

Springer is part of Springer Science+Business Media (www.springer.com)

Preface

Human rights are inalienable fundamental rights with which every human being is endowed. Moreover, human rights are *universal*, in that they are applicable everywhere, and *egalitarian*, in that they are the same for everyone without exception. These rights fundamentally exist as *natural rights* because they are not *granted* by law. The purpose of law is to guarantee and protect these pre-existing natural rights from any and all forces or agents that would accidentally or intentionally violate or encroach upon these rights to any degree.

The concept of the *Rights of the Child* has emerged, not as a subset of basic human rights—for every child has the same human rights as any adult—but in recognition of the fact that children, because of their dependence on adults, their vulnerability, and their powerlessness, are more liable than adults to having their human rights violated.

One of the most basic of human rights is the right of the individual to body ownership, that is, the right to physical intactness. Simply stated, every human has the right to keep every body part with which he or she was born. This right seems perfectly obvious and uncontroversial when speaking of a limb such as a foot, leg, hand, arm, ear, or nose. We can all agree that no one has the right to remove another person's leg except under the unusual and particular circumstance of medical necessity in the face of life-threatening disease or severe injury.

Unfortunately, this understandable exception of medical necessity creates a slippery slope down which less justifiable exceptions may slither. As many of the papers in this volume demonstrate, medical personnel regularly and routinely misuse the concept of *medical necessity* to infringe upon the human rights of the most vulnerable among us. One may well ask why doctors would want to do such a thing. The answer is that doctors, together with politicians, police, religious officials, and other members of the ruling elite, find themselves in the role of enforcer of cultural and religious norms. On the other side of the coin, individuals who have the urge to influence or enforce cultural norms have found it as expedient to wear a stethoscope as to wear a crown, a uniform, or a yarmulke.

These and other related issues were examined in the presentations made at the *Eleventh International Symposium on Circumcision, Genital Integrity, and Human Rights Genital Autonomy 2010*, held on 29–31 July 2010, at the University of California in Berkeley. Based on those presentations, the chapters in this book examine the problem of circumcision from medical, psychiatric, legal, ethical, cultural, political, religious, anthropological, and sociological perspectives.

This multi-disciplinary approach illuminates the cross fertilization that permeates and characterizes circumcision. For instance, many of the doctors who promote circumcision within an ostensibly medical context are revealed to have deep-seated, pre-existing religious bias in favor of circumcision. Or, as demonstrated by the analysis provided by Astrik Vardanyan, seemingly incomprehensible promotion of circumcision within the unlikely context of Armenian society occurs because of and despite powerful political and historical pressures brought about by Ottoman oppression. Similarly, J. Steven Svoboda's chapter demonstrates how covert and largely invisible religious and cultural pressures pervert and incapacitate the American judicial system, thereby thwarting the existing civil rights laws that, if applied, would protect every male and female from circumcision. The cherished doctrine of informed consent, as Svoboda argues, has been rendered ineffective so that male circumcision, which is in clear violation of the doctrine, can proceed unimpeded. The reasons for this are as interesting as they are worrisome.

While the reader may sink into pessimism in pondering the findings of many of these papers, Miriam Pollack's thoughtful essay provides a powerful and transformative analysis of the ways in which culture and religion do and can evolve. The slow march up from barbarism toward civilization may be fraught with setbacks and painful difficulties, but with the guidance of rational thinkers like Pollack, progress is inevitable. Because humans have the capacity to understand the concept of *human rights*, it is possible to work harder to guarantee that these rights will be protected so that every human will one day flourish in a world where the basic right to bodily integrity is universally regarded as inviolable.

George C. Denniston
Frederick M. Hodges
Marilyn Fayre Milos

Contents

Contributors

Gregory J. Boyle Faculty of Humanities and Social Sciences, Bond University, Queensland, Australia, e-mail: gregb@bond.edu.an

George C. Denniston Department of Family Medicine, University of Washington, Robbins Road 45, Nordland 98358, Washington, USA, e-mail: gcd@u.washington.edu

Erika Dionisio Anthropology, University of Padua, Padua, Italy

Christopher Fletcher School of Medicine, University of New Mexico, Santa Fe, NM, USA, e-mail: docfrodo@earthlink.net

Stefania Gazzea Psychology, University of Padua, Padua, Italia

Charles L. Geshekter Professor Emeritus, California State University, Chico, CA, USA, e-mail: charlesgeshekter@rethinkingaids.com

David Gisselquist Independent researcher and consultant, Hershey, PA, USA, e-mail: david_gisselquist@yahoo.com

Leonard B. Glick Professor Emeritus of Anthropology, Hampshire College, Amherst, Massachusetts, USA, e-mail: quabbin@rcn.com

Pia Grassivaro Gallo Psychology, University of Padua, Padua, Italia, e-mail: pia.grassivaro@uipd.it

Antonio Iaria Psychology, University of Padua, Padua, Italia

Paul Mason Former Tasmanian Commission of Children, Family Law Attorney, Brisbane, QLD, Australia, e-mail: pmmason@bigpond.net.au

Linda Massie NOCIRC of Northern Ireland, Glengormle, County Antrim, Northern Ireland, e-mail: nocircni@yahoo.co.uk

Miriam Pollack Educator in private practice, Boulder, CO, USA, e-mail: m3pollack@comcast.net

Elizabeth Reis Women's and Gender Studies, University of Oregon, Eugene, OR, USA, e-mail: lzreis@uoregon.edu

Hatem Kamal Saied Founder of the first Arabic online society opposing MGM, Alexandria, Egypt, e-mail: htm_kml@yahoo.com

David Smith General Manager, NORM-UK, Stone, Staffordshire, UK, e-mail: info@norm-uk.org

Michelle Storms Assistant Director and Research Director for the Marquette Family Medicine Residency Program, Marquette, MI, USA, e-mail: stormsmd@att.net

J. Steven Svoboda Attorneys for the Rights of the Child, Berkeley, CA, USA, e-mail: arc@postharvard.edu

John Taylor † Pathology, University of Manitoba, Winnipeg, Manitoba, Canada, e-mail: mtaylor.33@mymts.net

Robert S. Van Howe Clinical Professor, Michigan State University College of Human Medicine, pediatrician for Bell Memorial Hospital in Ishpeming, Michigan, USA, e-mail: rsvanhowe@att.net

Astrik N. Vardanyan Independent Anthropologist, California State University, Northridge, California, USA, e-mail: astrikvardanyan@yahoo.com

Franco Viviani FISPPA and Department of Human Movement Studies, University of Padua, Padua, Italy; Anthropology, University of Padua, Padua, Italy, e-mail: franco.viviani@unipd.it

B. Maurene White Nursing Consultant, Montreal, Quebec, Canada, e-mail: bmwhite41@hotmail.com

Hugh Young Pukerua Bay, New Zealand, e-mail: hugh@buzz.net.nz

Chapter 1
Tortured Bodies, Tortured Doctrines: Informed Consent as a Legal Fiction Inapplicable to Neonatal Male Circumcision

J. Steven Svoboda

Abstract The doctrine of informed consent functions reasonably within its area of applicability of competent adults, though even in that setting it suffers from some difficulties both theoretical and practical. When applied by proxy to incompetent persons such as mentally incapacitated adults and newborn babies, the doctrine becomes a legal fiction, i.e., a legal construct created to force-fit a set of facts into an established legal analysis that is not literally applicable. The conceptual, ethical and practical difficulties are maximized with proxy permission to authorize circumcision of neonates. "Proxy consent" for neonatal circumcision is a legal fiction that cloaks a usurpation of agency allowing ostensibly hallowed principles of autonomy and self-determination to be violated with impunity. Such legal fictions conceal our violations from ourselves and others under the pretenses of legal authorization and compliance with ethics and human rights, and—in the circumcision context—the further pretense of medical authorization, masking our failure to properly safeguard human dignity and autonomy.

Keywords Circumcision • Human rights • Law • Torture • Informed consent • Proxy consent • Medical ethics

1.1 Introduction

Legal fictions are artificial constructs created by the law to facilitate fitting the circumstances of a particular case into an established legal analysis to which the facts do not strictly conform. For example, the legal fiction of implied consent to a blood alcohol level test is imputed to drivers in certain states. No actual consent has been given, but according to this legal fiction, consent is deemed to have been given by the act of driving on the roads in one of these states. The doctrine of informed consent—the idea that the competent patient has the right to give or withhold permission for

J. S. Svoboda (✉)
Attorneys for the Rights of the Child, Berkeley, CA, USA
e-mail: arc@postharvard.edu

G. C. Denniston et al. (eds.), *Genital Cutting: Protecting Children from Medical, Cultural, and Religious Infringements*, DOI: 10.1007/978-94-007-6407-1_1,

proposed medical treatments or procedures based on full knowledge of relevant facts—is one of the foundations of modern medical ethics. This chapter analyzes informed consent as it is applied in its primary setting for competent adults, for incompetent adults, and for never competent children. I find informed consent to be a legal fiction in the latter two settings. The application of what is commonly called informed consent to neonatal male circumcision is analyzed in detail and shown to be the greatest legal fiction of all informed consent settings. When proxy consent is sought for neonatal circumcision, a thicket of conceptual, ethical, and practical difficulties are created. This legal fiction cloaks a usurpation of agency, thereby allowing supposedly respected ethical principles of autonomy and self-determination to be violated with little or no adverse consequences for the violators.

Informed consent is a legal doctrine that is only strictly applicable to a patient capable of consenting, that is, typically, a competent adult. In its intended setting of a competent adult patient, informed consent suffers from a number of theoretical and practical problems. Even basic information is often not effectively communicated to patients, a requirement to show actually damages effectively only protects reasonable patient consents, and a crucially important fourth element to informed consent—patient understanding—is omitted from most doctrinal formulations. Furthermore, informed consent is only applicable to incompetent adult patients via the legal fictions of proxy consent and substituted judgment, each of which introduces a host of distortions and discrepancies. In applying proxy permission to neonatal circumcision, we find ourselves confronted by a thicket of conceptual misapplications and theoretical distortions that stretches beyond the breaking point the ethical, moral, and human rights grounding of a parent's supposed medical permission for the procedure.

Schuck eloquently summarizes the somewhat unique power consent has in our culture:

> Consent is the master concept that defines the law of contracts in the United States. First, consent expresses the primacy of individualistic values in our culture.... Second, consent is instrumental to economic efficiency, a cherished value in American culture.... A third foundation for consent in American law more generally is our abiding, almost obsessive suspicion of state power (Schuck 1994 pp. 900–901).

Subject to certain exceptions—emergencies posing threats to life or danger of grievous bodily harm, self-defense, jostling in a crowd, and contact sports—a person who suffers a touching by another to which they did not consent is entitled to an action in battery. Since ancient times, consent has been the only defense to a cause of action for battery. In a medical context, since at least 1767, courts have agreed that liability for battery results from a completely unauthorized medical procedure or a procedure on a body part different from the one discussed with the patient.[1] Thus surgery is a technical battery that, regardless of the health-care provider's intentions, can be excused only when there is express or implied consent from the patient.[2] This is true even if the treatment proves to be beneficial or even necessary to preserve a

[1] Slater v. Baker and Stapleton, 95 Eng. Rep. 860 (1767).

[2] See Newmark v. Williams, 588 A.2d 1108, 1115–16 (Del. 1991).

patient's life.[3] A defendant who commits battery is liable for all consequences of his wrongful conduct, intended or not, and foreseeable or not.[4]

What liability exists if a procedure is consented to but the consent is not informed? For example, a procedure may be authorized but not properly explained so that the patient understands what he or she is agreeing to. In that event, battery seems not to provide the right analytical frame. According to Harrington, "Battery, with its connotations of violence and criminality, is seen as an inappropriately stigmatic label for doctors seeking in good faith to act in their patients' interests. Instead a duty of disclosure is imposed upon physicians, breach of which sounds in negligence. This requires that the doctor has been at fault by falling below the level of care expected of him by the law as a medical professional" (Harrington 1996, p. 352).

1.1.1 Changes in Doctor–Patient Relationship Usher in Informed Consent

Throughout the ages physicians believed that they, based on their training and expertise, were in the best position to make treatment decisions for their patients. This conviction inheres in the Hippocratic Oath, which does not mention the patient as a person whose ability and judgment deserve consideration. Indeed, in one of the few references to disclosure in the Hippocratic Corpus, physicians are admonished "to [conceal] most things from the patient…." Twenty-six centuries later, in the early 1950s the influential Harvard sociologist Talcott Parsons, who echoed physicians' views, stated that the physician's competence and specific judgments and measures cannot be competently judged by the layman and that the latter must take doctors' judgments and measures on 'authority' (Katz 1994, pp. 73–75).

The power imbalance between patients and doctors is clear. Jones notes, "Part of the imbalance between doctor and patient is due to the patient's lack of information, and, on one view, it is the function of the law to redress the imbalance by providing patients with the 'right' to be given that information, or perhaps more accurately imposing a duty on doctors to provide it" (Jones 1999, p. 129). A little over a half-century ago, American legal cases emerged to alter the relationship between patients and doctors by introduction of the informed consent doctrine.

1.1.2 Birth and Development of Informed Consent in Court Cases

Law, not medicine, drove change in the standards of communication between doctors and patients. In the US, as long ago as 1891, the United States Supreme Court recognized the right of all citizens to bodily integrity and self-determination. "No

[3] See Matter of Storar, 420 N.E.2d 64, 71 (N.Y. 1981).

[4] See Talmage v. Smith, 101 Mich. 370, 59 N.W. 656 (1894).

right is held more sacred, or is more carefully guarded by the common law, than the right of every individual to the possession and control of his own person free from all restraints or interference of others, unless by clear and unquestionable authority of law" (Feigenbaum 1992, p. 862).

Nearly a full century ago, in 1914, while still not requiring informed consent, Justice Cardozo famously proclaimed the importance of consent to medical treatment: "Every human being of adult years and sound mind has a right to determine what shall be done with his own body; and a surgeon who performs an operation without his patient's consent commits an assault for which he is liable in damages."[5]

In the US, the basis for the medical duty of *informed* consent first appeared in 1957 in the decision by the California Court of Appeal in *Salgo v. Leland Stanford, Jr, University Board of Trustees.* The court held that a physician violates a duty to his patient and subjects himself to liability if he withholds any facts that are necessary to form the basis of an intelligent consent by the patient to the proposed treatment.[6] According to Jay Katz, the new principle requiring doctors to share decision-making authority with their patients shocked the medical community and "constituted a radical break with the silence that had been the hallmark of physician-patient interactions throughout the ages" (Katz 1994, p. 72).

Continuing this trend in jurisprudence, *Canterbury v. Spence,* in 1972, held that any competent adult has a right to determine what shall be done with his or her own body, what we might today call a right to bodily integrity. The court held that genuine consent requires a choice that is properly informed. For the choice to be informed, there must be an opportunity to knowledgeably evaluate the alternatives and the risks entailed by each alternative. The court, presumably troubled by the concept of conferring liability simply for not being informed of an option, held that principles of self-determination permit liability only if nondisclosure would have affected the decision of a fictitious "reasonable patient."[7] The patient can only make a recovery if it can be shown that proper information would have produced a different decision, but not by the actual patient, but rather by a hypothetical reasonable patient. Some of the difficulties created by this analysis are discussed below.

In 1979, in *Scott v. Bradford*, the Oklahoma Supreme Court expanded on Canterbury by holding that a physician "has a duty to disclose to a patient all relevant material information his patient will need to make an informed decision on whether to consent to or reject physician's proposed treatment or surgery. This disclosure shall include alternatives to proposed treatment, and the risks of each course of action including those risks inherent in foregoing all treatment." Because of the critical interests at stake, consent must be "informed" in order to be valid: the individual must know to what he is consenting. If the physician has not given the patient all the information that the patient needs to make a knowledgeable

[5] Schloendorff v. Society of New York Hospital, 105 N.E. 92, 93 (N.Y. 1914).

[6] Salgo v. Leland Stanford Jr. University Board of Trustees, 154 Cal. App. 2d 560, 317 P.2d 170 (1957).

[7] Grounded in the ethical principle of respect.

decision regarding his medical care, any consent the patient gives is ineffectual.[8] Grounded in the ethical principle of respect for autonomy, informed consent protects the patient's rights to bodily integrity and self-determination, as well as promotes the patient's interest in rational decision-making (Annas 1977; Berg and Appelbaum 2001; Faden and Beauchamp 1986).

Unfortunately, as we will see, the ideal of informed consent is not always realized in clinical practice. Further, informed consent suffers from numerous shortcomings, both theoretical and practical, problems that exist even within its intended sphere of applicability to competent adults but which become even more intractable when attempts are made to apply informed consent to incompetent adults or to children.

1.2 How Informed Consent Plays Out with Competent Adults

According to Jackson, "Informed consent is commonly used as a shorthand for two distinct duties: the duty to obtain the patient's consent before treatment, and the duty to ensure that the patient has been properly informed about its risks and benefits" (Jackson 2006). Informed consent refers to a process of adequate *disclosure* of relevant information which may then be the basis for a decision to *voluntarily* give (or refuse) consent for medical treatment of a *competent* patient. Disclosure encompasses providing to the patient all information that is *material* to his or her decision regarding whether to agree to a proposed medical procedure including *alternatives* to the procedure. Voluntariness addresses the patient's ability to make health care choices free from manipulation or undue influence, which can include *timing, manner, or order* of disclosure designed to promote a particular decision by the patient. Competence refers to the patient's capacities to understand and process information and to reason about the consequences of possible medical courses of action. Competence relates to an often forgotten fourth element of informed consent—the patient's level of *understanding* of the information provided.

As we will see, even within the realm in which it is squarely applicable—competent adults—informed consent, while retaining some level of logical coherence, suffers from both conceptual and practical problems.

1.2.1 Disclosure

The physician's duty of disclosure arises from the patient's rights to autonomy and self-determination, which imply an entitlement to receive all relevant information prior to authorizing a procedure that otherwise would violate the person's human

[8] Scott v. Bradford, 1979 OK 165; 606 P.2d 554, 559 (1979).

rights and legal rights to privacy, autonomy, and bodily integrity. In addition to honoring the person's autonomy and self-determination, disclosure promotes a patient's ability to cope with the consequences—favorable or otherwise—of the selected procedure.

One widely noted study found that in practice "[o]nly 26 % of [consent] forms included all 4 basic elements" of disclosure (Bottrell et al. 2000, p.26). Similarly, Wu found that "clinicians infrequently communicate the four elements essential for informed consent "(Wu and Pearlman 1988, p. 12).

Numerous studies demonstrate that informed consent operationally fails to function as it is supposed to, even within its most fundamental context of competent adult patients. This breakdown occurs for a variety of reasons. First, physicians fail to satisfy the elements of informed consent. As summarized by Michael Jones, "[w]hatever the reason, many doctors are not good at communicating with patients and there are numerous studies in medical journals which demonstrate that in reality many if not most patients remain completely uninformed" (Jones 1999, p. 129). Moreover, doctors often do not disclose even the most obvious and crucial facts, such as major side effects of treatments (Bottrell et al. 2000, p. 26). One study found limited physician disclosure of side effects of nonsteroidal anti-inflammatory drugs other than epigastric discomfort (Katz et al. 1992, p. 1257).

Disclosure of adequate information is the first step in the informed consent process and review of the information disclosed is relatively tractable compared to less tangible issues such as voluntariness and competence. Accordingly, disclosure is often the primary feature of consent communication in the clinical setting.

On the other hand, courts often focus on disclosure at the expense of the other elements of the informed consent process, which contributes to what can be a counterproductive exercise of physicians disclosing all conceivably relevant information. Karako-Eyal summarizes the problems with this approach:

> First of all, piling vast amount of information onto patients detracts from their ability to understand the information given to them... Second, providing patients with information on *all* of the risks involved in the treatment, including rare risks, is likely to dissuade patients from obtaining needed medical treatment... Third, as the scope of the information given to patients increases, so does the amount of time devoted to the informed consent process and the costs involved therein (Karako-Eyal 2010, p. 20).

Materiality

Materiality as a criterion for disclosure addresses whether a patient would consider a given piece of information relevant to his or her process of evaluating the relative advantages and disadvantages of different treatment options. A physician has a duty to disclose all information that he or she knows—or *should* know—would be regarded as material by a reasonable person, which implies a duty of physicians to keep up to date with the relevant literature (Svoboda et al. 2000).

Naturally, there is a limit to how much and what kind of information medical professionals must provide. Even very slight risks generally must be disclosed to patients, particularly if the consequences may be severe. The High Court of Australia ruled that a physician was negligent for not disclosing a 1 in 14,000 chance that an elective eye operation would leave a patient blind in that eye, even though the risk was slight. The rare complication occurred, and the doctor was found liable.[9]

The Importance of Alternatives

As part of the process of obtaining informed consent prior to a proposed procedure, physicians are required to give patients all reasonably available, relevant information regarding alternative treatments, including the option of doing nothing (Berg and Appelbaum 2001; Wear 1998). The patient should be given enough information about the nature of each therapeutic option, and its advantages and disadvantages, to make a valid choice between alternatives. Informing the patient about options allows him to make decisions by weighing the potential implications of each—both medically and in terms of quality of life issues—based on his personal values, tolerance for risk, life goals, and the like. Ethically, this promotes the patient's autonomy as well as his human right of self-determination by promoting an informed, meaningful decision. Legally, health professionals are liable if alternatives are not adequately disclosed as this failure mitigates any consent thereby obtained as not truly informed.

At least in theory, the alternative of doing nothing always exists. Accordingly, at least in a non-emergency situation, the patient should always be informed of the prognosis with no treatment. As one court's opinion put it, "How can a patient give an informed consent to treatment for a condition if the patient is not informed that the condition might resolve itself without any treatment at all?".[10]

Studies show that alternatives are not being properly disclosed. One study found, "When examined across all decision categories, few decisions (9.0 %) met criteria for completeness of informed decision making." Moreover, "there was seldom discussion of alternatives (5.5–29.5 %) (Braddock et al. 1999, pp. 2317–2318). Another set of researchers determined that while 52 % of physicians mentioned the possibility of alternatives to the procedure in general terms, only 2.3 % specifically described alternatives (Bottrell et al. 2000, p. 29).

1.2.2 Voluntariness

In addition to proper disclosure of material information by health professionals, a second requirement for an informed consent to a procedure is that the decision be made voluntarily. The decision must be freely and autonomously made, absent coercive or unduly manipulative forces. For example, medical personnel must abstain from distorting or omitting information to promote a desired patient choice. The ethical goal of autonomy is thereby safeguarded. On the other hand, coercion or manipulation may

---

[9] Rogers v. Whitaker, 175 C.L.R. 479, 489–491 (Austl. 1992).

[10] Wecker v. Amend, 918 P.2d 658, 661 (Ka. Ct. App. 1996).

by definition alter a patient's decision from what she would have chosen of her own accord. Consent under the influence of such forces is legally and ethically invalid. Even full disclosure does not mitigate the effects of coercion or manipulation.

Timing, Manner, Order

Besides bald coercion and direct manipulation of information, the *process* of informing may be carried out in a range of ways that may impinge on voluntariness by restricting the autonomy of patient participation. The power imbalance between doctor and patient creates a great danger of undue influence. A patient often is for practical purposes restricted to responding to treatment options presented by the physician. Patients are of course often ill and anxious at the time informed consent is sought, rendering them even more vulnerable to influence by medical professionals. Because of this inherent imbalance of power, the timing, manner and order in which physicians present information can persuade the patient to select the option favored by the physician. Physicians should be sensitive to the likelihood that patients may interpret a suggestion, or even the mere mention of an option, as a recommendation.

The timing of disclosure is important. With an elective procedure that can be performed at any time, a physician must provide a patient with full disclosure far in advance to allow the patient sufficient time to reflect on whether to consent to undergo the procedure.

Regarding manner of disclosure, studies on preferable disclosure formats have produced mixed and in some cases surprising results, adding another obstacle of a more practical sort to the theoretical difficulties we reviewed above. Earlier studies seemed to suggest that some form of written disclosure, either alone or in combination with verbal disclosure, imparts greater knowledge than verbal disclosure alone (Etchells et al. 1996). More recently, at least one study suggested the opposite, with a form seemingly interfering with retention. "[P]atients remembered less of the information concerning anesthetic risks discussed during the preoperative interview if they received a preprinted, risk-specific anesthesia consent form at the beginning of the interview" (Clark et al. 1991, p. 13). In an early study producing counterintuitive results, a shorter form (mean score of 67 %) promotes greater understanding than a medium length form (mean score of 45 %), which in turn promotes greater understanding than a long form (mean of 35 %) (Epstein and Lasagna 1969, p. 684).

1.2.3 Competence/Capacity

Competence or capacity, the third element needed for legally and ethically valid informed consent, refers to the patient's ability to understand information regarding treatment decisions and to appreciate the consequences of a decision. This element protects patients' well being by ensuring that they have the cognitive capacities necessary to engage in rational decision-making. Accordingly, physicians must assess whether a patient is capable of both understanding the relevant medical information and making a rational decision based upon that information. While adults are presumed to be competent to give informed consent unless proven otherwise, parents are most often designated as surrogate decision makers for children. The same elements of competence, disclosure, voluntariness, and understanding are required for valid informed consent in the case of surrogates, as for informed consent by a competent patient for himself.

1.2.4 Understanding: The Forgotten Element

A fourth, usually omitted element is that in pursuing informed consent for medical treatment, a physician must provide the information in a manner conducive to a patient's *understanding* of the material. Without understanding, the patient is not in fact informed. Accordingly, she is unable to exercise her rights of self-determination and autonomy and to safeguard her own bodily integrity through an informed decision. Understanding is hard to determine empirically; legally, the predictable result becomes court cases fought over whether every possible complication was mentioned by the physician, often with no attention to the patient's actual comprehension of the material.

Numerous studies document the often strikingly low levels of patient comprehension. A 1988 study in Australia found that 77 % of patients said that they wanted more information about their treatment (Dunkelman 1979, p. 311). Of 100 patients having chemotherapy who were given a written information and consent form, 75 could not name any of their drugs, 26 did not know the goal of therapy and 17 remembered none of the four general side effects. In the author's terse appraisal, "Such forms may not satisfy the requirements of informed consent" (Olver et al. 1995). Robertson emphasizes that the "extent of the patient's comprehension of the disclosed information should... be a vital issue" (Robertson 1981, pp. 111–112). The exercise of informed consent becomes pointless regardless of information disclosed if the information is not understood.

1.2.5 Exceptions to Informed Consent with Competent Adults

Besides situations involving *incompetent* patients, there are several other legally accepted exceptions to the patient's right to informed consent. Several are based on the principle of beneficence and are applicable in cases where the best interests of the individual or society are deemed significant enough to take priority over the patient's right to self-determination. These exceptions include *public health emergencies*, such as when individuals with tuberculosis are legally required to be quarantined and treated, out of a need to promote public safety; and *medical emergencies*, in which a delay in order to obtain informed consent would place the patient at imminent risk of death or significant harm. Another exception that is becoming a relic of the past is the "therapeutic privilege" of the physician to withhold disclosure when the disclosure itself is deemed unduly harmful. A competent patient may voluntarily waive his right to information and/or cede decision making to the physician or someone else, but it is not clear that this "waiver" provides the physician any protection from a negligence suit.[11]

1.2.6 Problems with Informed Consent for Competent Adults

In addition to the practical problems mentioned above, the dictates of informed consent are simply not followed uniformly enough. Braddock found that "the ethical model of informed decision making is not routinely applied in office practice... By the most minimal definition consistent with an ethical framework, decision making in clinical practice may fall short of a basic level of patient involvement in routine decisions" (Braddock 1999, p. 2319).

Moreover, informed consent suffers from at least two glaring conceptual problems evident even in its intended regime of competent adult patients. As decided in *Canterbury v. Spence*, a claimant must typically show actual damage based on reference to a reasonable patient. Yet the right of informed consent obviously cannot logically require a "reasonable" decision as the right then becomes an empty letter. "Physicians, bioethicists, or the state need not agree with the patient's choice, nor even judge the choice reasonable" (Cherry 2010, p. 790).

Perhaps the Oregon Court of Appeals best summed up the self-contradictions of this still reigning approach, in a leading case interpreting and, on this point, questioning *Canterbury v. Spence*: "We are aware of no other context in which it has been suggested that the jury should resolve a question of causation on the basis of a hypothetical effect that a hypothetical defendant's act is likely to have on a hypothetical plaintiff, rather than base its decision on whether the actual defendant's act was the cause of harm to the actual plaintiff."[12] The Oklahoma Supreme Court went even further, rejecting *Canterbury* on this point and eloquently noting what is lost to patients:

> The *Canterbury* view certainly severely limits the protection granted an injured patient. To the extent the plaintiff, given an adequate disclosure, would have declined the proposed treatment, and a reasonable person in similar circumstances would have consented, a patient's right of self-determination is *irrevocably lost.* This basic right to know and decide is the reason for the full-disclosure rule. Accordingly, we decline to jeopardize this right by the imposition of the "reasonable man" standard .[13]

---

[11] Reibl v. Hughes, 114 D.L.R. 3d 1, 15–17 [1980].

[12] Arena v. Gingrich, 733 P.2d 75,76 (1987).

[13] Scott v. Bradford, 1979 OK 165; 606 P.2d 554, 559 (1979).

Nevertheless, this problem persists today as *Canterbury* and the contradictions pointed out in 1979 remain the law in most jurisdictions.

Maclean notes "the inconsistency between what the law claims to be the patient's right and what it is prepared to compensate. The law proclaims that the patient can make any decision regardless of reason. However, it is then only prepared to compensate those cases of a failure to disclose where claimants provide credible evidence that they would have made a different decision." To solve the conundrum, Maclean not unreasonably advocates "establishing a distinct liability for 'breach of consent to medical treatment'" (Maclean 2009).

Secondly, the important fourth element to informed consent—patient understanding—is omitted from most formulations of the doctrine, rendering it both legally and ethically invalid. As discussed above, numerous studies found that understanding is all too often absent from informed consent. Several authors conclude that informed consent seems primarily to be a legal self-protection exercise rather than a process genuinely designed to safeguard the patient's interests (Muss et al. 1979, p. 1556; Bottrell et al. 2000; Cassileth et al. 1980, p. 896).

1.2.7 Informed Consent and Non-therapeutic or Elective Surgery on Competent Adults

Elective surgery refers to surgery as a possible treatment option for non-emergent disease, in which there is not yet a medical consensus that surgery is the best course. Even with competent adults, the physician is under a stringent duty to guard against financial self-interest and to clarify the elective nature of the surgical route, while objectively presenting all reasonable alternatives and their likely benefits and burdens. Because of both the lack of clarity as to optimum treatment and also the longer time horizon for deliberation, Lustig and Scardino have argued that elective surgery demands a more extensive informed consent dialogue over a period of time. Such a process is more likely to give the patient an opportunity to fully absorb and meditate on all options, so as to optimize his autonomy and self-determination in reaching a plan that is best for his unique situation (Lustig and Scardino 1998).

Elective procedures may be subject to a stricter informed consent requirement than medically indicated procedures. A number of legal and medical scholars have suggested that the duty of care for disclosure should be higher when the procedure is elective (Berry 2005; Haberfield 1997; Schuck 1994). The usual practice of informed consent and disclosure of treatment alternatives is based on the premise that a medical problem exists that requires therapeutic intervention of some type for relief or correction of the problem. Somerville states, "a very full disclosure is needed when non-therapeutic medical intervention is involved," justifying this assertion on the grounds of giving patients a chance to more carefully consider deciding *against* procedures that have no therapeutic function (Somerville 1981).

1.3 Substituted Judgment for Incompetent Adults

Application of the doctrine of informed consent to incompetent adults requires use of a legal fiction—most commonly that of "substituted judgment"—as incompetents by definition cannot give informed consent. Under substituted judgment, a surrogate for an incompetent adult patient, typically a relative, is legally *permitted* to make decisions on behalf of the patient in furtherance of the rights *of the patient.* Surrogates are under a legal obligation to decide not on the basis of how *they* want the patient to be treated, but rather on the basis of how *the patient* would choose to be treated if he or she were capable of choosing. The more a surrogate seems influenced in her decision-making by his or her personal values and preferences, the less willing a physician should be to accept the surrogate's permission for a procedure. Substituted judgment typically requires the substitute decision-makers to present clear and convincing evidence as to the wishes of the patient before he or she became incompetent.[14]

Legal use of the substituted judgment doctrine dates to early nineteenth-century England, where it was initially invoked as a legal fiction allowing courts to distribute parts of a "lunatic's" or "idiot's" estate to relatives that were not owed any legal duty of support.[15] *In re Quinlan,* the first of the two US cases that are most identified with the doctrine, involved a once-competent woman in a persistent vegetative state. The New Jersey Supreme Court invoked the principle to reject a claim by the woman's parents that the hospital must withdraw life support because the claim was inconsistent with the parents' religious values.[16] In *Superintendent of Belchertown State School v. Saikewicz,* treatment for a severely retarded man with leukemia was withheld on the grounds that he himself would have refused treatment were he competent, but, at the same time, aware of his perpetual and irreversible incompetence.[17] Such a conclusion had no evidence to support it and again shows the tendency of paradoxes and inconsistencies to mount in applications of informed consent.

Even Judge Paul Liacos, the author of the opinion, admitted that attempting to implement substituted judgment in such a case "involves a legal fiction to some extent" (Liacos 1989). When no evidence of the patient's preferences or values is available, or when the patient has never been competent, surrogate decision-making often reverts to the *best interests* standard. Under the best interests standard, surrogates are directed to make necessary decisions based on what in their estimation would produce the highest net benefit to the incompetent patient, by careful and informed weighing of the patient's interests against the risks and costs of available treatment options. However, the ethical principle of best interests is problematic because it relies on the decision-maker referring to his or her own conception of quality of life, and then being able to appropriately apply this

---

[14] See Cruzan v. Director, Mo. Dept. of Health, 497 U.S. 261, 284–286 (1990).

[15] Ex Parte Whitbread in the Matter of Hinde, a Lunatic, 35 Eng. Rep. 878, 878 (Ch. 1816).

[16] In re Quinlan, 355 A.2d 647, 661-62 (N.J. 1976).

[17] Superintendent of Belchertown v. Saikewicz, 370 N.E.2d 417, 421, 431 (Mass. 1977).

conception to the patient and his future life. Because it is not their own bodies that are affected, there may be more of a tendency for surrogates to overlook or minimize harms that may result from decisions made for others.

An alternative approach that might be better founded ethically would follow Kant and Rawls in treating the infant as an end unto himself and never a means to an end. Under this approach, consideration would be given to the infant's position and the inherent value of his life and self-definition and using universal moral principles to guide decision-making in a manner more analogous to substituted judgment (Kant 1956; Rawls 1971, 1993).

1.3.1 Problems with Substituted Judgment for Incompetent Adults

One problem with substituted judgment is that it requires the acceptance of an oxymoron—that one's autonomy can be exercised by another. The notion that a court or any third person can decide for the incompetent person under a theory of substituted judgment denies the very autonomy from which the doctrine takes its life. "[T]hat decisions concerning a particular person's fate are better made *for* him than *by* him, because others wiser than he are more keenly aware of his best interests than he can be—conflicts with the notion of a right of self-determination."

A practical problem with decisions made by surrogates is that there is considerable evidence to show that surrogates do not always make choices that conform to what their wards would actually have chosen for themselves. A review of sixteen studies of still-competent patients and their designated surrogates found that nearly one third of the surrogates failed to correctly predict the treatment preferences of their designated wards in hypothetical end-of-life treatment decision scenarios (Shalowitz et al. 2006). An even greater lack of accuracy in surrogate decision-making—an abysmal 34 % agreement—has been found in research on hypothetical situations concerning elective surgery (Mantravadi et al. 2007).

Suhl found "patient surrogates guessed no better than would have been expected from random chance alone. This was true despite a generally long and close relationship between the patient and the surrogate, and the belief by virtually all pairs that the surrogate knew the patient's wishes" (Suhl 1994). Understandably, one such study concluded, "In light of these findings, it is apparent that this substituted judgment standard, intended to allow for an incompetent patient's right to autonomy, should be re-evaluated" (Seckler et al. 1991, p. 96).

1.4 Proxy Permission for Never Competent Children

Proxy permission for medical procedures on never competent children—most commonly provided by parents or other guardians—is itself a legal fiction but is at least linguistically accurate. By contrast, the widespread terminology "informed consent" in relation to never competent children is incorrect and misleading. Parents cannot "consent" based on an examination of their own values and preferences, as they would for a procedure on themselves, but rather can merely, as guardians, grant permission *on behalf of the child*, and only for procedures that are necessary to ensure the child's well-being (Committee on Bioethics 1995).

While one might assume that the grounding of informed consent in principles of autonomy and self-determination is inapplicable to incompetent children, the principle of autonomy should help guide parental decision-making for children. Citing Joel Feinberg's argument for the child's "right to an open future" (Feinberg 2007), Berg et al. have written:

> It may seem strange to speak of promoting the autonomy of incompetent patients. Yet some patients are only temporarily incompetent and non-autonomous, as when they are briefly unconscious or are infants. These patients will regain consciousness or mature; decisions made on their behalf should, therefore, safeguard their future autonomy and their opportunities to make future autonomous decisions. For this reason, for example, parents generally may not elect to sterilize their children; to do so would infringe on the future reproductive autonomy of their children (Berg and Appelbaum 2001, p. 94).

The British Medical Association (BMA) agrees on the need for "prioritising of options which maximize the patient's future opportunities and choices" (Medical Ethics Committee, British Medical Association 2006, p. 4).

A child's parents possess temporary authority to make health care decisions on behalf of their children, where the procedure is in the best interests of a child, and the child is incapable of consenting on his own behalf (Feigenbaum 1992, pp. 852, 875). Courts have recognized that parents do not possess an unrestricted authority to make decisions on behalf of their children. Parents are not permitted to make "martyrs" of their children.[18] Accordingly, the state can interfere via the *parens patriae* (parent of the nation) doctrine when serious harm or death to the child is likely to result from the parents' acts or omissions, which can create an "irreconcilable tension between child protection and parental deference" (Rosato 2000, p. 10).

1.4.1 Parent and Physician Duties in Proxy Permission for Never Competent Children

While the analysis of parental proxy consent for children is sometimes carried out under the principle of "substituted judgment," it is more commonly done as a best interests analysis. The physician's professional and legal duties in this context are at least as stringent as in the case of an autonomous adult. Physicians also have a duty to ensure that the surrogate is capable of understanding the information provided and of fully appreciating the consequences of a decision at the moment of decision-making. Likewise, physicians are obliged not to manipulate the surrogate

---

[18] Prince v. Massachusetts, 321 U.S. 158 (1944).

by presenting the information in a manner designed to secure permission, rather than facilitating an objective evaluation of the risks and benefits of the procedure. It is improper for a physician to suggest a procedure that is not medically indicated to parents who have not inquired about it. In addition to these requirements, which also arise in securing informed consent from a competent patient, a physician seeking permission for a surgical procedure on an incompetent adult must ensure that the substitute decision-maker is not acting out of self-interest but rather is deciding on the basis of what is best for the patient.

Parents, like substitute decision-makers for incompetent adult patients, should be viewed as agents for their never competent children, required to make decisions regarding medical interventions for their children in a manner consistent with their children's best interests. Surrogates should strive to maximize benefits while minimizing harms to the child patient. Factors to be considered in determining a child's best interests should include: the balance of the harms and benefits of treatment options; the evidence on long- and short-term outcomes of treatment options; long-term implications for the child's suffering and quality of life; how likely the proposed treatment is to improve or prevent deterioration of the child's condition; the child's chances of survival; and whether the proposed treatment is the least restrictive and least intrusive way to obtain the hoped-for benefits (Longley 2009).

Medical professionals owe a duty to their minor patients to assist parents in making decisions that conform to that standard. According to the American Academy of Pediatrics Committee on Bioethics, parental permission for medical intervention is authorized only in situations of clear and immediate medical necessity, such as disease, trauma, or deformity. Where parents request a procedure that is *not* medically indicated, courts have taken an even more child-protective stance than applies to medically justified procedures, requiring strong evidence that the procedure is in the patient-child's interests and does not entail parents inappropriately injecting their own preferences into the decision-making process. For example, even if a kidney transplant would save the life of a close relative, the decision must be made based exclusively on the patient's own interests.[19] The benefits of the proposed procedure must clearly outweigh short- and long-term disadvantages, and spiritual costs and benefits may not be incorporated into this analysis. The AAP Committee directs that for non-essential treatments, particularly those (such as neonatal circumcision) that can be deferred without loss of efficacy, the physician and family wait until the child's consent can be obtained (American Academy of Pediatrics Committee on Bioethics 1995, pp. 314–316). The AAP Committee and the United Kingdom Department of Health guidelines both stress that providers have legal and ethical duties to their child patients to render competent medical care based on what the patient needs, not what someone else expresses (Committee on Bioethics 1995, p. 315; Department of Health 1991).

While in certain circumstances patients may themselves be able to provide legally valid consent to prophylactic removal of their own healthy tissue, parents

---

[19] See Strunk v. Strunk, 445 S.W.2d 145, 148–149 (Ky. 1969); Hart v. Brown, 289 A.2d 386, 387-88 (Conn. Super. Ct. 1972).

can never grant permission for prophylactic removal of healthy tissue from their children and can only consent to medically necessary procedures. Because the foreskin is a normal, functional anatomical structure, and because routine neonatal circumcision has no recognized therapeutic benefit, parental consent for "routine" circumcision is invalid.

1.5 Proxy Permission for Neonatal Circumcision on Never Competent Baby Boys

We have seen that informed consent fails to protect patient's rights properly even for competent adults, and it fares worse within the realm of substituted judgment for incompetent adults. When proxy consent is to be granted to authorize neonatal circumcision on never competent baby boys, a plethora of interconnected conceptual, ethical, and practical problems arise. Proxy permission for an elective procedure that lacks medical indication conceals a usurpation of the child's agency, in violation of the ethical principles of autonomy and self-determination. Accordingly, the doctrine of proxy consent by parents for neonatal circumcision of their infants proves to be the most distorted legal fiction of all, ethically and legally unable to sustain its claims to legal authorization, medical authorization, and compliance with human rights.

We as a society thereby conceal from ourselves our failure to adequately protect the human rights and ethical entitlements of human dignity and autonomy whose importance we profess to recognize.

1.5.1 Background of Proxy Permission for Neonatal Circumcision

While the other English-speaking countries have since virtually abandoned neonatal circumcision, the United States has seen a slower but still precipitous drop in circumcision rates from a peak of approximately 90 % in the 1960s to—according to the Centers for Disease Control and Prevention (CDC)—33 % in hospital in 2009 (El Bcheraoui 2010). Longley notes: (colon) "it is interesting that the beginning of the shift coincided with the incorporation of informed consent into modern medical practice" (Longley 2009, p. 2).

Proxy consent stressed the ethical justification of parental permission for neonatal circumcision, in that information must be provided in a way that allows parents to make an autonomous decision, yet it is the child who is the patient and whose body and life will be affected by the decision. Indeed, because of this quandary, some authors have argued that non-therapeutic neonatal circumcision does not meet the legal criteria for valid parental consent (American Academy of Pediatrics Committee on Bioethics 1995; Canadian Paediatric Society Bioethics Committee 2004; Svoboda et al. 2000).

1.5.2 *Medicalization Helps Justify and Perpetuate Neonatal Circumcision*

A sleight of hand is lurking that is usually tacitly glossed over but whose significance should not be missed. As proxy consent to a procedure lacking medical justification is not possible, proxy consent is only relevant to circumcision based on its questionable status as an ostensibly medical procedure. No reputable medical organization maintains that neonatal circumcision has medical benefits justifying its performance (Circumcision Information and Resource Pages 2011). Circumcision has joined other originally non-medical practices that are now conceptualized as medical—for example, dying, alcoholism, drug addiction, and erectile difficulties (Carpenter 2010). Circumcision has followed a trajectory from being conceptualized as a religious procedure to a medical procedure. This explains why informed consent is applied to it. Under a pretense of legal authorization and compliance with human rights, we thereby mask our failure to properly protect human dignity and self-determination. Circumcision entails one further pretense that should not be overlooked—a suggestion of medical authorization where in fact none exists.

1.5.3 *Disclosure: Circumcision*

"[P]arental decisions to have infant sons circumcised are not based on adequate information" (McDermott et al 1982, p. 132). If doctors don't know this information themselves, they can't carry out their duties to inform their patients. One study found physicians' own knowledge regarding normal foreskin anatomy to be inadequate (Stein et al. 1982, p. 47). Predictably, this lack of information leads to harm to the doctors' child patients. Two studies completed in 1996 and 2001 respectively found that 25 and 37 % of mothers believed they had not been given enough information to make a meaningful decision regarding circumcision (Ciesielski-Carlucci et al. 1996; Adler et al. 2001). To further complicate matters, information does not always necessarily even help. Parents in one group that was provided with a written statement of the advantages and disadvantages of circumcision actually were slightly more likely (98–96 %) to authorize the circumcision of their newborn sons (Herrera et al. 1982).

Materiality: Neonatal Circumcision

Physicians who perform circumcisions have a legal and ethical duty to their infant patients to obtain and provide all available medical information to the patients' parents. This includes information about the nature and function of the foreskin, the pain that its removal causes even with pain relief, the risks of any pain relief, the risk of complications, any possible medical costs caused by its amputation, and a full examination of the alternative of not circumcising. Doctors rarely fulfill this duty, (Christensen-Szalanski et al. 1987; Fletcher 1999; Longley 2009, pp. 237–239) and thereby violate their ethical and legal obligations as well as the legal rights and human rights of their patients.

Because healthy, functional tissue is removed with every circumcision, the complication rate of circumcision arguably is 100 % (Svoboda et al. 2000). The risk of additional immediate complication is between 2 and 10 % (Williams and Kapila 1993). There is an additional 5–10 % likelihood of a later physical complication (Van Howe 1997a; Patel 1966; Van Howe 2006). The risk of a potentially lifelong psychological and/or sexual complication also exists (Boyle et al. 2002). A risk of death also exists, and sadly well over one hundred iatrogenic deaths from neonatal circumcision occur annually in the US (Bollinger 2010). Physicians are clearly obligated to make parents aware of these complication rates and the nature of the harms that might befall their son. No significant medical benefit has clearly been demonstrated to result from routine neonatal circumcision, and physicians have a duty to inform parents of that fact.

Importance of Alternatives: Circumcision

In the case of circumcision, alternatives that should be disclosed include type of pain relief if any, and the surgical method. However, the most significant alternative is simply that of doing nothing and allowing the boy to grow up with his natural genitals intact. One much cited study of circumcision disclosure found that doctors failed to discuss the alternatives, including no treatment (Ciesielski-Carlucci et al. 1996). Longley documents that the needed information on circumcision should be demystifying, normalizing, should give value, and should support (Longley 2009, pp. 237–239). "It is thus apparent that if parents, as guardians, consent to have their male neonates circumcised without a clear discussion of alternatives offered by the physician or hospital staff, and if at a later date they find the procedure to have been unnecessary or find that complications develop as a result of the procedure, they may successfully make the health-care providers liable for having failed to provide alternatives to the procedure" (McDermott et al. 1982, p. 135). Longley found that in North America, most handouts provided pursuant to the informed consent process did not provide adequate information on the option of *not* circumcising (Longley 2009, pp. 219–220). Accordingly, providers in the US and Canada fail to satisfy the important principle of providing adequate disclosure of viable alternatives.

1.5.4 Voluntariness: Neonatal Circumcision

Longley points out the wide range of forces that can distort parental decision-making, including unfamiliarity with the intact penis, widespread myths and misinformation about the foreskin, and social pressures including the (fading) notion of circumcision as a social norm. Parents are also subject to undue influence from power imbalances in the relationship between patients and health care providers; a simple question from a physician may be interpreted by parents as a recommendation for circumcision (Longley 2009, pp. 234–236). Accordingly, parental decisions about circumcision made under these conditions are unlikely to be either adequately informed or truly voluntary.

The voluntariness requirement demands that physicians provide information regarding circumcision to parents in an unbiased fashion well in advance of the birth and certainly that physicians do not solicit the procedure. Given the procedure's elective and non-therapeutic nature, a physician should assume, unless the parents indicate otherwise, that the baby is not to be circumcised. Unfortunately, current practice appears inconsistent with the voluntariness requirement. Even today, it is routine in the United States to ask a woman during one of the initial prenatal visits whether she desires circumcision for her child if it is a boy (Van Howe 2011). It is a subtle form of coercion; offering circumcision to a mother can easily be interpreted as a recommendation.

Timing, Manner, Order: Neonatal Circumcision

Timing, manner, and order of presentation of informed consent for circumcision can all be improved. Sixty-three percent of the parents in one study faced the issue for the first time at birth or shortly before, and they were forced to make a fast decision, which the authors found unfair for the parents and babies (Herrera and Trouern-Trend 1979, p. 1070). Regarding timing in circumcision informed consent, Van Howe observes, "Ethically it is probably best to wait for *parents* to initiate the circumcision discussion *before* dispensing information" (Van Howe 1997b, pp. 88–89).

In circumstances where a child's best interests are unclear, the Canadian Paediatric Society recommends that "when it is possible to defer or delay acute treatment, such a delay is encouraged while further information is gathered to clarify the issues" (Canadian Paediatric Society Bioethics Committee 2004, p. 100).

Even more troubling is the fact—still common today—of parents being presented with the circumcision question for the first time when a mother is in labor at a hospital.[20] Pediatric urologist George Kaplan notes what he considers the "inexcusable" fact that "all too often the consent to circumcise is included in a sheaf of papers that the mother signs hurriedly on her way to the delivery room. No discussion has been held regarding the merits of the procedure or of the inherent risks" (Kaplan 1977). Similarly, Ciesielski-Carlucci et al. found:

> Of the providers who perform circumcision, 22 % do not routinely provide care during the prenatal period. Of those who perform circumcisions and provide prenatal care, 26 % do not discuss circumcision prior to delivery. That is, nearly half of the providers who perform circumcisions do not discuss the medical pros and cons of circumcision with mothers prior to delivery (Ciesielski-Carlucci et al. 1996, p. 231).

---

[20] Private communications on July 12, 2011 with Robert S. Van Howe, MD, Marilyn Milos, and Amber Craig.

Raising the circumcision issue for the first time upon the mother's arrival at the hospital to give birth amounts to manipulation and coercion. Because the physician and the hospital benefit financially from the parent's decision, such a practice raises grave concerns about unethical profiteering.

The AAP Committee on Bioethics sensibly recommends delaying elective, cosmetic surgery until a child is old enough to give consent, and this would apply to circumcision (American Academy of Pediatrics Committee on Bioethics 1995, pp. 315, 316–317). The Australian Association of Pediatric Surgeons has taken this position specifically with respect to circumcision (Leditschke 1996). Because no sufficient reasons exist for not deferring the procedure, ethically and legally it *must* be deferred, given the harm caused by the procedure and the probability that as an adult the patient will most likely not desire it.

Regarding the manner of presentation of information, Longley showed that North American sources—but not sources from Australia or New Zealand—ignored the benefits of an intact penis or problematized the intact penis. Accordingly, providers in the US and Canada framed information so as to promote circumcision and so as to render unattractive the option of keeping the baby boy genitally intact (Longley 2009, pp. 219–220). Clearly this did not honor their obligations under principles of informed consent.

1.5.5 Competence/Capacity of Proxy Agents: Neonatal Circumcision

Medical personnel have a duty to the newborn child to ensure that parental surrogates have the capacity to make a rational, reflective decision about circumcision. They should fully disclose all relevant information about the procedure well in advance of the birth, and then evaluate whether the parents understood the information. If the parents do not appear to understand, the physician should attempt to convey the information in another way that is clearer to the parents. At least one scholar has contended that parents are less rational in medical decisions concerning their children than they are in medical decisions concerning themselves (Alderson 1993). Medical personnel may therefore have a heightened duty when dealing with parental surrogates to ensure the surrogate is capable of making a rational decision on behalf of the infant patient.

1.5.6 Understanding: The Forgotten Element Neonatal Circumcision

Studies show that risks of circumcision are inadequately disclosed (Christensen-Szalanski et al. 1987; Fletcher 1999). A 1979 study found that "80 % of mothers stated that the risks of circumcision had not been explained to them" (Lovell and Cox 1979, p. 811). Fully 25 % of mothers consenting to circumcision of their newborns believed there were no risks (Ciesielski-Carlucci et al. 1996, p. 233).

Care providers presumably avoid discussing the pain with parents because they fear it will be disturbing for the parents. But it *should be* disturbing, and physicians owe a duty to the infant patient to make his parents aware of this disquieting aspect of circumcision. They owe no duty to parents to make them feel better about granting permission for an unnecessary surgery.

1.5.7 Proxy Consent to Neonatal Circumcision: Conceptual Problems

The conceptual, ethical, and practical problems that crop up with "proxy consent" for neonatal circumcision underscore the difficulties that can arise from invocation of legal fictions, which by definition require fitting a fact situation into a legal analysis that is not designed to accommodate it. The AAP Committee evidently acknowledges this as its statement says the concept of "informed consent" does not apply to infant circumcision, because only a competent person can give consent (informed or otherwise) and an infant clearly is not competent. One commentator trenchantly observes, "The current inability of the medical community to differentiate between truly medically-necessary surgery and surgery performed for social and psychological reasons renders even fully-informed parents unable to consent to irreversible and unnecessary cosmetic genital surgery" (Lareau 2003, p. 151).

1.5.8 Proxy Consent to Neonatal Circumcision: Ethical Problems

In regard to circumcision, the BMA specifically states that "parents must explain and justify requests for circumcision, in terms of the child's interests" (Medical Ethics Committee, British Medical Association 2006, p. 4). While acknowledging the strong legal presumption against intervention into parental decision-making, various authors and professional organizations have voiced concerns about the ethical issues raised by pediatric proxy consent (American Academy of Pediatrics Committee on Bioethics 1995; Canadian Paediatric Society Bioethics Committee 2004; Svoboda et al. 2000).

The elective and non-therapeutic nature of neonatal circumcision, and the fact that it is undertaken by parental proxy consent, ethically requires a more stringent standard of information-giving than in other medical decision-making situations. Across the English-speaking world, the very validity of parental consent for neonatal circumcision is dubious. Bouclin finds that Canadian legal precedent limits parental authority to consent to "therapeutic" treatment only, or in situations of "imminent and serious danger requiring immediate treatment" (Bouclin 2005,

p. 214). The same principle applies in the US (Pappworth 1967). Recently, in Australia, the Tasmania Law Reform Institute has concluded that "there is uncertainty as to whether the consent of a parent for the circumcision of their child is sufficient to allow a circumciser to legally perform the procedure" (Marshall 2009). British pediatrician Jones argues that parental authority to consent to treatment is invalid "if it is not possible to demonstrate personal benefit to the child, or that the public interest is in any way served" (Jones 2000).

As an irreversible and medically unnecessary amputation that alters not only the appearance but also the function of the penis, neonatal circumcision can be seen as infringing on the future autonomy of the child to make his own decisions about how much of his natural penis he prefers to have. The approach that is most respectful of the child's future autonomy is to let the child be the definer of his own best interests, leaving the decision for him to make when he is old enough to give his own informed consent.

If the ultimate goal of medical decision-making for an incompetent person is to determine what the patient would decide for himself, if able, the best evidence may be what similarly situated competent persons actually decide for themselves. Only 1 in 200 intact males choose to have the surgery performed later in life, suggesting that the overwhelming majority believe that the risks and sequelae of becoming circumcised outweigh any supposed benefits (International Coalition for Genital Integrity 2011). Doctors should heed the AAP Committee's recommendation that the decision be deferred until the child can decide for himself whether to grant consent (Moore 1995, p. 320).

1.5.9 Proxy Consent to Neonatal Circumcision: Practical Problems and Considerations

Several practical problems with ethically obtaining proxy consent to circumcision are evident from experimental results. Physician under-reporting of risks and exaggeration of benefits seems to be the rule rather than the exception. Strong evidence suggests that a graphic depiction of the procedure—either a picture or a video—would be of significant help in educating parents about neonatal circumcision, and yet this is almost never done.

With respect to the risk of complications and the supposed medical benefits associated with circumcision, studies reveal that physicians under-report the risks and exaggerate the supposed benefits. A 1987 study found that physicians routinely inform parents about only three of the many possible complications of circumcision—namely, bleeding, infection, and pain (Christensen-Szalanski et al. 1987). Fletcher also found that bleeding, infection, and pain were the only complications to be discussed more than half of the time (Fletcher 1999). This is far below the standard level of disclosure for other surgeries, whether medically indicated or cosmetic. In circumcisions, the "principles of informed consent are often violated" (Ciesielski-Carlucci et al. 1996, p. 233).

We have already seen that presenting parents with video or pictorial images of the procedure helped inform parents of what circumcision entails. Yet this is almost never done. In 1980, one physician noted that use of printed educational materials clearly presenting advantages and disadvantages of circumcision led to a 30 % reduction in the neonatal circumcision rate (Gorske 1980). Solomon persuasively argues:

> parents have the right to see a video of a circumcision, if not at least a picture of a child restrained and being circumcised.... [B]ased on the fact that people's perception of what a circumcision is differs so radically from what actually happens during a circumcision, doctors are under an obligation to show parents a video, or if not, at least a photograph, of a baby being circumcised (Solomon 2007–2008, pp. 236, 238).

Seven studies have been performed to determine the effect of different informed consent procedures for neonatal circumcision such as verbal repetition of written disclosures, five of which found no difference in circumcision rates between the experimental and control groups (Binner et al. 2002; Christensen-Szalanski et al. 1987; Herrera et al. 1982; Maisels et al. 1983). This was attributed to the strength of social pressures, though obviously the importance of that factor has waned or even flipped now that in-hospital rates have—according to the CDC–declined to one in three nationwide (El Bcheraoui et al. 2010). Two of the seven studies found that circumcision rates were reduced in the group subject to an educational intervention. Rand et al. employed an experimental group comprised of obstetric patients who were given an accurate oral summary of risks as well as (supposed) advantages of circumcision. A substantial number of group members (28 % compared to 5.6 % of the control group) elected to keep their baby intact, and many of these parents had previously favored the procedure. The authors concluded that mothers who request circumcision do so based on inadequate medical information or strong social pressure (Rand et al. 1983, pp. 66, 64). Similarly, Enzenauer et al. found that the rate of circumcision in the experimental group dropped from the pre-study rate of over 90 % to about 70 % during the six-month intervention period. This study found that videotape counseling modestly reduced parental permission for circumcision from 75.9 to 70.5 % when compared with standard oral counseling (Enzenauer et al. 1986, p. 718). A factor that differentiates these two studies from the other five is that visual representations, either pictures or video, were employed to give parents an idea of what the procedure entailed.

1.5.10 Proxy Consent to Neonatal Circumcision as a Non-therapeutic, Elective Procedure

Because the foreskin is a normal, functional anatomical structure, and because routine neonatal circumcision has no recognized therapeutic benefit, parental consent for "routine" circumcision is invalid. Courts have uniformly held that surgical removal of any normal, healthy body part is not "treatment" and thus parental "consent" for such a procedure is invalid (Van Howe 1997b).

As mentioned above, the AAP Committee found that the concept of "informed consent" does not apply to infant circumcision. For the same reason, "patient assent" does not apply. Finally, the concept of "informed parental permission" cannot apply to infant circumcision because it only allows for medical interventions in situations of clear and immediate medical necessity, such as disease, trauma, or deformity.

Since neonatal circumcision is categorized as an elective procedure, we have already seen that a higher standard for informational disclosure is expected. When the procedure is, moreover, understood to be non-therapeutic, additional disclosure expectations are overlaid on this already elevated standard. The world's major medical organizations, having reviewed the evidence on the possible medical merit of neonatal circumcision acknowledge this fact, variously describing it as "non-therapeutic", (Council on Scientific Affairs, American Medical Association 1999) as lacking health benefits that justify its performance (Medical Ethics Committee, British Medical Association 2006) or likening it to a "cosmetic" procedure[21] done primarily for appearance rather than for health reasons.

According to bioethicist Somerville, the non-therapeutic nature of the procedure must be carefully made clear to the patient, particularly because "patients tend to identify physicians with therapy, and find it hard to believe that a physician would carry out a non-therapeutic procedure on them, even when they are expressly informed of this fact" (Somerville 1981). Moreover, the disclosure expectations generated by the non-therapeutic nature of neonatal circumcision are compounded to an additional degree by the fact that consent is provided by a proxy.

1.6 Conclusion

We have seen that while informed consent manages a degree of logical coherence when applied to competent adults, it fails to protect relevant concerns when applied by proxy to incompetent adults. This turns out to be more problematic when proxy consent is applied to never competent children for neonatal circumcision, which generates a hornet's nest of conceptual, ethical, and practical problems. Agency is thereby usurped, and ethical principles are violated without consequence to the violator. Physicians should approach decision-making on behalf of a newborn with the greatest caution and with a strong presumption against intrusive procedures. Amputating a highly sensitive and functional part of the body is extremely intrusive and should be undertaken only in situations of urgent necessity. Neonatal circumcision as it is routinely performed in this country clearly does not satisfy this criterion. It is therefore unethical and unlawful.

Infants do not have the capacity to give consent to any aspect of their medical care. Physicians may only obtain legally valid permission from parents to perform procedures on their incompetent children, provided full disclosure of all material

[21] American Academy of Family Physicians 2002.

information is made to parents who are able to understand the information and to appreciate the consequences of their decision, and provided that the parents are able to decide whether to grant their permission free from any manipulation or undue influence. Moreover, the only interventions for which parents may grant their permission are those conferring benefits that clearly outweigh the short- and long-term costs for the infant patient.

Because parents lack the power to give permission for prophylactic amputation of healthy tissue from their children, no parental permission for the procedure should be effective. Moreover, even if it were permissible for physicians to give effect to parental permission for circumcision, physicians would be under a stringent obligation to their infant patients to ensure that any such permission is informed—voluntarily given based upon competent review of all relevant information. Available evidence suggests that physicians today routinely fail to fulfill this duty. In doing so, they discredit their profession and expose themselves to legal liability. Video or at minimum photographs of a procedure should be routinely employed to educate parents as to the reality of the procedure.

The legal fiction of proxy consent to neonatal circumcision has not been directly considered by the courts. However, circumcision has gradually but steadily been falling out of favor in the past few decades, to the point where today more than two out of three boys leave the hospital intact. As the balance of public opinion shifts to opposing the practice, the legal system will become more accepting of lawsuits to protect baby boys. Consequently, the legal system will no longer be able to ignore the conflict between this practice and the legal and ethical duties of medical professionals relating to informed consent. The legal fiction of informed consent as applied to never competent newborns will crumble and genuine protection of the child's human rights, coupled with meaningful observation by practitioners of ethical principles of autonomy and self-determination, will become obligatory. Pretenses of legal and medical authorization and compliance with human rights and ethical requirements will dissolve forever.

References

Adler R et al (2001) Circumcision: we have heard from the experts; now let's hear from the parents. Pediatrics 107(2): e20

Alderson P (1993) Children's consent to surgery. Open University Press, Buckingham, p 30

American Academy of Pediatrics Committee on Bioethics (1995) Informed consent, parental permission, and assent in pediatric practice. Pediatrics 95:314–317 (here, pp 314–316)

Annas GJ (1977) Informed consent: the patient's most important right. Trustee 30(10):13–14

Berg JW, Appelbaum PS (2001) Informed consent: legal theory and clinical practice. Oxford University Press, New York

Berry RM (2005) Informed consent law, ethics, and practice: From infancy to reflective adolescence. HEC Forum 17(1):64–81

Binner SL et al (2002) Effect of parental education on decision-making about neonatal circumcision. South Med J 95(4):457–461

Bollinger D (2010) Lost boys: an estimate of U.S. circumcision-related infant deaths. Thymos: J Boyhood Stud 4:78–90

Bottrell MM et al (2000) Hospital informed consent for procedure forms. Arch Surg 135:26–33
Bouclin S (2005) An examination of legal and ethical issues surrounding male circumcision: the Canadian contest. Int J Men's Health 4(3):205–222
Boyle GJ et al (2002) Male circumcision: pain, trauma and psychosexual sequelae. J Health Psychol 7(3):329–343
Braddock CH et al (1999) Informed decision making in outpatient practice: time to get back to basics. JAMA 282(24):2313–2319
Canadian Paediatric Society Bioethics Committee (2004) Treatment decisions regarding infants, children, and adolescents. Paediatr Child Health 9(2):99–103
Carpenter L (2010) On remedicalisation: male circumcision in the Untied States and Great Britain. Sociol Health Illn 32(4):613–630
Cassileth BR et al (1980) Informed consent—why are its goals imperfectly realized. N Engl J Med 302(16):896–900
Cherry M (2010) Non-consensual treatment is (nearly always) morally impermissible. J Law Med Ethics 38(4):789–798
Christensen-Szalanski JJ et al (1987) Circumcision and informed consent: is more information always better? Med Care 25(9):856–867
Ciesielski-Carlucci C et al (1996) Determinants of decision making for circumcision. Camb Q Healthc Ethics 5:228–236
Circumcision Information and Resource Pages (2011) Circumcision policy statements. Available at URL: www.cirp.org/library/statements/. Updated 16 Jan
Clark SK et al (1991) A risk-specific anesthesia consent form may hinder the informed consent process. J Clin Anesth 3:11–13
Committee on Bioethics (1995) Informed consent, parental permission, and assent in pediatric practice. Pediatrics 95:314–317
Council on Scientific Affairs, American Medical Association (1999) Neonatal circumcision. American Medical Association, Chicago
Department of Health (1991) Local research ethics committees. § 4.4. Department of Health, London
Dunkelman H (1979) Patients' knowledge of their condition and treatment: how it might be improved. Br Med J 12:311–314
El Bcheraoui C et al (2010) Rates of selected neonatal male circumcision-associated severe adverse events in the United States, 2007–2009. In: 18th International AIDS Conference, Vienna, Austria
El Bcheraoui CE et al (2010) Rates of selected neonatal male circumcision-associated severe adverse events in the United States, 2007–2009. AIDS 2010. Presented on 22 July
Enzenauer RW et al (1986) Decreased circumcision rate with videotaped counseling. South Med J 79:717–720
Epstein LC, Lasagna L (1969) Obtaining informed consent. Arch Intern Med 123:682–688
Etchells E et al (1996) Bioethics for clinicians: 2. Disclosure. Can Med Assoc J 155:387–391
Faden RR, Beauchamp TL (1986) A history and theory of informed consent. Oxford University Press, New York
Feigenbaum MS (1992) Minors, medical treatment, and interspousal disagreement: should Solomon split the child? DePaul Law Rev 41:841–884
Feinberg J (2007) The child's right to an open future. In: Curren R (ed) Philosophy of education: an anthology, pp 112–123
Fletcher C (1999) Circumcision in America in 1998: attitudes, beliefs, and charges of American physicians. In Denniston GC et al (eds) Male and female circumcision: medical, legal, and ethical considerations in pediatrics practice, Kluwer Academic/Plenum, New York, pp 259–271
Gorske AL (1980) Circumcision and patient education [letter]. Am J Dis Child 134:527
Haberfield L (1997) Informed consent and infant male circumcision. Australasian Law Teachers Conference
Harrington JA (1996) Privileging the medical norm: liberalism, self-determination and refusal of treatment. Legal Stud 16(3):348–367

Herrera AJ, Trouern-Trend JBG (1979) Routine neonatal circumcision. Am J Dis Child 133:1069–1070
Herrera AJ et al (1982) The role of parental information in the incidence of circumcision. Pediatrics 70(4):597–598
International Coalition for Genital Integrity (2011) US adult circ rate. Available at URL: www.icgi.org/information/us-adult-circ-rate. Updated 10 June
Jackson E (2006) 'Informed consent' to medical treatment and the impotence of tort. In: McLean SAM (ed) First do no harm: law, ethics and healthcare. Ashgate, Burlington, pp 273–286 (here, pp 273–274)
Jones MA (1999) Informed consent and other fairy stories. Med Law Rev 7:103–134
Jones RB (2000) Parental consent to cosmetic facial surgery in Down's syndrome. Journal of Medical Ethics 26:101
Kant I (1956) Critique of practical reason. 1788. Bobbs-Merrill Educational Publishing, Indianapolis
Kaplan GW (1977) Circumcision—an overview. Curr Probl Pediatr 7:1–33
Karako-Eyal N (2010) Physicians' duty of disclosure: a deontological and consequential analysis. Quinnipiac Health Law J 14:1–47
Katz J (1994) Informed consent—must it remain a fairy tale. J Contemp Health Law Policy 10(4):69–91
Katz JN et al (1992) Informed consent and the prescription of nonsteroidal anti-inflammatory drugs. Arthritis Rheum 35(11):1257–1263
Lareau AC (2003) Who decides? Genital-normalizing surgery on intersexed infants. Georgetown Law J 92:129–151
Leditschke JF (1996) Guidelines for circumcision. Australasian Association of Paediatric Surgeons, Hersion
Liacos PJ (1989) Is 'substituted judgment a valid legal concept? Issues Law Med 5(2):215–224
Longley G (2009) Framing the foreskin: A content analysis of circumcision information handouts for expectant parents. Thesis, University of Colorado Denver
Lovell JE, Cox J (1979) Maternal attitudes toward circumcision. J Family Pract 9(5):811–813
Lustig A, Scardino P (1998) Elective patients. In: McCullough LB et al (eds) Surgical ethics, Oxford University Press, New York, pp 133–151
Maclean A (2009) Autonomy, informed consent and medical law. Cambridge University Press, New York, pp 198–209
Maisels MJ et al (1983) Circumcision: The effect of information on parental decision making. Pediatrics 71:453–455
Mantravadi AV et al (2007) Accuracy of surrogate decision making in elective surgery. J Cataract Refract Surg 33:2091–2097
Marshall W (2009) Non-therapeutic male circumciison. Tasmania Law Reform Institute, Hobart, p 6
McDermott RJ et al (1982) Neonatal circumcision. Patient Counselling Health Educ 3(4):132–136
Medical Ethics Committee, British Medical Association (2006) The law and ethics of male circumcision. British Medical Association, London
Moore DL (1995) Challenging parental decisions to overtreat children. Health Matrix 5:311–323
Muss HB et al (1979) Written informed consent in patients with breast cancer. Cancer 43(4):1549–1556
Olver IN et al (1995) Impact of an information and consent form on patients having chemotherapy. Med J Aust 162:82–83
Pappworth MH (1967) Human guinea pigs. Routledge & Kegan Paul, London, pp 31–32
Patel H (1966) The problem of routine circumcision. Can Med Assoc J 95:576–581
Rand CS et al (1983) The effect of an educational intervention on the rate of neonatal circumcision. Obstet Gynecol 62:64
Rawls J (1971) A Theory of justice. Harvard University Press, Cambridge
Rawls J (1993) Political liberalism. Columbia University Press, New York
Robertson G (1981) Informed consent to medical treatment. Law Q Rev 97:102–126

Rosato J (2000) Using bioethics discourse to determine when parents should make health care decisions for their children: is deference justified. Temple Law Rev 73(1):1–68
Schuck PH (1994) Rethinking informed consent. Yale Law J 103(4):899–959
Seckler AB et al (1991) Substituted judgment: how accurate are proxy predictions. Annals Intern Med 115(2):92–98
Shalowitz DI et al (2006) The accuracy of surrogate decision makers. Arch Intern Med 166:493–497
Solomon D (2007–2008) Informed consent for routine infant circumcision: a proposal. New York Law School Law Rev 52:215–245
Somerville M (1981) Structuring the issues in informed consent. McGill Law J 26(4):740–808
Stein MT et al (1982) Routine neonatal circumcision: the gap between contemporary policy and practice. J Fam Pract 15(1):47–53
Suhl J (1994) Myth of substituted judgment. Arch Intern Med 154:90–96
Svoboda JS et al (2000) Informed consent for neonatal circumcision: an ethical and legal conundrum. J Contemp Health Law Policy 17:61–132
Van Howe RS (1997a) Variability in penile appearance and penile findings: a prospective study. Br J Urol 80:776–782
Van Howe RS (1997b) Response to 'Determinants of decision making for circumcision' by C. Ciesielski-Carlucci, N. Milliken, and N.H Cohen. Cambridge Q Healthcare Ethics 6:88–92
Van Howe RS (2006) Incidence of meatal stenosis following neonatal circumcision in a primary care setting. Clin Pediatr 45:49–54
Van Howe RS (2011) Why does neonatal circumcision persist in the United States? In: DennistonGC, Milos MF (eds) Sexual mutilations: a human tragedy pp 111–119 [here, at p. 115] (Also private communications on July 12, 2011 with Robert S. Van Howe, MD, Marilyn Milos, and Amber Craig)
Wear S (1998) Informed consent: patient autonomy and clinician beneficence within health care, 2nd edn. Georgetown University Press, Washington
Williams N, Kapila L (1993) Complications of circumcision. Br J Surg 80:1231
Wu WC, Pearlman RA (1988) Consent in medical decision making: the role of communication. J Gen Intern Med 3:9–14

Author Biography

J. Steven Svoboda JD graduated *cum laude* from Harvard Law School in 1991 and founded Attorneys for the Rights of the Child (ARC) in early 1997. His publications include "A rose by any other name?: symmetry and asymmetry in male and female genital cutting," in *Fearful Symmetries*: *Essays and Testimonies Around Excision and Circumcision*; *ed. C. Zabus; Rodopi; 2008*, *Does Feminism Discriminate Against Men*?: *A Debate,* Oxford University Press; 2007, and "Neonatal Pain Relief and the Helsinki Declaration," in *The Journal of Law, Medicine & Ethics;* December 2008, coauthored with Robert S. Van Howe, MD. In 2002, Steven received the Human Rights Award for his work with ARC, which includes the first presentation and document ever accepted by the United Nations primarily focusing on male circumcision. Steven practices patent law in San Francisco. Berkeley, California, USA.

Chapter 2
Routine Infant Circumcision: Vital Issues that the Circumcision Proponents may be Overlooking

Robert S. Van Howe

Abstract Circumcision is not a mild, neutral medical intervention like a vaccination, but a culturally-loaded amputation of a highly significant and functionally valuable body part that the medical profession should be working to protect against pathological conditions. Instead, a small, vocal, influential group is calling for universal amputation of the foreskin, comparing it to a vaccination. While the average adult is willing to get himself vaccinated against diseases, the vast majority of adult males are not willing to get circumcised. Falling rates of circumcision in the United States may have prompted a surge in circumcision promotion. Demonstrating a circumcision benefit in the United States has been disappointing, so the research moved to Africa, where the latest health crisis, the AIDS epidemic, was at its zenith. Armed with a few studies performed by a handful of investigators, circumcision proponents (CPs) are saturating the medical literature with their opinions and calling on national medical organization to recommend universal infant male circumcision. Policies and recommendations should be evidence-based rather than relying on opinion pieces with selective bibliographies and a narrowly focused perspective (Schoen 2006; Flynn et al. 2007; Dickerman 2007; Morris 2007a; Weiss et al. 2008; Morris et al. 2006; Golden and Wasserheit 2009; Rennie et al. 2007; Gostin and Hankins 2008; Clark et al. 2007; Morris 2007b; Morris 2008; Sawires et al. 2007; Newell and Bärnighausen 2007a; Sullivan et al. 2007; Brusa and Barilan 2008; Katz and Wright 2008; Potts et al. 2006). The purpose of this chapter is to address the issues that the CPs have failed to mention, such as bioethics, human rights, the function of the foreskin, and conflicting information, to present the information their bibliographies selected out, and to itemize the barriers to making a convincing case for universal circumcision.

Keywords Circumcision • Amputation • Bioethics • Human rights • Foreskin function • Risks and harms • Penile problems • Cancer • Langerhans cells • HIV • T-cells • Immune system • Sexually transmitted diseases • Condoms

---

R. S. Van Howe (✉)
Clinical Professor, Michigan State University College of Human Medicine, pediatrician for Bell Memorial Hospital in Ishpeming, Michigan, USA
e-mail: rsvanhowe@att.net

G. C. Denniston et al. (eds.), *Genital Cutting: Protecting Children from Medical, Cultural, and Religious Infringements*, DOI: 10.1007/978-94-007-6407-1_2,

2.1 Bioethics and Human Rights

A number of international covenants provide that everyone, even minors, has a right to security of person, bodily integrity, and the freedom from cruel, inhumane, or degrading treatment.[1] Informed consent is based on this principle of individual autonomy (Svoboda et al. 2000). Because newborns do not have the capacity to give informed consent, proxy consent is sought from parents who are more likely to protect the child's best interest. There are limitations. The American Academy of Pediatrics (AAP) recommends that proxy consent only be given in situations of medical necessity, such as disease, trauma, or deformity. Since the healthy newborn male foreskin is without disease, trauma, or deformity (Committee on Bioethics 1995) and no national medical organizations have concluded that circumcision is medically necessary (American Academy of Pediatrics Task Force on Circumcision 1999; Fetus and Newborn Committee 1996; College of Physicians and Surgeons of British Columbia 2004; Medical Ethics Committee 2003; Beasley et al. 2002; Kendel 2002; American Medical Association Council on Scientific Affairs 1999), simple logic dictates that proxy consent for neonatal circumcision is not valid (Svoboda et al. 2000). The AAP further recommends that non-essential treatments, which can be deferred without loss of efficacy, be postponed until the child's consent can be obtained (Committee on Bioethics 1995). To justify infant circumcision, CPs need to demonstrate a compelling reason that respects the infant's autonomy and outweighs the infant's right to security of person and bodily integrity (Dekkers et al. 2005; Dekkers 2009). They have not found one. Making nebulous, general claims that infant circumcision benefits society and rarely the child (Darby and Svoboda 2008; Svoboda 2009) also runs afoul of the most basic Kantian ethics (Kant 1998) and indicates a lack of moral respect for the newborn (Alderson 1993). Interestingly, the Dutch Royal Medical Association recently recommended, in large part based on human rights concerns, that non-therapeutic infant circumcision not be performed (Royal Dutch Medical Association 2010; Sheldon 2010).

Because competent males rarely choose to be circumcised, CPs have recommended that infants be circumcised (Rennie et al. 2007). This underscores the weakness of their case favoring circumcision. If the benefits of circumcision were compelling, competent people would choose it. Taking advantage of the vulnerable infants too young to resist, to further an agenda is a clear case of exploitation.

The CPs do not want to acknowledge that as humans with a full complement of rights, males have the autonomy to make these choices (Rennie et al. 2007; Benatar and Benatar 2003a; Benatar and Benatar 2003b) or that the choices are

[1] Convention on the Rights of the Child. UN GA Resolution 44/25, November 20, 1989; International Covenant on Civil and Political Rights, GA res. 2200A (XXI), 21 UN GAOR Supp. (No. 16) at 52, UN Doc. A/6316 (1966), 999 UNTS 171, entered into force March 23, 1976; Universal Declaration of Human Rights. Article 25(2), G.A. Resolution 217A (III), UN Doc. No. A/810 (1948), adopted December 10, 1948; International Covenant on Civil and Political Rights, UN GA Resolution 2200 A [XXI], December 16, 1966.

straight-forward. If the financial resources normally allocated to an infant circumcision were invested at 5 % per annum for 14 years, the competent 14 year old would have the resources to buy 15,840 condoms (2¢ each) and still have all his penile fine-touch neuroreceptors. For the condoms not purchased, resources would be available for *effective* health care interventions.

Perhaps more important than considering the child's best interests is basing proxy choices on what the child would choose for himself if competent (Lebit 1992; Dwyer 2006). Given that adolescent and adult males rarely choose to be circumcised (Wallerstein 1980), it can be inferred that the infant would not choose circumcision if competent.

2.2 Foreskin Function

Anatomically, the foreskin is highly erogenous, pentalaminar, specialized, junctional (transitional) tissue. Other transitional tissues in the body include the lips and eyelids. These transitional tissues all have a high concentration of fine-touch neuroreceptors at the junction of internal (mucosal) surfaces with external (epidermal) surfaces.

The 12th Century Jewish physician and philosopher Moses Maimonides warned Jewish women not to have sex with an intact man, because it then becomes difficult to leave him (Maimonides 1963). In the 19th century, physicians, recognizing that the foreskin was the most sensitive portion of the penis, recommended its removal as a "cure" for masturbation (Darby 2005). Only recently was the ridged band of the prepuce, which is completely removed by circumcision, identified as containing nearly all of the penis's fine-touch neuroreceptors (Taylor et al. 1996; Cold and Taylor 1999).

Several small studies have surveyed adult men with medical indications for circumcision to determine differences in sexual response following surgery (Fink et al. 2002; Coursey et al. 2001; Collins et al. 2002; Shen et al. 2004). Although surgery was intended to be beneficial, a substantial number of these men failed to improve or worsened. They reported increases in erectile dysfunction, loss of sensitivity, and problems with intromission. Others studies have suggested that circumcised men have more trouble with premature ejaculation (O'Hara and O'Hara 1999; Kim and Pang 2007; Richardson and Goldmeier 2005).

Four studies have used objective physiologic measures of the penis. One underpowered study did not evaluate the foreskin but found no differences between circumcised and normal men (Payne et al. 2007). A second study measured fine-pressure thresholds on three locations and found normal men were significantly more sensitive on the glans, but the differences were no longer statistically significant when adjusted for age, diabetes mellitus, and hypertension (Bleustein et al. 2005). In a third study of 159 men taken from the general population, the circumcision scar was the most sensitive portion of the circumcised penis, whereas the most sensitive portion of the intact penis was the portion removed by circumcision. Also the glans of the normal penis was significantly more sensitive than the glans of the circumcised penis (Sorrells et al. 2007). Subsequently a fourth study found decreased vibratory sensation in the glans following circumcision (Yang et al. 2008).

The foreskin also provides protective and immunological functions. Through various secretions (Fleiss et al. 1998), the high concentration of fine-touch neuroreceptors at the transition between skin and mucosa (Taylor et al. 1996; Cold and Taylor 1999), and the structure of smooth muscle and elastic tissue in the dartos layer (Jefferson 1916), the foreskin is effective in keeping detritus and infection from affecting the glans and urethra. This may explain why normal men are less likely to develop sexually transmitted infections.

2.3 Harms and Risks

Several CPs believe that the neonatal period is the optimal time to circumcise, that the cosmetic outcome is superior, the complication rate is lower, and the financial costs are lower. There have been no studies to assess the cosmetic outcome of circumcisions performed neonatally as opposed to later in life; however, the cosmetic outcome in neonatal circumcision has a great deal of variability (Van Howe 1997a), including some horrific outcomes (Strimling 1996; Sherman et al. 1996; Bliss et al. 1997).

When directly compared, the complication rates in neonatal circumcision and those performed later in life, there has either been no difference in complication rates (Yegane et al. 2006), or a higher complication rate following neonatal circumcision (Machmouchi and Alkhotani 2007).

In developed nations, the cost difference is primarily from the anesthetic. While newborns often receive either no anesthetic or topical/local anesthetic, older children and adults are circumcised under general anesthetic (Holthusen et al. 1994).

While topical and local anesthetics reduce the pain of the procedure, the rise in cortisol levels and changes in vital signs from baseline levels during the circumcision with these agents indicate that the procedure is stressful and painful (Van Howe 1997b).

The AAP recommends that when administering anesthetic agents to newborns "the decision to withhold such medication should be based on the same medical criteria used for older patients (Poland et al. 1987)." Based on this, newborns should be circumcised using general anesthesia; however, the risks of general anesthesia in a newborn cannot be justified for an elective procedure.

To justify circumcising in the neonatal period, as opposed to later in life, many CPs argue that newborns have no memory of the event. Remarkably, perinatal events have been demonstrated in a plethora of studies to influence future behaviors (Jacobson et al. 1988; Jacobson et al. 1990; Nyberg et al. 1993; Nyberg et al. 1992; Jacobson et al. 1987; Jacobson and Bygdeman 1998; Zornberg et al. 2000; Anand et al. 2004). Males circumcised as infants cry longer and louder when being vaccinated than normal boys, which indicates that the main structures for memory are functional in neonates and that circumcision pain has long-lasting effects on pain response and perception (Taddio et al. 1995; Taddio et al. 1997).

The only clear advantage to circumcising the neonate is that he is easier to restrain.

2.4 Medical Issues

Breastfeeding: Circumcision interferes with early breastfeeding (Howard et al. 1994) and may explain why male infants in the United States did not breastfeed as long as female infants (Centers for Disease Control and Prevention 2004).

Complication rate: One prospective study found excessive bleeding following 8.9 % of circumcisions (Sutherland et al. 1967). Complication rates based on chart reviews have ranged from 2 to 6.8 % (O'Brien et al. 1995; Gee and Ansell 1976; Moreno and Realini 1989). Databases based on complications listed on discharge facesheets report the lowest complication rates, around 0.2 % (Wiswell and Geschke 1989; Christakis et al. 2000). These databases are often incomplete. For example, the discharge facesheet in the medical record of an infant who had a third of his glans amputated during a circumcision, listed no complications.[2]

These studies also will miss complications that take time to develop, primarily phimosis, webbed penis, and meatal stenosis. Meatal stenosis, which occurs in 5–8 % of boys circumcised neonatally, usually appears 2–5 years following the procedure (Van Howe 1997a; Van Howe 2006).

2.5 Penile Problems

Penile inflammation: In the three studies of children published, one study found no difference (Herzog and Alvarez 1986), two found that circumcised boys under three years of age were at greater risk (Fergusson et al. 1988; Van Howe 2007a). The only study in adults involved British men referred to a dermatologist (Mallon et al. 2000). The study suffers from referral bias and included a control group with a 47.8 % circumcision rate gathered from a country with a 21 % circumcision rate (Johnson et al. 1994).

Phimosis: The incidence of pathologic phimosis in normal boys is 0.6 % by a boy's fifteenth birthday (Shankar and Rickwood 1999). The most common cause is balanitis xerotica obliterans (BXO). The incidence of preputial stenosis as the result of a narrow circumcision scar is about 0.3–1.7 % (Van Howe 1997a; Kaweblum et al. 1984; Stenram et al. 1986). Four published studies provide direct

---

[2] *D.P.,Jr. v. Sonyika*, Fulton County, Georgia, 2009, Civil Action File No 2006EV001125-J.

comparisons of phimosis risk by circumcision status: none found a statistically significant difference (Van Howe 1997a; Herzog and Alvarez 1986; Fergusson et al. 1988; Metcalf et al. 1983).

Paraphimosis: The incidence of paraphimosis is unknown and rare (0.3 % of males referred for non-retractile foreskins) (Saxena et al. 2000). In children, it is nearly always iatrogenic, and simple reduction is sufficient to prevent recurrence (Rickwood 1992). The incidence of pseudoparaphimosis from a retained PlastiBell is between 0.27 and 1 % of circumcisions performed using a PlastiBell (Gee and Ansell 1976; Rubenstein and Bason 1968).

Urinary tract infections (UTIs): Males are more prone to have prenatal urinary tract anomalies: primarily vesicoureteral reflux (VUR) (Herndon et al. 1999; Anderson and Rickwood 1991; Yeung et al. 1997; Tsai et al. 1998). Fortunately, most VUR in newborn males resolves spontaneously (Yeung et al. 1997; Steele et al. 1989; Wennerstrom et al. 1998; Sillén et al. 1998); however, some males with more severe prenatal VUR have associated kidney damage (Yeung et al. 1997).

Nuclear renal imaging has disrupted the paradigm of VUR as a factor in renal scarring (Linshaw 1999; Garin et al. 1998; Ortigas and Cunningham 1997). Evidence has also accumulated that UTIs are rarely a cause of end-stage renal disease (Sreenarasimhaiah and Hellerstein 1998; Helin and Winberg 1980; Esbjörner et al. 1997; Esbjörner et al. 1990; Wennerström et al. 2000a), infections in the first 12 months of life are less likely to involve the kidneys (Pecile et al. 2009), and children with UTIs, renal scarring, and primary, uncomplicated VUR did not develop hypertension (Wolfish et al. 1993; Wennerström et al. 2000b). The net result is that UTIs in infant boys, which can be treated successfully with oral antibiotics (Hoberman et al. 1999), are very unlikely to have long-term sequelae.

There is no evidence of an association between circumcision, VUR, or renal damage (Mueller et al. 1997; Heldrich et al. 2000; Landau et al. 1994; Roth et al. 2009). A meta-analysis of the association of circumcision and UTI (Singh-Grewal et al. 2005) found that the UTI risk of having a foreskin is in a range that could be explained all or in part by confounding factors (Van Howe 2005).

2.6 Cancer

Penile cancer: The link between infant circumcision and penile cancer is tenuous. Two case-controlled studies of the risk factors associated with penile cancer found that phimosis, rather than just having a foreskin, was a significant risk factor (Tseng et al. 2001; Daling et al. 2005), consistent with growing evidence of a link between BXO and penile cancer (Pietrzak et al. 2006; Velazquez and Cubilla 2003; Powell et al. 2000).

Cervical cancer: Of the sixteen studies that have explored the relation between the risk of cervical cancer and the circumcision status of the male sexual partners, only one found a positive association (Castellsagué et al. 2002; Connon 1972; Aitken-Swan and Baird 1966; Abou-Daoud 1967; Wahi et al. 1972; Zarkovic 1985; Boyd and

Doll 1964; Jussawalla et al. 1985; Kjaer et al. 1991; Brinton et al. 1989; Terris et al. 1973; Agarwal et al. 1993; Rotkin 1973; Stern and Dixon 1961; Kmet et al. 1963; Jones et al. 1958)—which would have been expected by chance alone. Hopefully, the HPV vaccine will make discussions of penile and cervical cancer irrelevant.

Prostate cancer: Recently a couple of CPs have touted the impact of circumcision on prostate cancer, basing their promotion on the faulty assumptions that prostate cancer results from irritating infections and that circumcised men are less likely to have urethritis, and a selective bibliography (Morris et al. 2007; Van Howe 2007b). Such speculation is not evidence-based.

Community-acquired *Staphylococcus aureus* (CA-MRSA): Circumcised infants are known to be more prone to staphylococcal infections (Thompson et al. 1966; Enzenauer et al. 1985; Rush et al. 1990). Recently, in multiple reports of outbreaks of CA-MRSA in newborn nurseries, these infections were almost exclusively in boys with lesions primarily in the pubic area (Fortunov et al. 2006a; Fortunov et al. 2007; James et al. 2008; Fortunov et al. 2006b; Rothman 2006; Watson et al. 2006; Wen and Kowalczyk 2009; Van Howe and Robson 2007). In the only study offering a direct comparison, circumcised infants are at 12 times the risk for CA-MRSA infections (Nguyen et al. 2007).

2.6.1 Sexually Transmitted Infections

Unless they are sexually molested, infants and children are not at risk for sexually transmitted infections. Consequently, this issue does not apply until the child is at the age when he can be presumed to be competent.

Syphilis: A meta-analysis found syphilis to be more common in noncircumcised men, primarily in sexually transmitted disease (STD) clinics in Africa (Weiss et al. 2006); however, the meta-analysis excluded two large population surveys that did not find a difference in risk (Dave et al. 2003; Laumann et al. 1997). No difference in risk was found in three randomized clinical trials (RCTs) in Africa (Auvert et al. 2007; Tobian et al. 2009).

Herpes Simplex Virus Type 2 (HSV-2): A meta-analysis found no statistically significant difference in seropositivity for HSV-2 (Weiss et al. 2006). Two subsequent studies of HSV-2 likewise found no difference (Dickson et al. 2005; Xu et al. 2007). Initially the investigators of the three RCTs reported no difference in risk of HSV-2 seroconversion (Auvert et al. 2007); however, later one of the RCTs found men in the control group to be at greater risk for HSV-2 seroconversion (Tobian et al. 2009) and another found a non-statistically significant trend (Sobngwi-Tambekou et al. 2009). When the data are adjusted for the built-in lead time bias in both studies, the differences are not statistically significant (Storms 2009). These studies also confirmed that condom use and limiting number of sexual partners are more effective preventives (Mehta et al. 2008).

Chancroid: A meta-analysis found circumcised men, primarily in Africa, to be a lower risk for chancroid (Weiss et al. 2006); however, the meta-analysis included several studies in which the diagnosis was presumptive, so reaching a definitive conclusion is speculation (Van Howe 2007c).

Gonorrhea and Chlamydia: A meta-analysis found no difference in risk for gonorrhea or chlamydia (Van Howe 2007c). No difference in risk was found in three RCTs in Africa (Auvert et al. 2007).

Genital Discharge Syndrome: This is a non-specific, clinical diagnosis that includes gonorrhea, chlamydia, and non-specific urethritis. A meta-analysis has found that this is more common in circumcised men (Van Howe 2007c). One of the RCTs found no difference in risk (Tobian et al. 2009), while another found that the combined risk for laboratory evidence of gonorrhea, chlamydia, and trichomonas was significantly greater among those circumcised six months after the surgery, but there was no difference at 12 months (Mattson et al. 2008).

Genital Ulcerative Disease: This is non-specific, clinical diagnosis that includes syphilis, chancroid, and active genital herpes. Two meta-analyses have found that this is more likely in normal males (Weiss et al. 2006; Van Howe 2007c). This was confirmed in the RCTs in Africa (Auvert et al. 2007; Tobian et al. 2009).

HPV: A 2007 meta-analysis of studies looking for an association between HPV infection and circumcision status found that several studies had problems with sampling bias, small numbers, and misclassification bias (Van Howe 2007d). Five studies have found that HPV is more likely to be cultured on different parts the penis depending on circumcision status (Weaver et al. 2004; Cook et al. 1993; Aynaud et al. 1999; Hernandez et al. 2008; Nielson et al. 2009). For example, HPV is cultured primarily from the shaft of the circumcised penis and the glans of the normal penis. If only the glans is sampled, the risk of HPV in circumcised men will be underestimated by about 35 % (Weaver et al. 2004). Several studies sampled only the glans for HPV. Likewise, studies in which circumcision status is obtained by patient report, stronger associations between HPV and the foreskin are reported. When adjusted for these factors, there is no statistically significant association between HPV and circumcision status (Van Howe 2007d).

Subsequently, a birth cohort study from New Zealand found no difference in seroprevalence for HPV by circumcision status (Dickson et al. 2009). Two RCTs from Africa have reported a positive association between the foreskin and HPV infection (Tobian et al. 2009; Auvert et al. 2009). Since both findings only sampled the glans for HPV infection, their positive findings are not unexpected, but can be explained completely by sampling bias (Storms 2009; Van Howe 2009). Adding the studies published since the meta-analysis and employing meta-regression techniques (van Houwelingen et al. 2002), relying on patient report for circumcision status and sampling on the glans of the penis were both significant confounding factors. When adjusted for these factors there is no significant association between having a foreskin and being at risk for HPV infection (Van Howe and Storms 2009).

Overall STD Risk: A recent New Zealand study suggesting that normal men are at greater overall risk for STDs (Fergusson et al. 2006), but a birth cohort study in another part of New Zealand found no difference in risk (Dickson et al. 2008). When a meta-analysis is performed that incorporates the 13 studies that have assessed overall risk of STDs (Dave et al. 2003; Laumann et al. 1997; Dickson et al. 2005; Aynaud et al. 1999; Diseker et al. 2000; Parker et al. 1983; Schrek and Lenowitz 1947; Richters et al. 2006; Seed et al. 1995; Taylor and Rodin 1975; Urassa et al. 1997), circumcised men are at greater risk for contracting an STD [unpublished data].

A problem with recommending circumcision to prevent UTIs or STDs is that the intervention, removing an erogenous tissue on a non-consenting infant, is far out of proportion to the illness treated. In most cases, UTIs and STDs can be successfully treated with oral medications. STDs can be more effectively and less invasively prevented with condom use and limiting the number of sexual partners. The numbers needed to treat are large enough that the vast majority of those circumcised will never see any benefit from it.

Another problem is that the prevention of STDs, even if the numbers were to support the CPs' position, is not compelling enough to override violating the integrity and autonomy of the infant, who is not at risk for infection.

Human immunodeficiency virus (HIV): Three RCTs in Africa were recently halted prior to their completion because they found African men interested in being circumcised, but were willing to delay it for two years, were at greater risk of contracting HIV infection over a span of 24 months or less (Auvert et al. 2005; Bailey et al. 2007; Gray et al. 2007a). Although these were randomized trials, they shared several serious problems. It was impossible to blind the subjects, so the studies had an expectation bias. The study began when subjects randomized to the circumcision arm were circumcised, but the treatment arm was instructed to abstain from sexual contact while the circumcision healed (approximately four to six weeks) whereas the men in the control arm continued to be sexually active, thus introducing a lead-time bias, which was amplified by early termination of the trials. Early termination itself is more likely to result in an overestimate of the treatment effect (Mills and Siegfried 2006; Montori et al. 2005). The studies also suffered from attrition bias (700 men failed to complete the study, while only 205 became HIV infected), length bias (no long-term follow-up is planned), and selection bias (only men interested in circumcision were included). There were ethical concerns regarding the trials (Van Howe et al. 2005; Siegfried 2005), and the financial incentives to participate (a free circumcision, money equivalent to two-weeks' worth of employment, cash for recruiting additional subjects, unlimited access to free condoms, and free health care for 21–24 months) were coercive.

With the publication of the RCTs, those advocating circumcision have recognized this as their big opportunity, but they face a number of obstacles.

1. The RCTs have, as mentioned above, serious methodological problems.

2. National data from several African countries fail to confirm the RCT results (Garenne 2008; Connolly et al. 2008; Gisselquist 2008), and the data indicate other factors as being more influential (Talbott 2007). Public health officials in Africa recognize that circumcision is less effective and more expensive than what is currently available and would take resources away from these effective measures (Myers and Myers 2007; Myers and Myers 2008; Sidler et al. 2008).

3. The biological mechanism by which the normal penis increases the risk of HIV infection is based on pure speculation.

A. The inner lining of the foreskin is more susceptible to abrasions. There is no evidence to support this claim and some evidence to the contrary. The only study to address abrasions found a trend toward circumcised men having more penile abrasions (Bailey et al. 1999). More recently, a study found that the keratinization was similar on the internal and external portions of the foreskin (Dinh et al. 2010).

B. The subpreputial space acts as a breeding ground for sexually transmitted viruses. This is usually supported by the spurious claims that HSV-2 and HPV are more common in normal men.

C. Langerhans cells in the lining of the foreskin facilitate the transfer of HIV into the body. Such a claim has several problems.

a. The Langerhans cells are quite good at keeping HIV out of the body. Langerin, a C-type lectin specifically expressed by Langerhans cells, interferes with HIV transmission and inhibits T cell activation. Only when Langerhans cells are overwhelmed with high viral loads is HIV able to get into the body (de Witte et al. 2007). This explains the extremely low transmission rate per coital act for HIV compared to other STDs (Chin 2007).

b. Activated T cells are needed for HIV transmission to occur (Pope et al. 1997). This explains why concurrent STDs increase the risk of HIV transmission and the success of aggressive STD control programs in preventing HIV infections (Gilson et al. 1997; Grosskurth et al. 1995).

c. Langerhan's cells are the first line of defense in the immune system. Without them, the body would be overwhelmed with infections from garden-variety organisms (de Witte et al. 2007) and may also explain why the circumcised male is at greater overall risk for getting an STD.

d. There is no in vivo evidence to support this claim.

D. Keratinized epithelium is protective. Again, there is no evidence to support this claim.

4. Other methods of preventing HIV are more effective, less costly, and less invasive than circumcision. These include aggressive treatment of sexually transmitted infections (Gilson et al. 1997; Grosskurth et al. 1995), condoms (de Vincenzi 1994), and limiting the number of sexual partners. When compared to condoms, which decrease the risk of infection by 99 % or more (de Vincenzi 1994), the circumcision numbers are anemic. CPs speak of circumcision as though it were as effective as a vaccine (Morris 2007a; Clark et al. 2007; Morris 2007b; Auvert et al. 2005; Potts et al. 2008; Klausner et al. 2008; Berer 2008; Burrell 2008; Lie et al. 2006).[3] Typically vaccines that only reduce the risk by 40–50 % are often not used (Garenne 2008; Garenne 2006; Dennehy et al. 1998), and only very low complication rates are tolerated from vaccines. If a vaccine were released that only offered 50 % protection, but reduced condom usage, or increased other risky behaviors, it would likely result in a higher rate of HIV infections (Blower and McLean 1994).

---

[3] Male circumcision in some nations may be the best available HIV prevention tool. Evidence growing for safety, efficacy. AIDS Alert 2007; 22: 25–28.

5. The data from the RCTs have limited scope because of the short duration of the trials. The CPs have taken this short-term data and extrapolated them over several decades to estimate the savings in lives and dollars (Williams et al. 2006; Nagelkerke et al. 2007; Londish and Murray 2008; Podder et al. 2007; Kahn et al. 2006). These models make four assumptions that have no factual basis.

a. The results in a research setting from motivated, well-compensated volunteers can be duplicated in the real world. Generally, experience with RCTs is that the results are rarely replicated in the real world. (See obstacle 6)

b. The results seen in the short duration of the trial will continue in a linear fashion over the next couple of decades. The trajectory of the treatment effect over time is completely unknown and unlikely to remain linear as sexual behaviors change with age. It is unknown whether the protective effect of circumcision fades or reverses with time.

c. The low complication rates documented in a research setting will translate to the population at large. As discussed below [obstacle 6(c)], this is unlikely.

d. There are no delayed complications. As discussed above, meatal stenosis, often requiring meatotomy, occurs following 5–8 % of circumcisions.

At the very best, circumcision may delay infection, but it does not eliminate the risk (Myers and Myers 2007).

6. Treatment effects measured in a controlled, research setting often do not translate to "real world" situations. The "real world" problems are many.

a. Africa does not have enough medical providers to take care of medical needs of Africans, let alone circumcise half of them and take care of the circumcision complications.

b. The cost of circumcising in Africa represents a large portion of their average income. More importantly, the resources used to circumcise will not be available for other less expensive, more effective prevention strategies. For example, for the cost of one circumcision in Africa ($75), 3,500 condoms (2¢ each) can be purchased. Likewise, aggressive treatment of STDs is more cost effective in preventing HIV infection and also treats STDs (Gilson et al. 1997).

c. The low complication rates reported in the RCTs have not been replicated. For example, one African study found a 20.2 % complication rate in a hospital setting with 3.1 % having had part of the glans amputated (Okeke et al. 2006). Complication rates in Kenya have been reported as 35.2 % in a traditional setting and 17.7 % in a medical setting (Bailey and Egesah 2006). A trial of the Tara KLamp in South Africa reported bleeding in 21 %, infection in 32 %, swelling in 83 %, problems with urinating in 16 %, and injury to the penis in 21 % (Lagarde et al. 2009). The rate of moderate to severe adverse events was 8.8 % in the first 20 unsupervised circumcisions for novice practitioners in Africa and only after performing 100 supervised circumcisions were practitioners considered proficient with low complication rates (Kiggundu et al. 2009). It is not inconceivable and possibly likely that circumcisions performed outside the medical system in Africa could result in more deaths than the procedure has been speculated to prevent.

d. Unlike the RCTs, which were preceded with "feasibility" studies to stir up interest in pursuing circumcision (Bailey et al. 2002; Lagarde et al. 2003;

Kebaabetswe et al. 2003; Rain-Taljaard et al. 2003; Mattson et al. 2004; Mattson et al. 2005; Halperin et al. 2005; Scott et al. 2005; Madhivanan et al. 2008; Lukobo and Bailey 2007; Begley et al. 2008), there may not be funds for adequate preparation or education of either patients or providers.

7. A substantial number of HIV infections cannot be attributed to sexual transmission. In the RCTs a number of men became HIV-positive although denying any sexual conduct (Gisselquist 2008). There is an increasing body of evidence that iatrogenic spread of HIV in Africa may be responsible for a sizable portion of the epidemic (Gisselquist 2008; Brewer et al. 2007a; Potterat et al. 2006; Brody and Potterat 2005; Potterat and Brody 2001; Gisselquist et al. 2003; Brewer et al. 2003; Gisselquist et al. 2004; Deuchert and Brody 2007; Brewer et al. 2007b; Gisselquist et al. 2002; Gisselquist and Potterat 2003). One study found that boys circumcised before they became sexually active had greater risk for HIV (Brewer et al. 2007a), suggesting that they may have become infected during the procedure.

8. CPs need to demonstrate outside of a research setting that being circumcised will not give men the mistaken message that they no longer need to use condoms or practice safe sex. Promoting circumcision undercuts condom effectiveness in three ways.

a. With the most sensitive portion of the penis removed, condom use further reduces sexual pleasure in circumcised men, making them less likely to use one consistently.

b. Condoms are more likely to slip off the circumcised penis (Richters et al. 1995).

c. The difficulty in successfully convincing men that a condom is needed for every sexual encounter even after circumcision. Many men will be motivated to be circumcised because they believe after the procedure they will not need to wear a condom.

Models demonstrate that small decreases in condom use can undo any advantages gained from large increases in circumcision rates (Gray et al. 2007b).

Risk compensation has been noted in a number of settings (Blower and McLean 1994; Richens et al. 2000), and would likely occur with circumcision. Feeling that they had additional protection, circumcised men would engage in more risky behavior thus increasing their overall infection risk. While one of the RCTs has reported no signs of disinhibition (Mattson et al. 2008), the applicability of such numbers collected in a research setting with highly-motivated, well-compensated subjects to the general population, especially when circumcision is being promoted as a "natural condom (Fink 1989; Bonner 2001)," is uncertain.

CPs have floated the notion, without a shred of evidence to support it and evidence to the contrary (Laumann et al. 1997), that *infant* circumcision eliminates this disinhibition (Rennie et al. 2007; Clark et al. 2007).

9. CPs need to recognize that the heterosexual spread of HIV in sub-Saharan Africa is different than in the rest of the world. Sofia Gruskin identifies the two schools of thought in how best to control the AIDS epidemic (Gruskin 2007). The first school looks for a biological cure or preventive that will provide a quick, decisive solution. To date, vaccine trials have been disappointing. When the RCT

results became available, the quick fix camp instantly championed the circumcision cause, calling it a "vaccine" that they had been hoping for (Klausner et al. 2008).

The other school of thought professes that the epidemic can only change through behavioral changes (Chin 2007; Donovan and Ross 2000; Pisani 2009; Epstein 2008). The sexual-mixing pattern that predominates the epidemic in sub-Saharan Africa makes it unique. Having multiple concurrent sexual partners, coupled with a reliance on medication delivered parenterally (Gisselquist 2008), has allowed HIV to spread as quickly as it did through their communities. Early on, a similar heterosexual epidemic was predicted for Asia, but it never occurred because of the difference in sexual-mixing patterns (Chin 2007).

Applying the results to the United States is problematic. The United States has a much lower rate of HIV than in Africa, so the number needed to treat would be substantially greater [at least 4,500 (Van Howe 2004; Xu et al. 2009)]. The strain of HIV in Africa differs from the strain in the United States (Chin 2007). The epidemic in the United States is primarily in men having sex with men (MSM), while presumably the African epidemic is among heterosexuals. Applying the results to Europe is even more problematic, given that the HIV rates are several times lower than in the United States.

10. Circumcision would have a relatively small impact on HIV rates. Modeling has predicted that a universal circumcision program would reduce the HIV infection rate by between 3 and 22 % (Williams et al. 2006; Londish and Murray 2008). By comparison, behavior components are responsible for more than 85 % of HIV risk (Donovan and Ross 2000). This has been borne out by the experience in Uganda. With promotion of ABC (Abstinence, Be faithful (no grazing!), and Condoms), Uganda saw the national HIV infection rate drop by 47 % (Low-Beer and Stoneburner 2004).

11. CPs need to demonstrate the superiority of primary prevention over secondary prevention. For HIV, the most effective use of resources would involve identifying those who are HIV-infected, providing them a life-time supply of condoms, and/or treating them with anti-retroviral agents (Chin 2007). In HIV-infected individuals on anti-retroviral agents who do not have an active STD, their infectivity rate is considered to be zero (Vernazza 2008).

12. CPs need to explain what has happened in the United States, where the incidence of heterosexually transmitted HIV is several-fold higher than in Europe and Japan. The United States also has the highest rate of circumcision among Western nations. Among ethnic groups in the United States, blacks have the highest rates of heterosexually transmitted HIV (US Centers for Disease Control and Prevention 2007) and circumcision (O'Brien et al. 1995; Xu et al. 2007; Mor et al. 2007; Mansfield et al. 1995). Instead of an explanation, CPs have targeted blacks in the United States for even higher rates of circumcision (Gray et al. 2009).

13. Circumcision of males only protects males. Studies have failed to show that circumcision decreased the HIV risk of their female partners (Turner et al. 2007), and male circumcision may increase the risk for the female partner (Associated Press 2007; Wawer et al. 2009; Chao et al. 1994).

14. There is no evidence that the results in highly-motivated, well-compensated adults in Africa can be extrapolated to non-consenting, unmotivated, uncompensated infants. To date, there is no evidence that *infant* circumcision prevents HIV infection. To the contrary, infants and children are at very low risk for sexually transmitted HIV and by the time today's newborns begin having sexual contact they can decide for themselves how to protect themselves from HIV infection.

15. When all of the costs and health outcomes related to infant circumcision were combined in a cost-utility analysis, it was impossible with current conditions in developed countries, even with assumptions most favorable to circumcision, to manipulate the numbers to make the practice preserve health or save money. In the United States, it would cost between $1 and $11 million to avert one case of heterosexually transmitted HIV. In countries with lower incidences of HIV infection, the cost per averted case would be greater. Neonatal circumcision resulted in lifetime costs of $828.42 per person and a reduction in health of 15.30 quality-adjusted life-years per 1,000 males (Van Howe 2004).

16. Outside of circumcising cultures (primarily the United States), the CPs have to appear as though they are not fanatics promoting panic where there is no need to panic. Many of the prominent supporters of circumcision come from circumcising cultures. Over the past 150 years, circumcision has become so entrenched in American culture as a social norm, that rational discussions of the topic are rare, if not impossible (Waldeck 2003). With declining infant circumcision rates in the United States, CPs have resorted to the Chicken Little tactic of declaring that the epidemic is out of control and that desperate times call for desperate measures. Promoting circumcision also carries the stigma of unwelcomed paternalism. The procedure has been linked with controlling sexuality for millennia (Maimonides 1963; Hodges 1997; Immerman and Mackey 1997; Immerman and Mackey 1998; Hoffman 1996). Consequently, bringing the intervention to Africa by North Americans and Europeans rings of cultural colonialism (Van Howe et al. 2005).

2.7 Conclusion

The evidence on the "benefits" of circumcision always have been and continue to be contentious and contested. In the absence of a consensus, the most appropriate policy is to leave the decision to the individual to make when he is old enough to consider the evidence for himself and make an informed decision. If the CPs were confident in the merits of their case, believing that the evidence was so overwhelming that any rational person would willingly consent, they would adopt this policy. Instead, the CPs insist that the decision be taken out of the individual's hands and given to somebody else, imposing it by force on those too weak to resist.

Circumcision is an intervention out of proportion to the benefits hoped for: analogous to tapping in carpet tacks with a 16-pound sledgehammer. In every instance, more effective, less expensive, less invasive alternatives exist.

References

Abou-Daoud KT (1967) Epidemiology of carcinoma of the cervix uteri in Lebanese Christians and Moslems. Cancer 20:1706–1714

Agarwal SS, Sehgal A, Sardana S, Kumar A, Luthra UK (1993) Role of male behavior in cervical carcinogenesis among women with one lifetime sexual partner. Cancer 72:1666–1669

Aitken-Swan J, Baird D (1966) Cancer of the uterine cervix in Aberdeenshire. Aetiological aspects. Br J Cancer 20:642–659

Alderson P (1993) Children's consent to surgery. Open University Press, Buckingham

American Academy of Pediatrics Task Force on Circumcision (1999) Circumcision policy statement. Pediatrics 103:686–693

American Medical Association Council on Scientific Affairs (1999) Report 10: neonatal circumcision. American Medical Association, Chicago

Anand KJ, Runeson B, Jacobson B (2004) Gastric suction at birth associated with long-term risk for functional intestinal disorders in later life. J Pediatr 144:449–454

Anderson PAM, Rickwood AMK (1991) Features of primary vesicoureteric reflux detected by prenatal sonography. Br J Urol 67:267–271

Associated Press (2007) Circumcision may lift HIV risk for women. New York Times 7 Mar 2007

Auvert B, Taljaard D, Lagarde E, Sobngwi-Tambekou J, Sitta R, Puren A (2005) Randomized, controlled intervention trial of male circumcision for reduction of HIV infection risk: the ANRS 1265 trial. PLoS Med 2(11):e298

Auvert B, Bailey R, Gray R (2007) Results of the South African trial, the Kenyan trial, and the Rakai trial. Centers for Disease Control and Prevention consultation on public health issues regarding male circumcision in the United States for the prevention of HIV infection and other health consequences. Atlanta, Georgia, 26 Apr 2007

Auvert B, Sobngwi-Tambekou J, Cutler E, Nieuwoudt M, Lissaouba P, Puren A et al (2009) Effect of male circumcision on the prevalence of human-risk human papillomavirus in young men: results of a randomized controlled trial conducted in Orange Farm, South Africa. J Infect Dis 199:14–19

Aynaud O, Piron D, Bijaoui G, Casanova JM (1999) Developmental factors of urethral human papillomavirus lesions: correlation with circumcision. BJU Int 84:57–60

Bailey RC, Egesah O (2006) Assessment of clinical and traditional male circumcision services in Bungoma District, Kenya. Complication rates and operational needs. Special Report, Washington, DC: USAID, PSI Aidsmark, pp 1–39

Bailey RC, Neema S, Othieno R (1999) Sexual behaviours and other HIV risk factors in circumcised and uncircumcised men in Uganda. J Acquir Immune Defic Syndr Hum Retrovirol 22:294–301

Bailey RC, Muga R, Poulussen R, Abicht H (2002) The acceptability of male circumcision to reduce HIV infections in Nyanza Province, Kenya. AIDS Care 14(1):27–40

Bailey RC, Moses S, Parker CB, Agot K, Krieger JN, Williams CFM et al (2007) Male circumcision for HIV prevention in young men in Kisumu, Kenya: a randomised controlled trial. Lancet 369:643–656

Beasley S, Darlow B, Craig J, Mulcahy D, Smith G (2002) Position statement on circumcision. Royal Australasian College of Physicians, Sydney

Begley EB, Jafa K, Voetsch AC, Heffelfinger JD, Borkowf CB, Sullivan PS (2008) Willingness of men who have sex with men (MSM) in the United States to be circumcised as adults to reduce the risk HIV infection. PLoS ONE 3(7):e2731

Benatar M, Benatar D (2003a) Between prophylaxis and child abuse: the ethics of neonatal male circumcision. Am J Bioeth 3(2):35–48

Benatar D, Benatar M (2003b) How not to argue about circumcision. Am J Bioeth 3(2):W1

Berer M (2008) Male circumcision for HIV prevention: what about protecting men's partners? Reprod Health Matters 16(32):171–175

Bleustein CB, Fogarty JD, Eckholdt H, Arezzo JC, Melman A (2005) Effect of neonatal circumcision on penile neurologic sensation. Urology 65:773–777

Bliss DP, Healy PJ, Waldhausen JHT (1997) Necrotizing fasciitis after Plastibell circumcision. J Pediatr 131:459–462

Blower SM, McLean AR (1994) Prophylactic vaccines, risk behaviour change, and the probability of eradicating HIV in San Francisco. Science 265:1451–1454

Bonner K (2001) Male circumcision as an HIV control strategy: not a 'natural condom'. Reprod Health Matters 9(18):143–155

Boyd JT, Doll RA (1964) A study of the aetiology of carcinoma of the cervix uteri. Br J Cancer 18:419–434

Brewer DD, Brody S, Drucker E, Gisselquist D, Minkin SF, Potterat JJ, Rothenberg RB, Vachon F (2003) Mounting anomalies in the epidemiology of HIV in Africa: cry the beloved paradigm. Int J STD AIDS 14:144–147

Brewer DD, Potterat JJ, Roberts JM Jr, Brody S (2007a) Male and female circumcision associated with prevalent HIV infection in virgins and adolescents in Kenya, Lesotho, and Tanzania. Ann Epidemiol 17:217–226

Brewer DD, Potterat JJ, Brody S (2007b) Male circumcision and HIV prevention. Lancet 369:1597

Brinton LA, Reeves WC, Brenes MM, Herrero R, Gaitan E, Tenorio F et al (1989) The male factor in the etiology of cervical cancer among sexually monogamous women. Int J Cancer 44:199–203

Brody S, Potterat JJ (2005) HIV epidemiology in Africa: weak variables and tendentiousness generate wobbly conclusions. PLos Med 2(5):e137

Brusa M, Barilan YM (2008) Cultural circumcision in EU public hospitals: an ethical discussion. Bioethics; Epub ahead of print

Burrell C (2008) A low tech way to combat HIV-AIDS: the world is finally waking up to male circumcision. Harvey Public Health Review, Spring-Summer, pp 24–25

Castellsagué X, Bosch FX, Muñoz N, Meijer CJLM, Shah KV, de Sanjosé S et al (2002) Male circumcision, penile human papillomavirus infection, and cervical cancer in female partners. N Engl J Med 346:1105–1112

Centers for Disease Control and Prevention (2007) Breastfeeding practices: results from the National Immunization Survey. http://www.cdc.gov/breastfeeding/data/NIS_data/data_2004.html. Accessed 2 Dec 2007

Chao A, Bulterys M, Musanganire F, Habimana P, Nawrocki P, Taylor E et al (1994) Risk factors associated with prevalent HIV-1 infection among pregnant women in Rwanda. National University of Rwanda-Johns Hopkins University AIDS Research Team. Int J Epidemiol 23:371–380

Chin J (2007) The AIDS pandemic: the collision of epidemiology with political correctness. Radcliffe Publishing, Oxford

Christakis DA, Harvey E, Zerr DM, Feudtner C, Wright JA, Connell FA (2000) A trade-off analysis of routine newborn circumcision. Pediatrics 105:246–249

Clark PA, Eisenman J, Szapor S (2007) Mandatory neonatal circumcision in sub-Saharan Africa: medical and ethical analysis. Med Sci Monit 13(12):RA205–RA213

Cold CJ, Taylor J (1999) The prepuce. BJU Int 83(1):34–44

College of Physicians and Surgeons of British Columbia (2004) Policy manual: infant male circumcision Vancouver. BC, College of Physicians and Surgeons of British Columbia

Collins S, Upshaw J, Rutchik S, Ohannessian C, Ortenberg J, Albertsen P (2002) Effects of circumcision on male sexual function: debunking a myth? J Urol 167:2111–2112

Committee on Bioethics (1995) Informed consent, parental permission, and assent in pediatric practice. Pediatrics 95:314–317

Connolly C, Shanmugam R, Simbayi LC, Nqeketo A (2008) Male circumcision and its relationship to HIV infection in South Africa: results of a national survey in 2002. S Afr Med J 98:789–794

Connon AF (1972) Cancer detection survey gynaecological and epidemiological data. Med J Aust 1:738–741

Cook LS, Koutsky LA, Holmes KK (1993) Clinical presentation of genital warts among circumcised and uncircumcised heterosexual men attending an urban STD clinic. Genitourin Med 69:262–264

Coursey JW, Morey AF, Summerton DJ, Secrest C, White P et al (2001) Erectile function after anterior urethroplasty. J Urol 166:2273–2276

Daling JR, Madeleine MM, Johnson LG, Schwartz SM, Shera KA, Wurscher MA et al (2005) Penile cancer: importance of circumcision, human papillomavirus and smoking in in situ and invasive disease. Int J Cancer 116:606–616

Darby R (2005) A surgical temptation: the demonization of the foreskin and the rise of circumcision in Britain. University of Chicago Press, Chicago

Darby R, Svoboda JS (2008) A rose by any other name? symmetry and asymmetry in male and female genital cutting. In: Zabus C (ed) Fearful symmetries: essays and testimonies around excision and circumcision. Kenilworth, New Jersey (in press)

Dave SS, Fenton KA, Mercer CH, Erens B, Wellings K, Johnson AM (2003) Male circumcision in Britain: findings from a national probability sample survey. Sex Transm Infect 79:499–500

de Vincenzi I (1994) A longitudinal study of human immunodeficiency virus transmission by heterosexual partners. European Study Group on Heterosexual Transmission of HIV. N Engl J Med 331:341–346

de Witte L, Nabatov A, Pion M, Fluitsma D, de Jong MAWP, de Gruijl T et al (2007) Langerin as a natural barrier to HIV-1 transmission by Langerhans cells. Nat Med 13:367–371

Dekkers W (2009) Routine (non-religious) neonatal circumcision and bodily integrity: a transatlantic dialogue. Kennedy Inst Ethics J 19:125–146

Dekkers W, Hoffer C, Wils J-P (2005) Bodily integrity and male and female circumcision. Med Health Care Philos 8:179–191

Dennehy PH, Jost EE, Peter G (1998) Active immunizing agents. In: Feigin RD, Cherry JD (eds) Textbook of pediatric infectious diseases, 4th edn. WB Saunders Co, Philadelphia

Deuchert E, Brody S (2007) Lack of autodisable syringe use and health care indicators are associated with high HIV prevalence: an international ecologic analysis. Ann Epidemiol 17:199–207

Dickerman JD (2007) Circumcision in the time of HIV: when is there enough evidence to revise the Academy of Pediatric' policy on circumcision? Pediatrics 119:1006–1007

Dickson N, van Roode T, Paul C (2005) Herpes simplex virus type 2 status at age 26 is not related to early circumcision in a birth cohort. Sex Transm Dis 32:517–519

Dickson NP, van Roode T, Herbison P, Paul C (2008) Circumcision and risk of sexually transmitted infections in a birth cohort. J Pediatr 152:383–387

Dickson NP, Ryding J, van Roode T, Paul C, Hervison P, Dillner J et al (2009) Male circumcision and serologically determined human papillomavirus infection in a birth cohort. Cancer Epidemiol Biomarkers Prev 18:177–183

Dinh MH, McRaven MD, Kelley Z, Penugonda S, Hope TJ (2010) Keratinization of the adult male foreskin and implications for male circumcision. AIDS 24:899–906

Diseker RA 3rd, Peterman TA, Kamb ML, Kent C, Zenilman JM, Douglas JM Jr et al (2000) Circumcision and STD in the United States: cross sectional and cohort analyses. Sex Transm Infect 76:474–479

Donovan B, Ross MW (2000) Preventing HIV: determinants of sexual behaviour. Lancet 355:1897–1901

Dwyer JG (2006) The relationship rights of children. Cambridge University Press, Cambridge

Enzenauer RW, Dotson CR, Leonard T, Reuben L, Bass JW, Brown J III (1985) Male predominance in persistent staphylococcal colonization and infection of the newborn. Hawaii Medical Journal, vol 44, pp 389–390, 392, 394–396

Epstein H (2008) The invisible cure: why we are losing the fight against AIDS in Africa. Picador, New York

Esbjörner E, Aronson S, Berg U, Jodal U, Linne T (1990) Children with chronic renal failure in Sweden 1978–1985. Pediatr Nephrol 4:249–252

Esbjörner E, Berg U, Hansson S (1997) Epidemiology of chronic renal failure in children: a report from Sweden 1986–1994. Swedish Pediatric Nephrology Association. Pediatr Nephrol 11:438–442

Fergusson DM, Lawton JM, Shannon FT (1988) Neonatal circumcision and penile problems: an 8 years longitudinal study. Pediatrics 81:537–541

Fergusson DM, Boden JM, Horwood LJ (2006) Circumcision status and risk of sexually transmitted infection in young adult males: an analysis of a longitudinal birth cohort. Pediatrics 118:1971–1977

Fetus and Newborn Committee (1996) Canadian Paediatric Society. Neonatal circumcision revisited. Can Med Assoc J 154:769–780

Fink AJ (1989) Newborn circumcision: a long-term strategy for AIDS prevention. J R Soc Med 82:695

Fink KS, Carson CC, DeVellis RF (2002) Adult circumcision outcomes study: effect on erectile function, penile sensitivity, sexual activity and satisfaction. J Urol 167:2113–2116

Fleiss PM, Hodges F, Van Howe RS (1998) Immunological functions of the human prepuce: a review. Sex Transm Inf 74:364–367

Flynn P, Havens P, Brady M, Emmanuel P, Read J, Hoyt L et al (2007) Male circumcision for prevention of HIV and other sexually transmitted diseases. Pediatrics 119:821–822

Fortunov RM, Hulten KG, Hammerman WA, Mason EO Jr, Kaplan SL (2006a) Community-acquired Staphylococcus aureus infections in term and near-term previously healthy neonates. Pediatrics 118:874–881

Fortunov RM, Hulten KG, Hammerman WA, Mason EO, Kaplan SL (2006) Community-acquired *Staphylococcus aureus* infections in term and near term previously healthy neonates (Poster #2753.6). Poster presentation at: 2006 pediatric academic societies' annual meeting; San Francisco, California; 26 Apr 2006

Fortunov RM, Hulten KG, Hammerman WA, Mason EO Jr, Kaplan SL (2007) Infections in term and late-preterm previously healthy neonates: evaluation and treatment of community-acquired Staphylococcus aureus. Pediatrics 120:937–945

Garenne M (2006) Male circumcision and HIV control in Africa. PLoS Med 3:e78

Garenne M (2008) Long-term population effect of male circumcision in generalised HIVepidemics in sub-Saharan Africa. Afr J AIDS Res 7:1–8

Garin EH, Campos A, Homsy Y (1998) Primary vesicoureteral reflux: review of current concepts. Pediatr Nephrol 12:249–256

Gee WF, Ansell JS (1976) Neonatal circumcision: a ten-year overview: with comparison of the Gomco clamp and the Plastibell device. Pediatrics 58:824–827

Gilson L, Mkanje R, Grosskurth H, Mosha F, Picard J, Gavyole A et al (1997) Cost-effectiveness of improved treatment services for sexually transmitted diseases in preventing HIV-1 infection in Mwanza Region, Tanzania. Lancet 350:1805–1809

Gisselquist D (2008) Points to consider: responses to HIV/AIDS in Africa, Asia and Caribbean. Adonis & Abbey Publishers Ltd, London

Gisselquist D, Potterat JJ (2003) Heterosexual transmission of HIV in Africa: an empiric estimate. Int J STD AIDS 14:162–173

Gisselquist D, Rothenberg R, Potterat J, Drucker E (2002) Non-sexual transmission of HIV has been overlooked in developing countries. Br Med J 324:235

Gisselquist D, Pottarat JJ, Brody S, Vachon F (2003) Let it be sexual: how health care transmission of AIDS in Africa was ignored. Int J STD AIDS 14:148–161

Gisselquist D, Potterat JJ, Brody S (2004) Running on empty: sexual co-factors are insufficient to fuel Africa's turbocharged HIV epidemic. Int J STD AIDS 15:442–452

Golden MR, Wasserheit JN (2009) Prevention of viral sexually transmitted infections: foreskin at the forefront. N Engl J Med 360:1349–1351

Gostin LO, Hankins CA (2008) Male circumcision as an HIV prevention strategy in sub-Saharan Africa: sociolegal barriers. JAMA 300:2539–2541

Gray RH, Kigozi G, Serwadda D, Makumbi F, Watya S, Nalugoda F et al (2007a) Male circumcision for HIV prevention in men in Rakai, Uganda: a randomised trial. Lancet 369:657–666

Gray RH, Li X, Kigozi G, Serwadda D, Nalugoda F, Watya S et al (2007b) The impact of male circumcision on HIV incidence and cost per infection prevented: a stochastic simulation model from Rakai, Uganda. AIDS 21:845–850

Gray RH, Wawer MJ, Serwadda D, Kigozi G (2009) The role of male circumcision in the prevention of human papillomavirus and HIV infection. J Infect Dis 199:1–3

Grosskurth H, Mosha F, Todd J, Mwijarubi E, Klokke A, Senkoro K et al (1995) Impact of improved treatment of sexually transmitted diseases on HIV infection in rural Tanzania: randomised controlled trial. Lancet 346:530–536

Gruskin S (2007) Male circumcision, in so many words…. Reprod Health Matters 15(29):49–52

Halperin DT, Fritz K, McFarland W, Woelk G (2005) Acceptability of adult male circumcision for sexually transmitted disease and HIV prevention in Zimbabwe. Sex Transm Dis 32:238–239

Heldrich FJ, Barone MA, Spiegler E (2000) UTI: diagnosis and evaluation in symptomatic pediatric patients. Clin Pediatr (Phila) 39:461–472

Helin I, Winberg J (1980) Chronic renal failure in Swedish children. Acta Paediatr Scand 69:607–611

Hernandez BY, Wilkens LR, Zhu X, McDuffie K, Thompson P, Shvetsov YB et al (2008) Circumcision and human papillomavirus infection in men: a site-specific comparison. J Infect Dis 197:787–794

Herndon CDA, McKenna PH, Kolon TF, Gonzales ET, Baker LA, Docimo SG (1999) A multicenter outcomes analysis of patients with neonatal reflux presenting with prenatal hydronephrosis. J Urol 162:1203–1208

Herzog LW, Alvarez SR (1986) The frequency of foreskin problems in uncircumcised children. Am J Dis Child 140:254–256

Hoberman A, Wald ER, Hickey RW, Baskin M, Charron M, Majd M et al (1999) Oral versus initial intravenous therapy for urinary tract infections in young febrile children. Pediatrics 104:79–86

Hodges F (1997) A short history of the institutionalization of involuntary sexual mutilation in the United States. In: Denniston GC, Milos MF (eds) Sexual mutilations a human tragedy. Plenum Press, New York, pp 17–40

Hoffman LA (1996) Covenant of blood: circumcision and gender in Rabbinic Judaism. The University of Chicago Press, Chicago

Holthusen H, Eichwede F, Stevens M, Willnow U, Lipfert P (1994) Pre-emptive analgesia: comparison of preoperative with postoperative caudal block on postoperative pain in children. Br J Anaesth 73:440–442

Howard CR, Howard FM, Weitzman ML (1994) Acetaminophen analgesia in neonatal circumcision: the effect on pain. Pediatrics 93:641–646

Immerman RS, Mackey WC (1997) A biocultural analysis of circumcision. Soc Biol 44:265–275

Immerman RS, Mackey WC (1998) A proposed relationship between circumcision and neural reorganization. J Genet Psychol 159:367–378

Jacobson B, Bygdeman M (1998) Obstetric care and proneness of offspring to suicide as adults: case-control study. Br Med J 317:1346–1349

Jacobson B, Eklund G, Hamberger L, Linnarsson D, Sedvall G, Valverius M (1987) Perinatal origin of adult self-destructive behavior. Acta Psychiatr Scand 76:364–371

Jacobson B, Nyberg K, Eklund G, Bygdeman M, Rydberg U (1988) Obstetrical pain medication and eventual adult amphetamine addiction in offspring. Acta Obstet Gynecol Scand 67:677–682

Jacobson B, Nyberg K, Grönbladh L, Eklund G, Bygdeman M, Rydberg U (1990) Opiate addiction in adult offspring through possible imprinting after obstetric treatment. Br Med J 301:1067–1070

James L, Gorwitz RJ, Jones RC, Watson JT, Hageman JC, Jernigan DB et al (2008) Methicillin-resistant staphylococcus aureus infection among healthy full-term newborns. Arch Dis Child Fetal Neonatal Ed 93:F40–F44

Jefferson G (1916) The peripenic muscle; some observations on the anatomy of phimosis. Surg Gynecol Obst 23:177–181

Johnson AM, Wadsworth J, Wellings K, Field J, Bradshaw S (1994) Sexual Attitudes and Lifestyles. Blackwell Scientific, Oxford

Jones EG, MacDonald I, Breslow L (1958) A study of epidemiologic factors in carcinoma of the uterine cervix. Am J Obstet Gynecol 76:1–10

Jussawalla DJ, Yeole BB, Natekar MV (1985) Cancer in Indian Moslems. Cancer 55:1149–1158

Kahn JG, Marseille E, Auvert B (2006) Cost-effectiveness of male circumcision for HIV prevention in a South African setting. PLoS Med 3(12):e517

Kant I (1998) Critique of practical reason. Marquette University Press, Milwaukee

Katz IT, Wright AA (2008) Circumcision: a surgical strategy for HIV prevention in Africa. N Engl J Med 359:2412–2415

Kaweblum YA, Press S, Kogan L, Levine M, Kaweblum M (1984) Circumcision using the Mogen clamp. Clin Pediatr (Phila) 23:679–682

Kebaabetswe P, Lockman S, Mogwe S, Mandevu R, Thior I, Essex M et al (2003) Male circumcision: an acceptable strategy for HIV prevention in Botswana. Sex Transm Infect 79:214–219

Kendel DA (2002) Caution against routine circumcision of newborn male infants (Memo to physicians and surgeons of Saskatchewan). Saskatoon: College of Physicians and Surgeons of Saskatchewan; 20 February

Kiggundu V, Watya S, Kigonzi G, Serwadda D, Nalugoda F, Buwembo D et al (2009) The number of procedures required to achieve optimal competency with male circumcision: findings from a randomized trial in Rakai, Uganda. BJU International (Epub ahead of print)

Kim DS, Pang M-G (2007) The effect of male circumcision on sexuality. BJU Int 99:619–622

Kjaer SK, de Villiers EM, Dahl C, Engholm G, Bock JE, Vestergaard BF et al (1991) Case-control study of risk factors for cervical neoplasia in Denmark. I: role of the "male factor" in women with one lifetime sexual partner. Int J Cancer 48:39–44

Klausner JD, Wamai RG, Bowa K, Agot K, Kagimba K, Halperin DT (2008) Is male circumcision as good as the HIV vaccine we've been waiting for? Future HIV Ther 2(1):1–7

Kmet J, Damjanovski L, Stucin M, Bonta S, Cakmakov A (1963) Circumcision and carcinoma colli uteri in Macedonia, Yugoslavia. Results from a field study. Br J Cancer 17:391–399

Lagarde E, Dirk T, Puren A, Reathe RT, Bertran A (2003) Acceptability of male circumcision as a tool for preventing HIV infection in a highly infected community in South Africa. AIDS 17:89–95

Lagarde E, Taljaard D, Puren A, Auvert B (2009) High rate of adverse events following circumcision of young male adults with the Tara KLamp technique: a randomised trial in South Africa. S Afr Med J 99:163–169

Landau D, Turner ME, Brennan J, Majd M (1994) The value of urinalysis in differentiating acute pyelonephritis from lower urinary tract infection in febrile infants. Pediatr Infect Dis J 13:777–781

Laumann EO, Masi CM, Zuckerman EW (1997) Circumcision in the United States: prevalence, prophylactic effects, and sexual practice. JAMA 277:1052–1057

Lebit LE (1992) Compelled medical procedures involving minors and incompetents and misapplications of the substituted judgment doctrine. J Law Health 7:107–130

Lie RK, Emanuel EJ, Grady C (2006) Circumcision and HIV prevention research: an ethical analysis. Lancet 368:522–525

Linshaw MA (1999) Controversies in childhood urinary tract infections. World J Urol 17:383–395

Londish GJ, Murray JM (2008) Significant reduction in HIV prevalence according to male circumcision intervention in sub-Saharan Africa. Int J Epidemiol 37:1246–1253

Low-Beer D, Stoneburner RL (2004) Behaviour and communication change in reducing HIV: is Uganda unique? Africa Journal of AIDS Research, p 12

Lukobo MD, Bailey RC (2007) Acceptability of male circumcision for prevention of HIV infection in Zambia. AIDS Care 19:471–477

Machmouchi M, Alkhotani A (2007) Is neonatal circumcision judicious? Eur J Pediatr Surg 17:266–269

Madhivanan P, Krupp K, Chandrasekaran V, Karat SC, Reingold AL, Klausner JD (2008) Acceptability of male circumcision among mothers with male children in Mysore, India. AIDS 22:983–988

Maimonides M (1963) The guide of the perplexed (Tr. Pines S). University of Chicago Press, Chicago

Mallon E, Hawkins D, Dinneen M, Francics N, Fearfield L, Newson R et al (2000) Circumcision and genital dermatoses. Arch Dermatol 136:350–354

Mansfield CJ, Hueston WJ, Rudy M (1995) Neonatal circumcision: associated factors and length of hospital stay. J Fam Pract 41:370–376

Mattson CL, Muga R, Poulussen R, Onyango T, Bailey RC (2004) Feasibility of medical male circumcision in Nyanza Province, Kenya. East Afr Med J 81:230–235

Mattson CL, Bailey RC, Muga R, Poulussen R, Onyango T (2005) Acceptability of male circumcision and predictors of circumcision preference among men and women in Nyanza Province, Kenya. AIDS Care 17:182–194

Mattson CL, Campbell RT, Bailey RC, Agot K, Ndinya-Achola JO, Moses S (2008) Risk compensation is not associated with male circumcision in Kisumu, Kenya: a multi-faceted assessment of men enrolled in a randomized controlled trial. PLoS ONE 3(6):e2443

Medical Ethics Committee (2003) The law and ethics of male circumcision: guidance for doctors. British Medical Association, London

Mehta SD, Moses S, Agot K, Agingu W, Parker C, Ndinya-Achola JO et al (2008) Herpes simplex virus type 2 infection among young uncircumcised men in Kisumu, Kenya. Sex Transm Infect 84:42–48

Metcalf TJ, Osborn LM, Mariani EM (1983) Circumcision. A study of current practices. Clin Pediatr (Phila) 22:575–579

Mills E, Siegfried N (2006) Cautious optimism for new HIV/AIDS prevention strategies. Lancet 368:1236

Montori VM, Devereaux PJ, Adhikari NK, Burns KE, Eggert CH, Briel M et al (2005) Randomized trial stopped early for benefit: a systematic review. JAMA 294:2203–2209

Mor Z, Kent CK, Kohn RP, Klausner JD (2007) Declining rates in male circumcision amidst increasing evidence of its public health benefit. PLoS ONE 2(9):e861

Moreno CA, Realini JP (1989) Infant circumcision in an outpatient setting. Tex Med 85:37–40

Morris B (2007a) Why circumcision is a biomedical imperative for the 21(st) century. Bioessays 29:1147–1158

Morris BJ (2007b) Circumcision facts trump anti-circ fiction. Australia Skeptic (Summer), pp 52–56

Circumcision and circumspection. Lancet Infect Dis 2007; 7:303

Morris BJ (2008) Circumcision: who should you believe? Australia Skeptic (Winter), pp 55–58

Morris BJ, Bailis SA, Castellsague X, Wiswell TE, Halperin DT (2006) RACP's policy statement on male circumcision is ill-conceived. Aust N Z J Public Health 30:16–22

Morris BJ, Waskett J, Bailis SA (2007) Case number and the financial impact of circumcision in reducing prostate cancer. BJU Int 100:5–6

Mueller ER, Steinhardt G, Naseer S (1997) The incidence of genitourinary abnormalities in circumcised and uncircumcised boys presenting with an initial urinary tract infection by 6 months of age [Abstract 121]. Pediatrics 100:580

Myers A, Myers J (2007) Male circumcision: the new hope? S Afr Med J 97:338–341

Myers A, Myers J (2008) Rolling out male circumcision as a mass HIV/AIDS intervention seems neither justified nor practical. S Afr Med J 98:781–782

Nagelkerke NJ, Moses S, de Vlas SJ, Bailey RC (2007) Modelling the public health impact of male circumcision for HIV prevention in high prevalence areas in Africa. BMC Infect Dis 13(7):16

Newell M-L, Bärnighausen T (2007a) Male circumcision to cut HIV risk in the general population. Lancet 369:617–619

Newer approaches to HIV prevention. Lancet 2007; 369:615

Nguyen DM, Bancroft E, Mascola L, Guevara R, Yasuda L (2007) Risk factors for neonatal methicillin-resistant Staphylococcus aureus infection in a well-infant nursery. Infect Control Hosp Epidemiol 28:406–411

Nielson CM, Schiaffino MK, Dunne EF, Salemi JL, Giuliano AR (2009) Associations between male anogenital human papillomavirus infection and circumcision by anatomic site sampled and lifetime number of female sex partners. J Infect Dis 199:7–13

Nyberg K, Allebeck P, Eklund G, Jacobson B (1992) Socio-economic versus obstetric risk factors for drug addiction in offspring. Br J Addict 87:1669–1676

Nyberg K, Allebeck P, Eklund G, Jacobson B (1993) Obstetric medication versus residential area as perinatal risk factors for subsequent adult drug addiction in offspring. Paediatr Perinat Epidemiol 7:23–32

O'Hara K, O'Hara J (1999) The effect of male circumcision on the sexual enjoyment of the female partner. BJU Int 83(1):79–84

O'Brien TR, Calle EE, Poole WK (1995) Incidence of neonatal circumcision in Atlanta, 1985–1986. South Med J 88:411–415

Okeke LI, Asinobi AA, Ikuerowo OS (2006) Epidemiology of complications of male circumcision in Ibadan, Nigeri. BMC Urol 6:21

Ortigas AP, Cunningham AS (1997) Three facts to know before you order a VCUG. Control Pediatric, vol 14(9), pp 69, 73–74, 79

Parker SW, Stewart AJ, Wren MN, Gollow MM, Straton JA (1983) Circumcision and sexually transmissible disease. Med J Aust 2:288–290

Payne K, Thaler L, Kukkonen T, Carrier S, Binik Y (2007) Sensation and sexual arousal in circumcised and uncircumcised men. J Sex Med 4:667–674

Pecile P, Miorin E, Romanello C, Vidal E, Contardo M, Valent F et al (2009) Age-related renal parenchymal lesions in children with first febrile urinary tract infections. Pediatrics 124:23–29

Pietrzak P, Hadway P, Corbishley CM, Watkin NA (2006) Is the association between balanitis xerotica obliterans and penile carcinoma underestimated? BJU Int 98:74–76

Pisani E (2009) The wisdom of whores: bureaucrats, brothels and the business of AIDS, 2nd edn. Granta Books, London

Podder CN, Sharomi O, Gumel AB, Moses S (2007) To cut or not to cut: a modeling approach for assessing the role of male circumcision in HIV control. Bull Math Biol 69(2447–2466):244

Poland RL, Roberts RJ, Guitierrez-Mazorra JF, Fonkalsrud EW (1987) Committee on Fetus and Newborn, Committee on Drugs, Section on Anesthesiology, Section on Surgery. Neonatal anesthesia. Pediatrics 80:446

Pope M, Frankel SS, Mascola JR, Trkola A, Isdell F, Birx DL et al (1997) Human immunodeficiency virus type 1 strains of subtypes B and E replicate in cutaneous dendritic cell-T-cell mixtures without displaying subtype-specific tropism. J Virol 71:8001–8007

Potterat JJ, Brody S (2001) Does sex explain HIV transmission dynamics in developing countries? Sex Transm Dis 28:730

Potterat JJ, Brewer DD, Muth SQ, Brody S (2006) The protective effect of male circumcision as a faith lift for the troubled paradigm of HIV epidemiology in sub-Saharan Africa. PLoS Med 3:e64

Potts M, Prata N, Walsh J, Grossman A (2006) Parachute approach to evidence based medicine. Br Med J 333:701–703

Potts M, Halperin DT, Kirby D, Swidler A, Marseille E, Klausner JD et al (2008) Reassessing HIV prevention. Science 320:749–750

Powell J, Robson A, Cranston D, Wojnarowska F, Turner R (2000) High incidence of lichen sclerosus in patients with squamous cell carcinoma of the penis. Br J Dermatol 145:85–89

Rain-Taljaard RC, Lagarde E, Taljaard DJ, Campbell C, MacPhail C, Williams B et al (2003) Potential for an intervention based on male circumcision in a South African town with high levels of HIV infection. AIDS Care 15:315–327

Rennie S, Muula AS, Westreich D (2007) Male circumcision and HIV prevention: ethical, medical and public health tradeoffs in low-income countries. J Med Ethics 33:357–361

Richardson D, Goldmeier D (2005) Premature ejaculation: does country of origin tell us anything about etiology? J Sex Med 2:508–512

Richens J, Imrie J, Copas A (2000) Condoms and seat belts: the parallels and the lessons. Lancet 355:400–403

Richters J, Gerofi J, Donovan B (1995) Why do condoms break or slip off in use? An exploratory study. Int J STD AIDS 6:11–18

Richters J, Smith AMA, de Visser RO, Grulich AE, Rissel CE (2006) Circumcision in Australia: prevalence and effects on sexual health. Int J STD AIDS 17:547–554

Rickwood AM (1992) The unkindest cut of all? J Ir Coll Physicians Surgeons 21(3):179–181

Roth CC, Hubanks JM, Bright BC, Heinlen JE, Donovan BO, Kropp BP et al (2009) Occurrence of urinary tract infection in children with significant upper urinary tract obstructions. Urology 73:74–78

Rothman P (2006) Infections prevalent in boys may come from mothers. Infect Dis Child 19(7):17

Rotkin ID (1973) A comparison review of key epidemiological studies in cervical cancer related to current searches for transmissible agents. Cancer Res 33:1353–1567

Royal Dutch Medical Association (2010) Non-therapeutic circumcision of male minors. KNMG

Rubenstein MM, Bason WM (1968) Complication of circumcision done with a plastic bell clamp. Am J Dis Child 116:381–382

Rush J, Fiorino-Chiovitti R, Kaufman K, Mitchell A (1990) A randomized controlled trial of a nursery ritual: wearing cover gowns to care for healthy newborns. Birth 17:25–30

Sawires SR, Dworkin SL, Flamma A, Peacock D, Szekeres G, Coates TJ (2007) Male circumcision and HIV/AIDS: challenges and opportunities. Lancet 369:708–713

Saxena AK, Schaarschmidt K, Reich A, Willital GH (2000) Non-retractile foreskin: a single center 13 years experience. Int Surg 85:180–183

Schoen EJ (2006) Ignoring evidence of circumcision benefits. Pediatrics 118:385–387

Schrek R, Lenowitz H (1947) Etiologic factors in carcinoma of penis. Cancer Res 7:180–187

Scott BE, Weiss HA, Viljoen JI (2005) The acceptability of male circumcision as an HIV intervention among a rural Zulu population, Kwazulu-Natal, South Africa. AIDS Care 17:304–313

Seed J, Allen S, Mertens T, Hudes E, Serufilira A, Carael M et al (1995) Male circumcision, sexually transmitted disease, and risk of HIV. J Acquir Immune Defic Syndr Hum Retrovirol 8:83–90

Shankar KR, Rickwood AMK (1999) The incidence of phimosis in boys. BJU Int 84:101–102

Sheldon T (2010) Dutch medical alliance moves to change thinking on male circumcision. Br Med J 340:c2987

Shen Z, Chen S, Zhu C, Wan Q, Chen Z (2004) Erectile function evaluation after adult circumcision. Zhonghua Nan Ke Xue 10:18–19

Sherman J, Borer JG, Horowitz M, Glassberg KI (1996) Circumcision: successful glanular reconstruction and survival following traumatic amputation. J Urol 156:842–844

Sidler D, Smith J, Rode H (2008) Neonatal circumcision does not reduce HIV/AIDS infection rates. S Afr Med J 98:762–766

Siegfried N (2005) Does male circumcision prevent HIV infection? PLoS Med 2(11):e393

Sillén U, Bachelard M, Hansson S, Hjälmas K, Jodal U, Hanson E (1998) Resolution rate in infantile dilating vesicoureteral reflux diagnosed after UTI [Abstract 109]. Pediatrics 102:869

Singh-Grewal D, Macdessi J, Craig J (2005) Circumcision for the prevention of urinary tract infection in boys: a systematic review of randomized trials and observational studies. Arch Dis Child 90:838

Sobngwi-Tambekou J, Taljaard D, Lissouba P, Zarca K, Puren A, Legarde E et al (2009) Effect of HSV-2 serostatus on acquisition of HIV by young men: results of a longitudinal study in Orange Farm. South Africa. J Infect Dis 199:958–964

Sorrells ML, Snyder JL, Reiss MD, Eden C, Milos MF, Wilcox N et al (2007) Fine-touch pressure thresholds in the adult penis. BJU Int 99:864–869

Sreenarasimhaiah S, Hellerstein S (1998) Urinary tract infections per se do not cause end-stage kidney disease. Pediatr Nephrol 12:210–213

Steele BT, Robitalle P, Demaria J, Grignon A (1989) Follow-up evaluation of prenatally recognized vesicoureteric reflux. J Pediatr 115:95–96
Stenram A, Malmfors G, Okmian L (1986) Circumcision for phimosis–indications and results. Acta Paediatr Scand 75:321–323
Stern E, Dixon WJ (1961) Cancer of the cervix: a biometric approach to etiology. Cancer 14:153–160
Storms MR (2009) Male circumcision for the prevention of HSV-2 and HPV infections. N Engl J Med 361:307
Strimling BS (1996) Partial amputation of glans penis during Mogen clamp circumcision. Pediatrics 97:906–907
Sullivan PS, Kilmarx PH, Peterman TA, Taylor AW, Nakashima AK, Kamb ML et al (2007) Male circumcision for prevention of HIV transmission: what the new data mean for HIV prevention in the United States. PLoS Med 4(7):e223
Sutherland JM, Glueck HI, Gleser G (1967) Hemorrhagic disease of the newborn: breast feeding as a necessary factor in the pathogenesis. Am J Dis Child 113:524–533
Svoboda JS (2009) "Three-fourths were abnormal": Misha's case, sick societies, and the law. In: Denniston GC, Hodges FM, Milos MF (eds) Circumcision and human rights. Springer, New York
Svoboda JS, Van Howe RS, Dwyer JG (2000) Informed consent for neonatal circumcision: an ethical and legal conundrum. J Contemp Health Law Policy 17:61–133
Taddio A, Goldbach M, Ipp M, Stevens B, Koren G (1995) Effect of neonatal circumcision on pain responses during vaccination in boys. Lancet 345:291–292
Taddio A, Katz J, Ilersich AL, Koren G (1997) Effect of neonatal circumcision on pain response during subsequent routine vaccination. Lancet 349:599–603
Talbott JR (2007) Size matters: the number of prostitutes and the global HIV/AIDS pandemic. PLoS ONE 2(6):e543
Taylor PK, Rodin P (1975) Herpes genitalis and circumcision. Br J Vener Dis 51:274–277
Taylor JR, Lockwood AP, Taylor AJ (1996) The prepuce: specialized mucosa of the penis and its loss to circumcision. Br J Urol 77:291–295
Terris M, Wilson F, Nelson JH Jr (1973) Relation of circumcision to cancer of the cervix. Am J Obstet Gynecol 117:1056–1066
Thompson DJ, Gezon HM, Rogers KD, Yee RB, Hatch TF (1966) Excess risk of staphylococcal infection and disease in newborn males. Am J Epidemiol 84:314–328
Tobian AAR, Serwadda D, Quinn TC, Kigozi G, Gravitt PE, Laeyendecker O et al (2009) Male circumcision for the prevention of HSV-2 and HPV infections and syphilis. N Engl J Med 360:1298–1309
Tsai JD, Huang FY, Tsai TC (1998) Asymptomatic vesicoureteral reflux detected by neonatal ultrasonographic screening. Pediatr Nephrol 12:206–209
Tseng HF, Morgenstern H, Mack T, Peters RK (2001) Risk factors for penile cancer: results of a population-based case-control study in Los Angeles County (United States). Cancer Causes Control 12:267–277
Turner AN, Morrison CS, Padian NS, Kaufman JS, Salata RA, Chipato T, Mmiro FA, Mugerwa RD, Behets FM, Miller WC (2007) Men's circumcision status and women's risk of HIV acquisition in Zimbabwe and Uganda. AIDS 21:1779–1789
Urassa M, Todd J, Boerma JT, Hayes R, Isingo R (1997) Male circumcision and susceptibility to HIV infection among men in Tanzania. AIDS 11:73–80
US Centers for Disease Control and Prevention (2007) Racial/ethnic disparities in diagnoses of HIV/AIDS—33 states, 2001–2005. MMWR Morbidity and Mortality Weekly Report, vol 56, pp 189–193
van Houwelingen HC, Arends LR, Stijnen T (2002) Advanced methods in meta-analysis: multivariate approach and meta-regression. Stat Med 21:589–624
Van Howe RS (1997a) Variability in penile appearance and penile findings: a prospective study. Br J Urol 80:776–782

Van Howe RS (1997b) Anesthesia for neonatal circumcision: who benefits? J Prenatal Perinatal Psychol Health 12(1):3–18
Van Howe RS (2004) A cost-utility analysis of neonatal circumcision. Med Decis Making 24:584–601
Van Howe RS (2005) Effect of confounding in the association between circumcision status and urinary tract infection. J Infect 51:59–68
Van Howe RS (2006) Incidence of meatal stenosis following neonatal circumcision in a primary care setting. Clin Pediatr (Phila) 45:49–54
Van Howe RS (2007a) Neonatal circumcision and penile inflammation in young boys. Clin Pediatr (Phila) 46:329–333
Van Howe RS (2007b) Case number and financial impact of circumcision in reducing prostate cancer [letter]. BJU Int 100:1193–1194
Van Howe RS (2007c) Genital ulcer disease and sexually transmitted urethritis and circumcision: a meta-analysis. Int J STD AIDS 18:799–809
Van Howe RS (2007d) Human papillomavirus and circumcision: a meta-analysis. J Infect 54:490–496
Van Howe RS (2009) Sampling bias explains association between human papillomavirus and circumcision. J Inf Dis 200:832
Van Howe RS, Robson WLM (2007) The possible role of circumcision in newborn outbreaks of community-associated methicillin-resistant Staphylococcus aureus. Clin Pediatr (Phila) 46:356–359
Van Howe RS, Storms MR (2009) Circumcision to prevent HPV infection. Lancet Oncol 10:746–747
Van Howe RS, Svoboda JS, Hodges FM (2005) HIV infection and circumcision: cutting through the hyperbole. J R Soc Health 125:259–265
Velazquez EF, Cubilla AL (2003) Lichen sclerosus in 68 patients with squamous cell carcinoma of the penis: frequent atypias and correlation with special carcinoma variants suggests a precancerous role. Am J Surg Pathol 27:1448–1453
Vernazza P (2008) La prévention du sida devient plus simpl, mais aussi plus complexe! Bull Med Suisses 89:163–164
Wahi PN, Luthra UK, Mali S, Mitra AB (1972) Religion and cervical carcinoma in agra. Indian J Cancer 9:210–215
Waldeck SE (2003) Using male circumcision to understand social norms as multipliers. U Cinn L Rev 72:455–526
Wallerstein E (1980) Circumcision: an American health fallacy. Springer, New York
Watson J, Jones RC, Cortes C, Gerber SI, Golash RG, Price J et al (2006) Community-associated methicillin-resistant Staphylococcal aureus infection among healthy newborns: Chicago and Los Angeles County, 2004. MMWR 55:329–332
Wawer MJ, Makumbi K, Kigozi G, Serwadda D, Watya S, Nalugoda F, Buwembo D et al (2009) Circumcision in HIV-infected men and its effect on HIV transmission to female partners in Rakai, Uganda: a randomised controlled trial. Lancet 374:229–237
Weaver BA, Feng Q, Holmes KK, Kiviat N, Lee SK, Meyer C et al (2004) Evaluation of genital sites and sampling techniques for detection of human papillomavirus DNA in men. J Infect Dis 189:677–685
Weiss HA, Thomas SL, Munabi SK, Hayes RJ (2006) Male circumcision and risk of syphilis, chancroid, and genital herpes: a systematic review and meta-analysis. Sex Transm Infect 82:101–110
Weiss HA, Halperin D, Bailey RC, Hayes RJ, Schmid G, Hankins CA (2008) Male circumcision for HIV prevention: from evidence to action? AIDS 22:567–574
Wen P, Kowalczyk L (2009) Beth Israel faulted for staph outbreak in mothers, babies. Boston Globe 10 Apr 2009. http://www.boston.com/lifestyle/family/articles/2009/04/10/beth_israel_faulted_for_staph_outbreak_in_mothers_babies/. Accessed 11 May 2009
Wennerstrom M, Hansson S, Jodal U, Stokland E (1998) Disappearance of vesicoureteral reflux in children. Arch Pediatr Adolesc Med 152:879–883

Wennerström M, Hansson S, Jodal U, Stokland E (2000a) Primary and acquired renal scarring in boys and girls with urinary tract infection. J Pediatr 136:30–34
Wennerström M, Hansson S, Hedner T, Himmelmann A, Jodal U (2000b) Ambulatory blood pressure 16–26 years after the first urinary tract infection in childhood. J Hypertens 18:485–491
Williams BG, Lloyd-Smith JO, Gouws E, Hankins C, Getz WM, Hargrove J et al (2006) The potential impact of male circumcision on HIV in sub-Saharan Africa. PLoS Med 3:e262
Wiswell TE, Geschke DW (1989) Risks from circumcision during the first month of life compared with those for uncircumcised boys. Pediatrics 83:1011–1015
Wolfish NM, Delbrouck NF, Shanon A, Matzinger MA, Stenstrom R, McLaine PN (1993) Prevalence of hypertension in children with primary vesicoureteral reflux. J Pediatr 123:559–563
Xu F, Markowitz LE, Sternberg MR, Aral SO (2007) Prevalence of circumcision and herpes simplex type 2 infection in men in the United States: the National Health and Nutrition Examination Survey (NHANES), 1999–2004. Sex Transm Dis 34:479–484
Xu X, Patel DA, Dalton VK, Pearlman MD, Johnson TRB (2009) Can routine neonatal circumcision help prevent human immunodeficiency virus transmission in the United States? Am J Men's Health 3:79–84
Yang DM, Lin H, Zhang B, Guo W (2008) Circumcision affects glans penis vibration perception threshold. Zhonghua Nan Ke Xue 14:328–330
Yegane RA, Kheirollahi AR, Salehi NA, Bashashati M, Khoshdel JA, Ahmadi M (2006) Late complications of circumcision in Iran. Pediatr Surg Int 22:442–445
Yeung CK, Godley ML, Dhillon HK, Gordon I, Duffy PG, Ransley PG (1997) The characteristics of primary vesico-ureteric reflux in male and female infants with pre-natal hydronephrosis. Br J Urol 80:319–327
Zarkovic G (1985) Alterations of cervical cytology and steroid contraceptive use. Int J Epidemiol 14:369–377
Zornberg GL, Buka BL, Tsuang MT (2000) Hypoxic-ischemia-related fetal/neonatal complications and risk of schizophrenia and other nonaffective psychoses: a 19 years longitudinal study. Am J Psychiatry 157:196–202

Author Biography

Robert S. Van Howe MD, MS, is a Clinical Professor at Michigan State University College of Human Medicine and a full-time pediatrician for Bell Memorial Hospital in Ishpeming, Michigan. He graduated from Loyola-Stritch School of Medicine, completed a Pediatrics residency at the Children's Hospital of Wisconsin in Milwaukee, Wisconsin, and received a Masters of Science in Clinical Research Design and Statistical Analysis from the University of Michigan School of Public Health. Dr. Van Howe has researched and published extensively on neonatal circumcision. He has lectured worldwide and provided expert testimony in court cases involving circumcision. His goal is to provide an evidence-based and scientific appraisal of the medical literature on this topic. He is considered a leading expert on neonatal circumcision, which led to his being a consultant for the World Health Organization, the Centers for Disease Control, and the American Academy of Pediatrics. Marquette, Michigan, USA.

Chapter 3
The Smart Penis

John Taylor

Abstract The human penis is usually seen, by anatomists, as a patchwork of tissues with distinct and separate functions. Each function makes intuitive good sense; for instance, its skin covering facilitates sliding movement. The glans is seen as touch-sensitive and, therefore, an important source of erogenous sensation, which Guyton, in his standard book on human physiology, informs us is the main trigger of sexual reflexes. The frenulum, like the glans, is thought to have touch-sensory functions; at the same time it helps retain the foreskin on the supposedly sensitive glans. Corpus spongiosum surrounds and supports the long male urethra and may facilitate ejaculation. The question is whether this is the only function of the longest part of the penis, which forms the bulb of the penis at one end and glans at the other. From all this, it is reasonable to suppose that the penis is structured to physically support the glans and its function, namely, the generation of touch and then erogenous sensation which, in turn, is thought to be the main trigger of sexual reflexes including erection and ejaculation. Maybe so, maybe not.

Keywords Penis • Glans • Foreskin • Frenulum • Corpus spongiosum • Sexual reflexes • Erection • Ejaculation

3.1 The Smart Penis

The main problem with the idea that one tissue does one thing and another tissue something entirely different is the fact that the construction of the penis, like that of all organs, is extremely uniform across different species, including humans, suggesting close links between the shape and function of its various named parts. Despite its apparent importance, the glans has not run away with its lion's share of penile development. So, we have to answer questions about the precise nature of the links, or ties, between it and other penile tissues: what it is that keeps the glans

---

This author is deceased

J. Taylor (✉)
Pathology, University of Manitoba, Winnipeg, Manitoba, Canada
e-mail: mtaylor.33@mymts.net

G. C. Denniston et al. (eds.), *Genital Cutting: Protecting Children from Medical, Cultural, and Religious Infringements*, DOI: 10.1007/978-94-007-6407-1_3,

and other tissues in harmonious union. To take an example, if the glans were, for instance, pure sensory tissue acting independently of other penile tissues it might not have remained so uniform in construction, if only because touch sensation alone does not demand the highly uniform structure possessed by three billion or so males. Another question: what is the link between penile shaft skin and corpus spongiosum, and how might such a linkage affect glans function? What is it about structure that keeps penile tissues in lockstep with one another? What is the developmental importance of shapes and positions of penile tissues?

This essay, then, focuses on sexual reflexes generated by anatomically precise reflexogenic tissues, that is, by the penis itself rather than by external forces such as touch. It sees the penis as a true organ with interconnected parts and internal functions required for the generation of sexual reflexes geared specifically to reproduction.

The activation of reflexes for muscle contraction depends upon stretching mechanisms activated by movement of perhaps distant tissues. How, then, is the penis shaped to respond, as a single unit, to all its various structures? The ridged band of the prepuce is a good starting point, if only because it is distant from the musculature it activates at the base of the penis. An early observation, confirmed by Internet volunteers, is that stretching of the ridged band of the prepuce produces sharp reflex contraction of bulb muscles (bulbospongiosum and bulbocavernosum) around the base of the penis. The significance of this finding with respect to erection and ejaculation is obvious. The ridged band of the prepuce facilitates erection and ejaculation. The prepuce is much more than a simple cover for the glans.

Our next observation switches to corpus spongiosum, which at first sight is totally unrelated to the prepuce and its reflexogenic function. Bulb-muscle contraction, whether voluntary, as after urination, or involuntary, squeezes the bulb of the penis, which sends a pressure wave via corpus spongiosum to the glans. The glans, especially the wide-radius corona of glans, appears to be structured, according to the Law of LaPlace, to respond to a mild increase in intraglanular pressure by expansion, thereby triggering a 'glanular reflex' for secondary or repeat bulb-muscle contraction. Suppression of the bulbar pressure wave, as by gentle compression of corpus spongiosum and, at the same time, penile urethra, was found to interfere with reflex bulb muscle contraction, presumably by suppressing hydraulic expansion of the corona of the glans. This observation conflicts with the old idea that the function of the glans is touch sensory, long-since abandoned, thanks to the knowledge, easily tested, that the glans is in fact insensitive to light, if not to deep, touch. In summary, we hypothesize that the glans, like the ridged band of the prepuce, is a trigger of reflex-bulb muscle contraction, which is itself erogenous. The benefit of dual contractions of bulb muscles, with the glanular reflex following rapidly on the ridged-band reflex, helps prolong and intensify bulb-muscle contraction and accompanying erogenous sensation.

Corpora cavernosa, the main erectile bodies of the penis, have one other function; they lodge corpus spongiosum in a deep groove, protecting it from external compressive forces during vaginal intercourse, thus preserving its hydraulic function and essential sexual reflexes.

Last, I come to by far the least understood but most obvious penile tissue, its skin. Far from its popular description as loose and highly mobile, it stiffens during erection thanks to its smooth muscle content, thus providing a relatively non-stretchy connection between the ridged band of the prepuce and skin of the now deeply wrinkled and hence shortened scrotal skin (pars scrotalis) surrounding the first inch or so of the base of the penis. Shortening of the scrotum, as well as skin of the rest of the penis, plays an important role in the activation of sexual reflexes. Dartos muscle of penile and scrotal skin extends into skin of the pubic region of the anterior abdominal wall, providing an additional penile skin-shortening mechanism This is not all: we found that skin of the dorsum of the penis, the main sexual contact area of the intact penis, becomes rugose during erection, with forward pointing, stiffened, skin ridges. In short, the intact penis becomes modestly frictional during erection, adding to the ability of muscularized shaft skin to prod, or pull, the ridged band into action.

The frenulum attracts a lot of attention as sensory tissue but it appears to be little more than a structural link between penile shaft skin and tip of glans. Backward retraction of the frenulum, it might be noted, distorts the corona of glans, triggering the glanular reflex in much the same way as the hydraulic expansion of the corona and its stretch-sensitive nerve endings from the inside. Again, this reflex activation mechanism is easily confirmed.

Of course, this is not all there is to the penis, but reflexes are easier to ignite and check than sensory sensations, as Marilyn Milos and her colleagues who did the Touch Test Sensitivity Study well know. So, we took the easy road.

I am sorry I could not be with you at this important NOCIRC meeting in beautiful California. In particular, I thank the many members who sent their good wishes. Marilyn Milos has been a great help to me as she has to all of you. Harry Meislahn of Winnetka, Illinois, provided much of the information and confirmations summarized in this essay. Dennis Harrison of British Columbia, Canada, took care of the Interneting. The faults are all mine

John R. Taylor (26 July 1932–27 October 2010), MB, ChB MRCPEd, FRCPC. Pathologist. Health Sciences Centre, Winnipeg, Manitoba, Canada.

References

Cold CJ, Taylor JR (1999) BJU International 83(Suppl. 1):34–44

Taylor JR, Lockwood AP, Taylor AJ (1996) British Journal of Urology I(77):291–295

Author Biography

John R. Taylor MB, ChB, MRCPEd, FRCPC. (1932–2010), spent 27 years at the Health Sciences Centre, Winnipeg, Manitoba, Canada, as a forensic pathologist, teacher, and researcher. He was an Associate Professor of Pathology at the University of Manitoba. Dr. Taylor received international recognition with his work to support a growing opposition to routine infant circumcision. His landmark publication (1996) in the *British Journal of Urology*, "The prepuce: specialized mucosa of the penis and its loss to circumcision," identified what is now known as *Taylor's Ridged Band,* the specialized sensory mucosa located at the junction of true penile skin with smooth preputial mucosa. The important work of Dr. Taylor can be found at http://research.cirp.org.

Editors' note: In 1996, Dr. John Taylor published his landmark anatomical paper, "The prepuce: specialized mucosa of the penis and its loss to circumcision," in the *British Journal of Urology* (Cold and Taylor 1999). Dr. Taylor identified and named what is now known as Taylor's Ridged Band, a vitally important structure that encircles the opening of the prepuce and houses 20,000–70,000 fine-touch sensory, erogenous nerve endings. These are the nerve endings that provide sensory and erogenous feedback to the brain and play a significant and dynamic role in the ejaculatory reflex of the intact penis.

Following further research, Dr Taylor, in collaboration with researcher Dr. Christopher Cold, published a follow-up paper entitled: "The prepuce." This was also published by the *BJU International* (Taylor et al. 1996) (successor to the *British Journal of Urology*). The last sentence of this study reads, "As physicians and parents learn the normal anatomy and functions of the external genitalia, there will be greater understanding of its essential nature, and more attempts to limit its removal".

Dr. Taylor's work provided new and ground-breaking information about the anatomy and physiology of the intact human penis, thereby underscoring the importance of genital integrity to health and well-being.

Dr. Taylor was scheduled to deliver yet another paper on the same topic at the 11th International Symposium on Circumcision, Genital Integrity, and Human Rights at the University of California at Berkeley in 2010, but was unable to attend because of a terminal illness. Marilyn Milos delivered the paper at the symposium for Dr. Taylor. This chapter represents Dr. Taylor's last contribution to the Genital Integrity Movement. His paper is included in this volume to honor Dr. John Taylor and his contributions to science, medicine, and human rights.

Chapter 4
The Harm of Circumcision

George C. Denniston

Abstract Advocates for circumcision employ the veneer of science in an attempt to conceal that they are apologists for the procedure rather than impartial researchers. Furthermore, unlike genuine scientists who would welcome all evidence about circumcision's consequences, advocates ignore and actively work to suppress scientific evidence demonstrating the short-term and long-term negative sequelae of the surgical alteration of the penis. Consequently, the public is largely ignorant of the extent of the harm caused by circumcision. While the reality of immediate surgical error, such as injury to the glans, loss of the entire penis, gangrene, severe hemorrhage, and even death are grudgingly acknowledged, though downplayed as rare, advocates for circumcision refuse to acknowledge the large body of scientific research showing long-term and permanent negative sequelae to the penis and to sexual function caused by destruction and amputation of the prepuce. Moreover, in addition to the physical and sexological consequences, a body of research now documents that the surgery also has psychological and cultural consequences. This would naturally be expected when such a psychologically significant part of the body such as the penis is surgically altered. These deleterious physical, sexological, psychological, and cultural sequelae of circumcision not only affect the individual, but also affect human relationships and the ethics and mores of the afflicted society, as is demonstrated by the peculiar dynamics of societies that tolerate, encourage, or enforce circumcision.

Keywords Circumcision • Harm • Sexology • Ethics

G. C. Denniston (✉)
Department of Family Medicine, University of Washington, Robbins Road 45, Nordland 98358, Washington, USA
e-mail: gcd@u.washington.edu

G. C. Denniston et al. (eds.), *Genital Cutting: Protecting Children from Medical, Cultural, and Religious Infringements*, DOI: 10.1007/978-94-007-6407-1_4,

4.1 Introduction

Circumcision can be simply, accurately, and impartially defined as the deliberate amputation of the prepuce, which encompasses at least half of the penile skin system, from another person. The justifications for this act, which are offered by the perpetrators are varied, change from decade to decade and from culture to culture. The justifications range from primitive superstition, appeasement of supernatural beings, anti-sexualism, social control, and even supposed medical necessity. As a procedure performed by doctors for supposed medical reasons, circumcision has existed for only approximately one-hundred years, even though it existed and was practiced by a small number of non-Western cultures, most especially by Jews, Muslims, and some African animist tribes, for thousands of years prior to this. Most interestingly, the most ardent advocates for the medicalization of circumcision are, in fact, individuals from these traditionally circumcising cultures who either now live in the Western World or whose cultures have undergone varying degrees of westernization, such as the introduction and application of modern, western science and medicine over the existing culture. As such, what passes for science in this instance is heavily distorted by pre-existing cultural norms and practices. Indeed, it can be postulated that whenever science is used to support or justify culture or religion, it is no longer science. Science is the impartial and thorough search, collection, and examination of data. While scientific inquiry may start with a hypothesis, the process continues with an attempt to disprove the hypothesis in order to test the validity of the hypothesis. All studies performed by circumcision advocates violate this fundamental scientific principle by beginning not with a hypothesis but with a desired conclusion and design "tests" that will prove the foregone conclusion. This is called "confirmation bias." Evidence of confirmation bias automatically invalidates any results and calls into question the motivations of the researchers. Indeed, in all other spheres of science, evidence of confirmation bias is taken quite seriously by governing bodies and results in scandal, loss of position and reputation, and frequently in legal action. One of the most obvious cultural harms caused by the existence of circumcision in a society is that these scientific checks are dismantled in the case of circumcision. Bad science is not only unpunished but rewarded. This attests to the psychological damage caused by circumcision that can accrue to the minds of men who are perhaps in all other respects perfectly rational.

During the past one-hundred years, both circumcisers and survivors of circumcision have typically denied the harm of circumcision and have used science to promote the non-therapeutic amputation of a normal body part of a non-consenting minor. This situation is strikingly akin to the Stockholm Syndrome, in which the victims come to identify with the objectives of their victimizers. In the case of circumcision, it results in a vicious cycle, in which victims of circumcision become the next generation of circumcisers and circumcision advocates, perpetuating a cycle that is difficult to stop.

The circumcision of a child represents a violation of medical ethics and is, in fact, a criminal act. In law, it is clear that forceful non-therapeutic amputation of any other healthy part of another person's body, no matter how slight, constitutes a criminal act. Indeed, as a parallel, it is illegal in the United States for anyone, even a doctor, to amputate any amount of tissue from the genitals of a minor female for nontherapeutic reasons. One of the cultural harms of circumcision is that only the penis is exempt from legal protection. A person can evade prosecution or censure if he cuts into the penis of a male child for nontherapeutic reasons. Indeed, the perpetrator is rewarded for his actions. Such an irrational situation can only exist in cultures where circumcision is the norm. Advocates of circumcision claim to use science to justify their actions, whereas they are actually violating all the tenets of science.

One tactic of circumcision advocates is to claim that circumcision prevents various fatal diseases that are otherwise incurable. Beginning with the conclusion that circumcision prevents these diseases, scientific-looking studies are published that purport to prove the conclusion. Evidence to the contrary is never sought and is certainly discarded or attacked. In every case, impartial scientists have performed genuinely scientific studies that prove that circumcision does not, in fact, prevent the disease in question. Unfortunately, millions of innocent victims are nevertheless circumcised for the false reasons originally offered by circumcisers (Denniston 1999). By the time the original justification has been disproven, circumcisers typically have shifted their argument and claim the prevention of another deadly disease as the justification for imposing mass circumcision on the society. The presumption is that their claims of efficacy are true unless later disproved. This, of course, is a violation of the scientific method. This reductionist attitude adopted by circumcisers—that all claims are true unless later disproven—fails to take into account that there is much that has not yet been proven or disproven by science. Forcing circumcision on males, before a thorough examination of the claims has been made, is a violation of medical ethics and is a classic example of the a priori religious, i.e., non-scientific motivations of the perpetrators.

It is axiomatic of circumcision cultures that most individuals in that culture, especially the majority of victims, prefer to remain ignorant of the scientific facts and consequences of the amputative alteration of the penis. Certainly circumcisers have a vested interest in ignoring or suppressing the facts, as their careers, authority, power, income, and egos depend on the continuation of the status quo.

Human values are at stake, as are the basic tenets of medical care. The treatment of one person by another entails a sacred trust, which is violated by the existence and performance of circumcision. It has been observed that those doctors who actively and aggressively campaign for mass circumcision and who perform it, are immune to ethical and scientific arguments. They cannot and will not stop. In the case of male circumcisers, we can infer that they are motivated by their own victimhood and are psychologically unequipped to process the shame and horror that they would feel if they were to recognize the harm they are causing.

4.2 Consequences of Circumcision

This chapter will describe some of the harmful effects of circumcision. It includes information encountered over the past twenty years of unbiased and rational scientific inquiry. It is necessary to understand the scope and magnitude of the harm if we are to defend science against incursions of superstition, religion, and undiagnosed psychiatric disorder.

4.3 Physical Consequences

A six-pound newborn has about twelve ounces of blood in his body. A loss of 20 % of that, or 2.4 ounces, is only 5 tablespoons of blood. A loss of five tablespoons of blood in a six-pound infant can kill the baby. Pediatricians are not, by training, surgeons, so they know little about controlling blood loss. Rarely do they pinch bleeding blood vessels with a hemostat and then tie them off with a suture during circumcision, as is done in routine surgery. The tiny, wounded, bleeding penis is simply wrapped in Vaseline gauze, and it is hoped that excessive bleeding will not occur. It only takes five tablespoons of blood loss to initiate shock, coma, and, sometimes, death (Newell 2004).

Infections, which are far too common, would never occur without the circumcision wound. Infections are readily treated with antibiotics, but infections in delicate newborns also result in death (Scurlock and Pemberton 1977; Paediatric Death Review Committee 2007).

By far, the most common circumcision complication (100 %) is the removal of half of the normal skin from the normal penis (Taylor et al. 1996). The consequence of this complication is that the circumcised male will never experience a normal sex life (O'Hara and O'Hara 1999). Since circumcision does not fit into the definition of surgery, it cannot be considered a procedure with genuinely medical objectives. All of the short-term and long-term sequelae of circumcision are complications of an unnecessary amputation (Grimes 1978).

Accidentally removing all the skin from the penis during circumcision of a six-pound infant is not difficult. The skin is pulled up through the circumcision clamp, and the shaft of the penis sinks into the fat pad. When the clamp is applied, all the skin on the entire penis may be removed (Sotolongo et al. 1985). I have testified as an expert witness in such cases.

Amputation of the foreskin decreases the size of the penis. Circumcision cuts through many arteries, veins, and nerves. There is always some bleeding. When this is stopped, healing of the wound begins, but a massive disruption of blood flow has occurred in this six-pound infant (Persad et al. 1995). As the boy grows, much less blood is delivered to his penis, leading to impaired growth. One study documented that circumcised men's erect penises are eight millimeters shorter than the penises of intact men, on average (Richters et al. 1995).

Amputation of the entire penis is a well-documented injury. All or part of the penis is amputated by surgical negligence (Sherman et al. 1996). An electrocautery machine is often involved. Recently there have been three multi-million dollar awards of damages, varying from $2 million up to $10.8 million (Tagami 2010). Some years ago, a similar lawsuit was settled for an amount in excess of $23.8 million (Seabrook 1991). This money does little to improve the child's life.

Circumcision prevents normal erections because a major function of the foreskin is to cover the elongated shaft of a tumescent penis. As the circumcised penis erects, the tight skin may pull the penis to one side or the other, giving it an abnormal curvature. Often the scrotal skin and hair is pulled onto the shaft of the penis, in a futile attempt to permit the shaft to achieve its full length.

There are many additional physical complications of circumcision (Ritter and Denniston 2002).

4.4 Psychological Consequences

Circumcision is a primal wound that happens before a baby is capable of understanding the profound pain and wounding that is forced upon him without his consent in the tender, vulnerable first days of life. Circumcision interferes with the maternal/infant bond, disrupts breastfeeding and normal sleep patterns, and undermines a male's first developmental task of establishing trust.

Circumcision leaves psychological scars, and men who have been circumcised against their will are harmed in many ways. An accurate and impartial observer of the harm inflicted on circumcised men was the psychiatrist John Rhinehart. Regarding the level of trauma experienced by a circumcised male, Rhinehart noted:

> It is helpful to note that, in considering the levels of defense, whenever the two earlier levels (relational and fight or flight) are experienced by the mind as ineffective, the mind tends not to use them later. This means that a mind patterned in this way jumps right to terror, rage, and/or dissociation when confronted with situations that are interpreted as threatening, even though to the rational mind or cortex these situations may not be significant.
>
> In other words, when an event occurs in a man's life that resembles any aspect of the original circumcision experience, the chances that the extreme forms of panic, rage, violence, or dissociation might result are much more likely–just as they are in any other post-traumatic stress situation (Rhinehart 1999).

Every sexual experience a male has after circumcision is on a neuronal background of pain, even if the male does not remember or recognize it. What the mind forgets, the body remembers. Hyper-reactivity, defensiveness, or the inability to cope when faced with threatening or frightening situations are evidence of early trauma caused by neonatal circumcision.

In my practice, I have seen how circumcision can be posited as the untoward cause of many abortions. Adult neonatally circumcised males frequently exhibit an irrational terror at the prospect of a vasectomy. They finally go reluctantly, after their wife has had at least two abortions. They knew that they did not want more children, but their fear of a genital operation was so great from the early trauma of circumcision that they refused vasectomy and thus let their wives suffer needlessly. Multiply these experiences by the 500,000 vasectomies that are performed every year in the United States, and there is the potential for one million abortions caused by circumcision every year.

One of the saddest and most troubling aspects about the psychological wounding that occurs with neonatal circumcision is that, when a male represses an emotion, he is often unable to recognize the expression of that same emotion in someone else. This is what induces a new father to subject his own son to circumcision. He fails to recognize the pain and trauma experienced by the infant, and shows no compassion or empathy to or for the suffering infant. It is this process that has allowed genital wounding to be passed from one generation to the next.

While some circumcision advocates claim that amputation of the foreskin helps "perfect" the man or free him from base, sexual drives, in truth, it is the wounding of the genitals that causes men to focus on the wounded part. With the loss of normal, satisfying sexual function, a male works more diligently to experience what has been lost, something he can never reclaim. As C. J. Falliers wrote in the *Journal of the American Medical Association,* in 1970, "The fundamental biological sexual act becomes, for the circumcised male, simply the satisfaction of an urge and not the refined sensory experience it was meant to be" (Falliers 1963).

4.5 Cultural Consequences

The short- and long-term harmful consequences of circumcision adversely affect personal, social, and cultural well-being in a number of ways. Some of the latter are discussed here.

Men who have been circumcised have a permanently decreased sexual sensitivity. This results from the loss of the erogenous nerve receptors in the prepuce and in the buildup of sclerotic tissue over the mucous membrane of the surgically externalized glans penis. Consequently, affected men do not want to decrease any remaining sensitivity by wearing a condom. Condoms have been shown to reduce the risk of sexually transmitted diseases, including HIV/AIDS. No one knows how many circumcised men have gotten AIDS because they did not wear a condom, but we do know that circumcised American men have the highest rate of AIDS in the industrialized world, despite the fact that condoms are more available in the USA than elsewhere. This implies that condoms are not worn as much by circumcised men, and it also implies that circumcision does not prevent AIDS but, instead, contributes to its spread.

There is another way that circumcision contributes to the spread of HIV/AIDS. We know that at least 30 % of AIDS cases in Africa are caused by the dirty needles and dirty medical/surgical equipment being used by practitioners (Deuchert and Brody 2007). If adult males are to be circumcised, they will require anesthesia. African practitioners, who have already caused so much unnecessary disease through inadequately sterilized equipment or even carelessness, will *not* be capable of suddenly changing their habits. They will continue to use dirty needles.

Circumcision also causes the transmission of HIV/AIDS when it is used as an attempt to prevent the spread of AIDS. Circumcision advocates have relied on flawed studies that only show AIDS prevention over the short term (Auvert et al.

2005; Bailey et al. 2007; Gray et al. 2007). Because newly circumcised men were recovering from their circumcisions, they were unable to engage in sexual activity. Consequently, they were not exposed to AIDS over the short term. Further, the alleged 60 % reduction is a relative reduction. The absolute reduction is only 1.4 %, which is not statistically significant (Van Howe and Storms 2011; Boyle and Hill 2011). As soon as hundreds of thousands of black African victims get circumcised, they will begin to get AIDS at the rates of circumcised Americans. In fact, the rates could become much higher due to unsterilized instruments, the lack of condoms, and the decrease in condom use.

Another hypothesized cultural consequence of circumcision is that it may contribute to divorce. While the number of divorces in which circumcision plays a role is unknown, we do know that sexual intercourse is generally recognized as an important variable in marriage as well as divorce. If a wife is continually suffering from dyspareunia (painful intercourse) because the artificially externalized glans penis is hard and callused, irritating the delicate mucosal membrane on her vaginal walls, she is often discouraged from wanting sex. When the corona of the externalized glans acts like a piston ring, stripping all lubrication from the vaginal walls, and irritating and tearing the delicate mucosal membrane of the vagina, many women lose interest in satisfying themselves or their partner. How many marriages are disrupted as a result? It is likely that the abnormal, callused glans penis adversely affects virtually every marriage (See Chap. 8).

Another way in which circumcision contributes to divorce is when a mother and father disagree about circumcision for their son. I have witnessed a mother divorcing the father in order to protect her son. Recently, we have seen a number of lawsuits where parents disagree during divorce proceedings and the son's foreskin is used as a pawn to upset or punish the other partner.

Circumcision also harms doctors (Goldman 2004). As I described in my paper presented at Keele University in England (proceedings of the 10th International Symposium on Genital Integrity in 2010, *Genital Autonomy: Protecting Personal Choice*), doctors are greatly harmed by being allowed to participate in an unethical act without being stopped by their professional societies or the law.

In fact, circumcision harms the entire medical profession. Just as pedophile priests, under the protection of the Catholic Church, play with the child's penis, some doctors, practicing under the protection of the medical profession, torture (by definition) an infant and mutilate (by definition) him permanently by removing half of the normal skin system from his organ of pleasure and procreation, his penis. Both priests and doctors damage the child psychologically. National and international laws already are in place to prevent this human rights violation—e.g., the UN Declaration on Human Rights, the UN Convention on the rights of the Child, the UN International covenant on Civil and Political Rights, the First (freedom of religion), Fourth (security of person), and Fourteenth (equal protection under the law) Amendments, and the laws against battery and false imprisonment–must be recognized, honored, and upheld.

One of the great ironies of circumcision, is that in those cultures that practice it, the intact, natural, unmodified, non-circumcised penis is stigmatized and demonized. The stigma of the intact penis caused by circumcision may adversely affect intact males in these cultures. In Africa, intact men have been ruthlessly circumcised because those in circumcising tribes cannot tolerate the fact that others are intact. Members of the non-circumcising Luo tribe in Kenya are being forcibly circumcised by men in circumcising tribes and are erroneously being blamed for causing the AIDS pandemic in Africa.

The stigma has affected boys in American schools, too. Bullying of one boy by others is a huge problem. One middle-aged man told me about his experiences in Norfolk, Virginia, as a teenager. So far as he knew, he was the only boy in his class who was intact. Many of the circumcised boys harassed him regularly. They would point at him and make derogatory statements. One day in a store, a circumcised boy with his father pointed at the intact boy, and jeeringly told his father who he was (the boy who was not circumcised). A year later, things had gotten so bad that he fought one of his circumcised tormenters and broke his arm, putting him in the hospital for a few weeks. Only then did things begin to get better for him. We do know that bullying in schools is widespread and is harmful to many young people, and we may never know how much is related to circumcision status.

As we can see by the example of the forced circumcision of members of the Luo tribe in Africa, circumcision plays a major role in human warfare. In the Bible, when David first heard of the Philistine giant, Goliath, he asked, "Who is this uncircumcised Philistine, that he should defy the armies of the Living God?" (King James version, I Samuel 17: verse 26).

Later—"And Saul said, 'Thus shall ye say to David, The King desireth not any dowry, but an hundred foreskins of the Philistines, to be avenged of the king's enemies.' But Saul thought to make David fall by the hand of the Philistines. [He was jealous of David.] And when his servants told David these words, it pleased David well to be the king's son in law. Wherefore David arose and went, he and his men, and slew of the Philistines two hundred men; and David brought their foreskins, and they gave them in full tale to the king, that he might be the king's son in law. And Saul gave him Michal his daughter to wife." (King James version, I Samuel 18: verse 25–27) These are two of the early examples of circumcision having an important part of warfare.

A more recent example is the first Gulf War. The main protagonists were the United States and Iraq, both circumcising nations. Contributing the most troops were the United States, the United Kingdom, Saudi Arabia, and Egypt, all, with the exception of the United Kingdom, circumcising nations. One sixth of all troops were the 100,000 Turks massed along their southern border with Iraq. The Turks are also a circumcising nation, usually forcing it on boys during late childhood, which, like neonatal circumcision, has been demonstrated to impair the trust between mother and son (Cansever 1965). Israel would certainly have been in the war had it not been that the United States specifically requested that they remain neutral. Here is an example of circumcising nations pitted against circumcising nations. If circumcision is not a direct cause of war, certainly it is a correlate and exacerbating factor (DeMause 1996). If we are to reduce warfare, then we must reduce the incidence of circumcision for, as Karl Menninger said, "What we do to children, they will do to society."

Sigmund Freud observed that circumcision was a major cause of anti-Semitism. The irony of this is that one is considered to be fully Jewish if one's mother is Jewish, and not by whether or not he is circumcised. I personally know Jewish men who are proud to be Jewish and delighted not to be circumcised.

Last, but not least, circumcision interferes with spiritual functioning. Circumcision lowers self-esteem (Goldman 1997) and thus contributes to a man's inability to think for himself, an ability which is necessary to free himself from organized religion, and to develop his spirituality.

Circumcision can be postulated to be a contributing factor to major global problems—lowered self-esteem, divorce, abortions, human perversions, and war. That should be enough to condemn the procedure, which could never be introduced as a new procedure into medical practice today. Even if we could document scientifically all of the harms induced by circumcision, it probably would not be enough to stop the circumcisers. We must recognize the truth about the harm of circumcision, the importance of genital integrity, and the inherent right of all children—male, female, and intersex alike—and to implement the laws that are in place to protect the child and to prohibit this unconscionable practice, which has no place in civilized society.

References

Auvert B, Taljaard D, Lagarde E, Sobngwi-Tambekou J, Sitta R et al (2005) Randomized, controlled intervention trial of male circumcision for reduction of HIV infection risk: the ANRS 1265 trial. PLoS Med 2:e298

Bailey RC, Moses S, Parker CB et al (2007) Male circumcision for HIV prevention in young men in Kisumu, Kenya: a randomised controlled trial. Lancet 369(9562):643–656

Boyle GJ, Hill G (2011) Sub-Saharan African randomised clinical trials into male circumcision and HIV transmission: methodological, ethical and legal concerns. J Law Med (Melbourne) 19:316–334

Cansever G (1965) Psychological effects of circumcision. Br J Med Psychol 38(4):321–331

DeMause L (1996) Restaging fetal traumas in war and social violence. Pre Per Psychol J 10(4):227–258

Denniston GC (1999) Tyranny of the victims: an analysis of circumcision advocacy. In: Denniston GC, Hodges FM, Milos MF (eds) Male and female circumcision: medical, legal, and ethical considerations in pediatric practice, Kluwer Academic/Plenum Publishers, NY

Deuchert E, Brody SA (2007) Lack of autodisable syringe use and health care indicators are associated with high HIV prevalence: an international ecologic analysis. Ann Epidemiol 17(3):199–207

Falliers CJ (1963) Routine circumcision. Am J Dis Child 106(12):47

Goldman R (1997) Circumcision the hidden trauma. Vanguard Publications, Boston

Goldman R (2004) Circumcision policy: a psychosocial perspective. Paediatr Child Health 9(9):630–633

Gray RH, Kigozi G, Serwadda D et al (2007) Male circumcision for HIV prevention in men in Rakai, Uganda: a randomised trial. Lancet 369(9562):657–666

Grimes DA (1978) Routine circumcision of the newborn: a reappraisal. Am J Obstet Gynecol 130(2):125–129

Newell TEC (2004) Judgment of inquiry into the death of McWillis, Ryleigh Roman Bryan, B.C. Coroner's Service, Burnaby, 19 Jan 2004

O'Hara K, O'Hara J (1999) The effect of male circumcision on the sexual enjoyment of the female partner. Br J Urol Suppl 1:79–84
Paediatric Death Review Committee (2007) Office of the chief coroner of ontario. Circumcision: a minor procedure? Paediatr Child Health 12(4):311–312
Persad R, Sharma S, McTavish J et al (1995) Clinical presentation and pathophysiology of meatal stenosis following circumcision. Br J Urol 75(1):91–93
Rhinehart J (1999) Neonatal circumcision reconsidered. Transactional Anal J 29:215–221
Richters J, Gerofi J, Donovan B (1995) Why do condoms break or slip off in use? An exploratory study. Int J STD AIDS 6(1):11–18
Ritter TJ, Denniston GC (2002) Doctors re-examine circumcision. Third Millennium Publishing, London
Scurlock JM, Pemberton PJ (1977) Neonatal meningitis and circumcision. Med J Aust 1(10):332–334
Seabrook C (1991) $22.8 million in botched circumcision. Atlanta Const
Sherman J, Borer JG, Horowitz M, Glassberg KI (1996) Circumcision: Successful glanular reconstruction and survival following traumatic amputation. J Urol 156:842–844
Sotolongo JR, Hoffman S, Gribetz ME (1985) Penile denudation injuries after circumcision. J Urol 133:102–103
Tagami TY (2010) Atlanta lawyer wins $11 million lawsuit for family in botched circumcision. Atlanta J Const (19 July 2010)
Taylor JR, Lockwood AP, Taylor AJ (1996) The prepuce: specialized mucosa of the penis and its loss to circumcision. Br J Urol 77:291–295
Van Howe RS, Storms MS (2011) How the circumcision solution in Africa will increase HIV infections. J Public Health in Africa 2:e4. doi:10.4081/jphia.2011.e4

Author Biography

George C. Denniston MD, MPH,a graduate of the Harvard School of Public Health, is the founder and President of Doctors Opposing Circumcision (D.O.C.), the first group of medical professionals to uphold their premier tenet, First, Do No Harm! *and* to defend the inalienable right of citizens to intact genital organs. He is co-author of *Doctors Re-Examine Circumcision,* co-editor of the Proceedings of the International Symposia on Circumcision, Genital Integrity, and Human Rights,including *Sexual Mutilations: A Human Tragedy, Male and Female Circumcision: Medical, Legal, and Ethical Considerations in Pediatric Practice, Understanding Circumcision: A Multi-Disciplinary Approach to a Multi-Dimensional Problem, Flesh and Blood: Perspectives on the Problem of Circumcision in Contemporary Society, Bodily Integrity and the Politics of Circumcision: Culture, Controversy and Change, Circumcision and Human Rights,* and *Genital Autonomy: Protecting Personal Choice.* He is a former Associate Medical Director of the Planned Parenthood Federation of America, and he is a co-producer of the landmark documentary, *Birth As We Know It,* by Elena Tonetti-Vladimirova (birthintobeing.com). Olympic Peninsula, Washington, USA.

Chapter 5
Evolution of Circumcision Methods: Not "Just a Snip"

Hugh Young

Abstract A survey of circumcision methods and instruments is presented from an evolutionary perspective. Instruments for circumcising have evolved, but not in any coherent or consistent manner. Nor, after more than 4,000 years, has any consistent ("best") method emerged for circumcising. This underlines fundamental problems with the operation. The instruments have been fetishized along with the operation.

Keywords Instruments • Circumcision devices • Bible • Spear • Knife • Superincision • Dorsal slit • Accu-circ • Milah • Periah • Metzitzah • Scalpel • Gomco • Mogen clamp • Plastibell • Fistula • Necrosis

All my means are sane, my motive and my object mad.
Herman Melville, Moby Dick.

5.1 Introduction

Machines evolve. They are intelligently designed, but artificially selected by commercial pressures and feedback from users to makers. Unlike living organisms, modifications made during the lifetime of one machine may be incorporated into the next generation of machines, in a kind of mechanistic Lamarckism. Thus, over time, successive generations of machines become more fit for their purposes and, depending on commercial factors, more durable, longer lasting, efficient, easy to use, etc.

The evolution of circumcision devices contrasts sharply with that of some household items.

1. The hurricane lantern is said to be unchanged since 1840—certainly since 1898.[1] It quickly became as good as it could get, readily manufactured by pressing and spinning, light, sturdy, simple, and doing what it's meant to—giving light and resisting wind.

[1] A picture of an 1898 hurricane lantern is at http://www.lanternnet.com/faqs.htm accessed July 9, 2010.

H. Young (✉)
Pukerua Bay, New Zealand
e-mail: hugh@buzz.net.nz

G. C. Denniston et al. (eds.), *Genital Cutting: Protecting Children from Medical, Cultural, and Religious Infringements*, DOI: 10.1007/978-94-007-6407-1_5,

2. Scissors have changed but once, from sprung shears to pivoted crossover blades, perhaps in the first century CE.[2] Shears continue in specialized applications, such as gardening and shearing sheep.
3. The car door handle has progressed steadily in one direction, from a turning handle screwed on, similar to a house door handle, towards being flush with the door, for safety and for streamlining. The gradual change tracked user familiarity: while present designs seem obvious today, they would have baffled and frustrated drivers and passengers presented with them ab initio.

The evolution of circumcision devices, on the other hand, far from being any kind of steady progress, has been intermittent, inconsistent, and sometimes retrograde:

1. Vacillating between straight-line clamps and circular crushing.
2. Tending from shields that were removed immediately to clamps that remained for days—with a retrograde move in the Accu-circ, back to shielding, clamping, and a circular chop, with immediate removal.
3. From re-usable to disposable, but not necessarily to non-reusable (self-destroying).

I argue that the reason for this is fundamental problems with circumcision itself, problems that those who want to mechanize the operation have acknowledged only partially and intermittently.

5.2 History

Proponents of circumcision are fond of referring to its great antiquity, as if that somehow proved its worth.

Tribal circumcision is of unknown antiquity. The commonest method today is to pull out the foreskin and chop with a spear or slice with a knife against some hard substrate. Nelson Mandela of the Xhosa reports the first method, Brian Morris describes the second among the Maasai (Mandela et al. 1995; Morris 2010). The terror and pain of this seems to be part of its appeal (to the adults). In the Philippines and Eastern Polynesia, the practice was superincision (at least until the missionaries arrived), the hard substrate having been placed under only the upper integument of the foreskin and a dorsal slit made from the sulcus to the tip.

The first record of a circumcision instrument is from the Bible:

> So Joshua made flint knives and circumcised the Israelites at the Hill of Foreskins.
> —Joshua 5:3

---

[2] "Among the earliest surviving shears is a pair, Egyptian in origin, attributed to the Third Century B.C...." ... "Sir Flinders Petrie ascribes the development of cross-bladed shears [with a center pivot] to the First Century" (Wiss 1948).

The Jewish method was codified in the Babylonian Talmud (Nedarim 31) c. 500 CE:

> The proper way to perform the Mitzvah of Milah is to cut the foreskin with an iron knife and afterwards to separate the skin of the Periah with the nails and to pull it back to this side and that side (And not cut the skin together with the foreskin), and after that is done The Mohel has to suck the blood from the cut with his mouth (The Metzitza) (Yitzchak 2010).

"The skin of the Periah" apparently refers to the inner mucosa.

Traditional Jewish circumcision introduced two instruments, the *izmel* (Heb. scalpel) and the *barzel* (Heb. iron), sometimes called a *mogen* (Heb. shield).[3]

The izmel is a double-bladed knife, to ensure that a nervous mohel cannot choose the wrong side and thereby hurt the baby elsewhere than intended. (One might think that the wrong side could be made distinctive, and thereby remove the greater risk of cutting some other part of the baby or the mohel himself with the back blade.) Some circumcision kits include a whetstone to ensure that both blades are as sharp as possible.

The barzel is a slotted, flat metal shield to protect the glans, which it may or may not do, depending on the glans' size and conformation. The foreskin is pulled out–tearing it from the glans if that has not been done already–and the barzel slid across it, then the iszmel slices the foreskin off, distal to the barzel. In some extant examples, the slot is so narrow a knife would hardly be needed.

In the late 19th century, when non-religious circumcision of adults became a commonplace, Sir Frederick Treves used scissors (Dunsmuir and Gordon 1999).

[The next section is greatly in debt to an essay by Grossman (Grossman 1982).]

The problem with cutting without clamping is how to keep an even tension on the foreskin to give a straight cut. Grossman points out that, as the cut proceeds, the same amount of tension is concentrated in less and less skin, "so the incision at the frenulum was often deeper and uneven".[4]

For that reason, surgeons began using bone forceps in an attempt to isolate the glans and give hemostasis. In Paris, Doyen used a lockable hemostat-like clamp he called an écraseur (crusher).[5]

The first specialized instrument for secular circumcision seems to have been the circumcision forceps invented by a Dr. Moskovich in 1920, apparently for adult circumcision.[6] The blades of a locking hemostat are expanded into two flattened, radially grooved rings with seven notches each. They look as though they should be used to blow bubbles.

---

[3] Devices mentioned in this article may be seen at http://www.circumstitions.com/methods.html.

[4] Ibid, p. 29.

[5] Dunsmuir and Gordon, loc. innom.

[6] Grossman, p. 17.

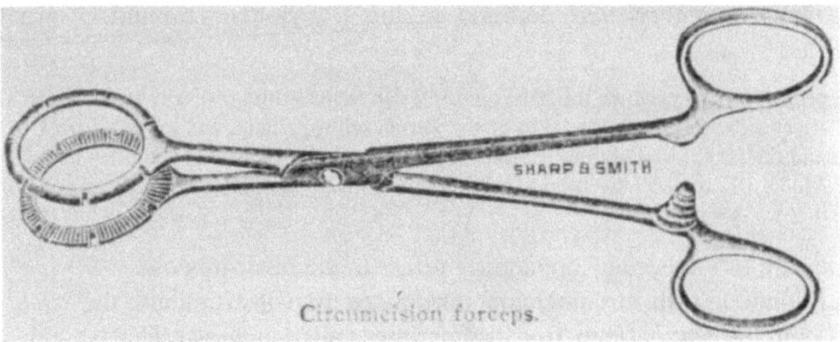

5.2.1 Circumcision Forceps

The top ring was introduced into the preputial cavity–somehow–and the foreskin fanned out between the two rings, which were then locked together. After cutting round the outside, seven sutures could be made in the notches. It had the obvious problem of where to put the foreskin at the place where the forceps met the rings. The rings also left a collar of skin round the glans. Less obviously, it could not apply much pressure over so large an area, but it was the first circumcision device to acknowledge that the prepuce is more or less circular.

The Harris Clamp of 1932 certainly did not.[7] Like an elaborate pair of scissors, but with three thumbholes, it suggests three thumbs were needed to work it. The first two lock a flat clamp together, then the third jaw drives an angled blade up through aligned narrow slits in both jaws of the clamp, somewhat reminiscent of a guillotine. A problem is that the blade grows blunt with repeated use.

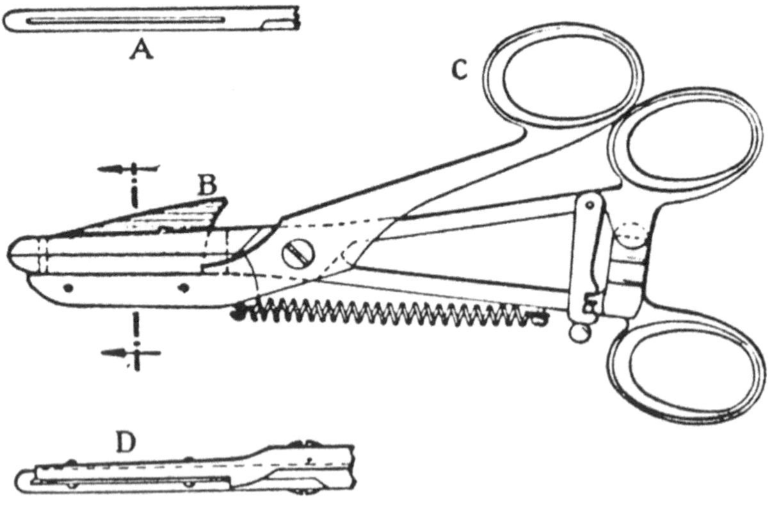

[7] Grossman, p. 29.

5.2.2 *Harris Clamp*

In 1934, Dr Hiram "Inch" Yellen and Aaron Goldstein added leverage to the circumcision forceps.

The Gomco clamp (from "Goldstein Manufacturing Company") was based on the tyre-lever used for Model T Fords, according to Julian Wan's sycophantic history of the device (Wan 2002). A metal bell is placed over the glans (requiring a slit in the foreskin first) and a flat plate with a hole in it is placed over both. Then both are brought up through the hole by a lever whose far end is screwed toward the plate to apply circular crushing and fusing force (of 8,000–20,000 pounds, according to Wan). The fulcrum of the lever and the plate is a low post or posts (see the Tomlinson modification below) on the plate, mating with a hole or holes on the underside of the lever. A crossbar through the shaft of the bell seats in two depressions in a notch on the lever transmitting the tension down the shaft to the bell. The Gomco leaves a characteristic dark line at the excision scar. Lowenstein says its disadvantages are that "it involves more parts, requires more steps in the procedure, and it takes more time." (Lowenstein 1997) Under that enormous pressure and prolonged use, a groove wears in the bell, making it ineffective.

Grossman adds:

> The bell has been found to develop grooves and nicks following repeated use with the surgical blades. There have been reports of the bell breaking....A ring of metal breaks off and is left in the prepucial cavity and the clamp is rendered useless.[8]

Grossman's concern for the *clamp* is touching–the *baby* doesn't much like it either.

There have also been reports of glans injury as a result of the scalpel cutting through the bell.[9]

The clamp is made in a set with different-sized bells and plates and there is a danger of mixing parts of different sizes. In 2001, the FDA issued a warning against clamp injuries caused by this mismatch. (Reuters 2001) In 2009, Dr David Tomlinson produced a version intended to reduce this risk by adding:

- Coded holes in the lever and matching posts on the plate (one size with a single hole and post, one with two close together, one with two further apart), and
- differently sized shafts on the ring, matched to differently sized notches on the lever (Tomlinson et al. 2009).

The Gomco can obviously not be left on the penis; in fact, it is removed as soon as the skin is cut off, giving a risk of bleeding.

The Nutech Clamp, invented by Rabbi Harry Bronstein, is much bigger and heavier, a long lockable lever replacing the screw.[10]

---

[8] Grossman p. 19.

[9] See footnote 8

[10] Grossman, p. 24.

A more obvious descendent of the Gomco is the Circumstat, invented by Rabbi Irving Grossman in 1962, with a cam replacing the screw, apparently quicker and simpler.[11]

Even simpler was the Tibone clamp of 1944, operating like a G-clamp in reverse, to pull the bell and crush the foreskin into the sharp-edged hole.[12] This lost the leverage provided by the arm of the Gomco, and was more awkward to fit. Also, says Grossman, the side arm of the C was too close to the bell, and got in the way of the scalpel. (One would have thought that was easy to fix). The device never gained any popularity. A similar device, the Winkelman clamp, invented in 1935, has a wingnut instead of the Tibone's knurled nut.[13] It was still in use in 2011.

Another variant on the Gomco, again lacking leverage, was the Improved Bloodless Circumcision Clamp invented by a Dr. H. O. Maryan in 1954.[14] This has three interchangeable bells and three corresponding holes in the base, and supports the screw on a tiny lintel, like an early printing press, one that pulls instead of pushing, at one of three positions over the appropriate hole.

The Turner Clamp of 1952 is similar, but operates in the reverse direction, the bell crushing the prepuce down on the aperture.[15] It also has three interchangeable bells, but all operating through the same hole, into three correspondingly sized inserts. Both the Turner and the Bloodless have the problem of the Tibone twice over, the supports of the bell getting in the way of the scalpel on both sides. Neither eclipsed the Gomco.

A cross between the Circumcision Forceps and the Gomco was the Preputome, invented in 1945 by a Brooklyn doctor called Al Akl.[16] It was not actually a preputome because it did not cut, but actually a "prepustat." With an olive-shaped bell as one jaw of a hemostat pressing into a ring on the other, it looks as though it should be used to pit olives. It thoughtfully provided a hole through the "olive" through which the baby could urinate on the doctor. Since the bell pressed the glans downward, it could wedge some of the corona against the ring as the clamp was closed, allowing it to be cut along with the foreskin. The Preputome never became popular.

Flat clamping continued with the Leff Clamp, invented in 1950, which looked and worked like a large paper clip, used in conjunction with a barzel.[17]

It led to the first incarnation of the Sheldon Clamp, in which the spring was augmented by a screw in order to achieve haemostasis.[18] With a slot in the clamp for the scalpel, this has the obvious problem of awkwardness in making the cut, but

[11] Grossman, p. 21.
[12] Grossman, p. 24.
[13] Dunsmuir and Gordon, loc. innom.
[14] Grossman, p. 23.
[15] Grossman, p. 22.
[16] Grossman, p. 20.
[17] Grossman, p. 30.
[18] Grossman, p. 31.

apparently for Sheldon, the problem was not enough pressure, and the next version applied pressure with leverage (Gluckman et al. 1995). The design seems, simply unfortunate, making it quite hard not to capture the glans, difficult to make a clean straight cut through the hole in the top, and–though this is a mixed curse–impossible to give a "tight" (close to the glans) cut. Except that Sheldon seems to have taken the idea of "jaws" and "biting" very literally, it's hard to understand how this ever left the drawing-board. Its lever action was similar to a Vise-grip clamp.

W. G. Rathmann's instrument for female genital cutting *was* a modified Vise-grip (Rathmann 1959). It crushed the clitoral prepuce between two heart-shaped jaws, and the prepuce was cut around the inner outline. A flat shield on the lower jaw protected the clitoris. (This was the only instrument I found specifically for female cutting. The photographs suggest it was used only on adults.)

In 1953, a Texas physician called Kantor mounted a hemostat behind a bisected barzel in a device that looks like a guitar.[19] Grossman points out that, with the Kantor, linear cuts result in crushed "dog ears" at the front and back of the penis, as with all linear devices.

In 1954, Rabbi Bronstein, who'd previously invented the annular, locking Nutech clamp, invented the Mogen clamp.[20] It resembles a barzel, but one whose two blades are hinged together at one end, and brought together at the other with a cam. This is a step backward to straight-line cutting, but mohelim like it because it's quick and resembles the traditional method. The glans, below and completely out of sight of the operator, can be trapped in the locked slit and, as Grossman points out, the meatal lips often project from the glans and into the clamp.

In 2010 in New York, a boy was awarded $10 million against Mogen Circumcision Instruments, Ltd. in settlement of a claim for partial amputation of his penis, the second such case.[21] As a result, the Mogen company went out of business, but the Mogen clamp was still being used and recommended in 2013 (Bowa et al. 2013, Plank et al. 2013).

A doctor called Melges invented the plastic straight-line Glansguard as late as 1972.[22] It resembled a miniature modern kitchen plastic-bag sealer and had a built in knife. It did *not* guard the glans, especially if it was put on upside down, hence a clear message on one side, "This Side Up."

The first of the tourniquet devices that dealt with the foreskin by necrosis was the reusable metal Ross ring, developed in 1939 (Anonymous 2010). In five sizes and made of metal (sold in sets in a handsome art deco walnut case), it included one groove for the ligature and one to catch the scalpel as it cut off the foreskin. It had a tiny handle distal to the glans, on an angle, perhaps to place the ring at an angle with respect to the axis of the penis and follow the line of the sulcus. An enclosed leaflet says the device is to be left in place for 24–72 h.

---

[19] Grossman, p. 32

[20] Grossman, p. 33.

[21] L.G. v. Mogen Circumcision Instruments, Ltd., Civil Action File No. CV06-5864, United States District Court for the Eastern District of New York.

[22] Grossman, p. 34.

5.3 Disposable Devices

Come the 1950s, plastics and the age of disposables, and the Plastibell–developed out of the Ross Ring in 1950—became the method of choice.[23] Like the Gomco, it requires a dorsal slit and tearing of the foreskin from the glans before it can be fitted. Then the foreskin is pulled up over the bell, and a ligature tied to crush it into the groove. Everything distal to the ligature dies and, to stop this from upsetting parents too much, the foreskin may be cut off first.

One risk of the Plastibell is that the ring may slip down the penis and become trapped. Another is that it can block the urethra. A death occurred in Ontario, Canada, from this cause (Paediatric Death Review Committee 2007). It can also lead to some horrendous complications, including urethral fistulae and necrosis of the glans (Bode et al. 2010; Samad et al. 2010).

From the Gomco almost to the present day, the penis is treated as if its cross-section at the sulcus is a perfect circle and no provision is made for the frenulum; the membrane connecting foreskin and glans, and often the last remnant of Taylor's ridged band left after circumcision, hence of significant erogenous value (Taylor et al. 1996).

The Circumcision Centre in the UK says the frenulum is not touched by shield methods, such as the barzel (Circumcision Centre 2010).

It says the forceps-guided method "does not cut the frenulum but it can be removed before or after the circumcision if desired."

In sleeve resection, "The glans and frenulum are not protected. The frenulum can be included in the main cutting or can be cut separately if desired."

With the Gomco, "The glans and frenulum are protected. The frenulum can be removed before or after the circumcision if required." Desired and required by whom it does not say.

With the Plastibell, "The glans and frenulum are protected by the bell. The frenulum will never be cut when using the Plastibell."

The claim that circumcision reduces the risk of HIV/AIDS has brought a flurry of invention in the circumcision industry. The emphasis has been on plastic construction, adult sizes, simplicity, disposability, and low cost. Most of these devices originate from South East Asia and have not been subjected to Western regulation or testing.

The Tara KLamp from Malaysia and the Smart Klamp are very similar (Anonymous 2010a, b). Both involve pulling the foreskin up over a conical bell with an open end for urination, then a ring-shaped clamp is pushed down over the outside and held in place by leverage and locking catches, to crush the prepuce by leverage.

A trial comparing the Tara KLamp (TK) with forceps found almost 40 % (N = 34) of those circumcised with the TK reported adverse effects, including infection, delayed wound healing, swelling, and problems with penis appearance (Lagarde et al. 2009).

[23] Grossman, p. 25.

Ali's clamp is similar to the TK, but crushes at a tilt, to follow the line of the sulcus more closely–the only device to do so (Anonymous 2010).

The Ismael clamp is similar to the TK, but uses a screw to apply pressure instead of levers (Anonymous 2010). It claims to be "readily removable." That would make it re-usable, which introduces the risk of cross-infection.

The Sunathrone uses a separate plastic device like a jar-opener to squeeze a divided ring onto the foreskin over a conical bell similar to those of the Tara and the Ismael. The ring then locks on like a handcuff (Sunathrone 2010).

The Chinese Shangring has a sharp-edged outer ring, which crushes the foreskin into the soft insert of the inner ring (Weihai Zhenxi Medical Equipment Corporation 2010). It provides no protection to the glans when the foreskin is trimmed off. It comes in 22 different sizes!

The Korean–Chinese Zhenxi ring works differently, though it looks similar (Anonymous 2010). It claims it does not require an incision or suture, and "features a tying type of simple operation." It comes in 13 sizes, 7 for babies, 6 for adults.

The Accu-circ, announced in 2006, is a radical departure from all previous instruments, though Dr. David Tomlinson developed it out of the Plastibell (Anonymous 2010). An intermediate stage, which he called an improved Plastibell, included a small disposable blade mounted at the top of the handle to trim the foreskin (Tomlinson et al. 2009).

The Accu-circ, which Tomlinson optimistically calls an atraumatic circumcision device, is disposable, self-contained, and does everything. It reverts from crushing and necrosis to clamping and cutting. Its action is annular, but still assumes the penis is circular, and makes no provision for the frenulum. It resembles a cork puller. Two hemostats are provided to pull the foreskin away from the glans. A probe on one end of the multipurpose tool is used to complete the lysis, then a broken ring on the other end is twirled into the foreskin without the need of a dorsal slit, and the "shielding ring" slid down the probe onto the circular "chopping block" (not their term) to hold the foreskin in place. A video on the Accu-circ website shows the acroposthion hanging out the sides of the clamp, with the potential of impeding the cut. The "cork-puller" is then slid down the probe, where it locks, enclosing the whole penis. Closing the handle then brings down the blade past the clamping ring, through the foreskin, and onto the "block." Like the Glansguard, it is a blind procedure with no guarantee that the glans will stay out of harm's way. Then,

1. If it fails to cut completely, the operator has no way of seeing that, and is at risk of pulling the instrument off, and a random amount of the rest of the penis with it.
2. If the operator does see that in time, there appears to be no way to dismantle the instrument simply and safely. (If there is, the Accu-circ is likely to be reused in poor countries, with consequent risk of cross-infection.)

What happens to the frenulum with the Accu circ is very much a matter of chance, depending on what the blunt probe did, and where the frenulum ends up, between the inner ring and the outer. This raises a grave risk of hemorrhage from the frenular arteriole, and no way to reach it if the device fails to re-open. BP's oil well at the bottom of the Gulf of Mexico springs to mind.

The Accu-circ has been cleared by the Food and Drug Administration for use in the US, on babies up to 10 days old, on the basis that it is "substantially equivalent … to legally marketed … devices" but in fact it is radically different.[24] It is the only one that:

- conceals the penis,
- puts a chopping block inside the foreskin,
- grasps the chopping block through the foreskin,
- cuts in a circle,
- chops instead of slicing.

Tomlinson has treated circumcision as if it were a kitchen chore like crushing garlic, and invented a device to do it like that. But, the issues involved in crushing garlic well or badly are of much less moment than those involved in circumcision.

Since this paper was presented, a new device, the PrePex, has come on the market with much publicity. Like the Plastibell, the PrePex crushes the foreskin into a grooved ring and is left on while the foreskin, or what has not been trimmed away, necroses. Like the Plastibell, it is disposable. It is not clear that it is *not* re-usable. Instead of a ligature, it uses an elastic ring, like the Elastrator used for castrating sheep and docking their tails. It is so far made only in adult sizes. It claims to have FDA approval and to be bloodless, painless, and non-surgical. If those claims are true, it can no longer be said that "adult circumcision is much more painful, complicated, and dangerous than infant circumcision" and that, therefore, males should be circumcised before they can give–or withhold–their consent.

5.4 Summary of Methods

Here is a timeline of the invention of methods of circumcision, based on the shape of the cut and disposability of the instrument. (Linear methods all use reusable instruments.)

Linear (Re-usable)	Annular Re-usable	Annular Disposable
BCE Flint knife		
CE Izmel		
CE Barzel		
CE Pocket knife		
18XX Bone forceps		
1903 Scissors		
1920 Écraseur Écraseur	1920 Circumcision forceps	

(continued)

[24] http://www.accucirc.com/documents/AccuCirc_501k.pdf (accessed January13, 2011).

(continued)

1932 Harris clamp		
	1934 Gomco clamp	
	1939 Ross ring	
	19XX Nutech clamp	
	1944 Tibone clamp	
	1945 Preputome	
1950 Leff clamp		1950 Plastibell
	1952 Turner clamp	
1953 Sheldon clamp (1)		
195X Sheldon clamp (2)		
1954 Kantor Clamp	1954 Improved bloodless	
1954 Mogen clamp		
	1962 Circumstat	
1972 Glans guard		
		1995 Tara KLamp
		199X Smart clamp
		199X Ismail clamp
		199X Sunathrone
		2003 Shang ring
		2003 Zhengi rings
		200X? Ali's clamp
		2004 Kirve clamp
		2006 Accu-circ
	2009 Improved gomco	2009 Improved plastibell
		2011 Pre Pex

The only consistent development is that all recent devices are disposable, but that will have as much to do with modern medical practice and plastics as with circumcision.

The devices may also be sorted according to what they do;

Cutting	Holding and cutting (brief crushing for hemostasis)	Holding (brief crushing for hemostasis)	Crushing (prolonged for necrosis)
BCE Flint knife			
CE Izmel		CE Barzel	
CE Pocket knife			
18XX Scalpel		18XX Bone forceps	
1903 Scissors			
		1920 Écraseur	
		1920 circumcision forceps	
	1932 Harris Clamp		
		1934 Gomco Clamp	
			1939 Ross ring
		19XX Nutech clamp	
		1944 Tibone clamp	
		1945 Preputome	

(continued)

(continued)

Cutting	Holding and cutting (brief crushing for hemostasis)	Holding (brief crushing for hemostasis)	Crushing (prolonged for necrosis)
		1950 Leff clamp	1950 Plastibell
		1952 Turner clamp	
		1953 Sheldon clamp (1)	
		195X Sheldon clamp (2)	
		1954 Kantor clamp	
		1954 Improved bloodless	
		1954 Mogen clamp	
		1962 Circumstat	
	1972 Glansguard		
			1995 Tara KLamp
			199X Smart clamp
			199X Ismail clamp
			199X Sunathrone
			2003 Zhengi rings
			2003 Shang ring
			200X? Ali's clamp
	2006 Accu-circ		
		2009 Improved Gomco	2009 Improved plastibell
			2011 Pre Pex

Unlike the hurricane lantern, they did not find the best method and stick with it; unlike the scissors, there was no great leap forward; unlike the car door handle, there was no smooth progression, from linear to annular to disposable, Instead, inventors have jumped back and forth, apparently having some nostalgia for the linear barzel, and perhaps some dislike of the necrosis of the Plastibell.

It took the designers of the devices thousands of years to work out how to compress in a circle. They still have not accommodated the frenulum because the frenulum intractably complicates the cutting. And though it is common knowledge that the frenulum, the last remnant of Taylor's ridged band, is the male G-spot, circumcisers have not yet formulated a consistent policy towards it and hence their devices do not treat it consistently.

What this exposes is that no way of circumcising is without problems because the foreskin has not evolved in a way that lends itself to being removed.

The best method of circumcision is not doing it.—Sarah Strandjord, MD, FAAP

5.5 Instruments and Fetishism

The various circumcising devices are often bright and glittering–the kind of thing a jackdaw would use to decorate its nest. They are also attractive to circumcision fetishists. According to the Encyclopedia of Psychiatric Disorders:

> Fetishism is a form of paraphilia, a disorder that is characterized by recurrent intense sexual urges and sexually arousing fantasies generally involving non-human objects, the suffering or humiliation of oneself or one's partner (not merely simulated), or children or other non-consenting persons. The essential feature of fetishism is recurrent intense sexual urges and sexually arousing fantasies involving specific objects. While any object may become a fetish, the distinguishing feature is its connection with sex or sexual gratification (Fetishism 2010).

A circumcision fetishist, or circumfetishist for short, is a person who gets sexual pleasure from the act of circumcision.

Women may fetishize apparently non-sexual objects, such as large structures (Simpson 2010), though their attraction seems more like falling in love than a purely sexual involvement. Circumfetishists appear to be virtually all men–though being circumcised by a scornful woman is a common circumfetishist fantasy.

Circumfetishism should be distinguished from just eroticizing the circumcised penis (accucullophilia), as many women and gay men may do, just from familiarity (and unfamiliarity with the intact version), and then it should be considered in the context of apotemnophilia (the wish to be an amputee) and acrotomophilia (sexual interest in amputees).

Circumfetishism may involve fantasies of power and control, which may be ritualistically acted out. They may be active (sadistic) fantasies of circumcising, or passive (masochistic) fantasies of being circumcised, and the rituals, when they occur, of course involve both. Circumfetishists have several websites (Anonymous 2010; Anonymous 2010; Anonymous 2010). Until June 2010, the Circlist website (Circlist 2010) linked to a Google discussion group that said

> Circlist has always permitted, and will continue to permit, circumcision-related fetish/ sexual postings/materials, straight, gay, or otherwise. Individuals may use CIRCLIST to make contact with one another, including for sexual purposes. The list is not just a medical interest list, but rather all things circumcision, including circ-fetish, sexual info, medical info and a place to meet up with fellow circumcision enthusiasts and proponents.

Circumsexuals held the first International Circumsexual Symposium, in Washington, DC, in June 2005, and another in Las Vegas in May 2010.

Circumfetishist "Ben Winkie" blogs about it. ("Interests: Being masturbated whilst circumcision is being discussed. Watching circumcisions with others. Etc.") and features a Gomco and a Mogen clamp on his avatar (Blogger Ben Winkie 2010).

The extent of circumfetishism among doctors and others who perform infant circumcisions is unknown. It warrants further research.

Hugh Young, B.Sc., is a retired broadcaster and editor with a science background. He has published two dictionaries, of Solomon Islands Pijin and New Zealand Maori place name pronunciation (oral, now online at http://nga-ingoa.notlong.com). He has presented three papers at Genital Integrity Symposia, on the rise and fall of circumcision in New Zealand (with Ken McGrath), on circumcision as a memeplex, and on the foreskin and circumcision in popular media, subsequently published. For more than 14 years he has maintained the Intactivism Pages, www.circumstitions.com, a pro-intact website. Pukerua Bay, New Zealand.

Acknowledgments Thanks to Marilyn Milos for scanning the Grossman essay and sending it to me, to my husband, Tim, for his unfailing support, and to Circlist for alerting me to the existence of the Ross rings, and whose obsessive interest in the details of the operation saved me from having to think about it too much.

References

Anonymous (2010) Ross circumcision ring. Circlist http://www.circlist.com/instrstechs/rossring.html Accessed 8 July 2010

Anonymous (2010) Alisklamp: Advanced technology for perfect male circumcision http://www.alisklamp.com/english/sorularla_alisklamp.html Accessed 22 July 2010

Anonymous (2010) Why Use Isamail Clamp http://www.ismailclamp.com/index_files/Whyuseismailclamp.htm)Accessed 22 July 2010

Anonymous (2010) The Shangring circumcision device http://medgadget.com/archives/2008/08/the_shangring_circumcision_device.html Accessed 22 July 2010

Anonymous (2010) Accu-Circ single-action circumcision device http://www.accucirc.com Accessed 22 July 2010

Anonymous (2010) Inter-circ http://groups.yahoo.com/group/Inter-Circ Accessed 24 July 2010

Anonymous (2010) Roundheads UK http://uk.groups.yahoo.com/group/RoundHeads/ Accessed 24 July 2010

Anonymous (2010) Circumcision images http://www.icon.co.za/~hugot/circum/circum.htm Accessed 22 July 2010 (circlist)

Anonymous (2010) Circlist http://www.circlist.com/news.html Accessed 24 July 2010

Anonymous (2010a) Tara KLamp for non-invasive male circumcision http://www.cirp.org/library/procedure/tara-klamp/booklet.doc Accessed 20 July 2010

Anonymous (2010b) The SmartKlamp® a new invention http://www.smartcircumcision.com/smartklamp.html Accessed 22 July 2010

Ben Winkie (2010) Blogger Ben Winkie http://www.blogger.com/profile/11085999452260195794 Accessed 22 July 2010

Bode CO, Ikhisemojie S, Ademuyiwa AO (2010) Penile injuries from proximal migration of the Plastibell circumcision ring. J Ped Urol 6:23–27

Bowa K et al. (2013) A controlled trial of three methods for neonatal circumcision in Lusaka, Zambia. JAIDS, vol 62(1), pp e1-6. http://journals.lww.com/jaids/Fulltext/2013/01010/A_Controlled_Trial_of_Three_Methods_for_Neonatal.12.aspx Accessed April 3,2013

Circumcision Centre (2010) Circumcision methods and techniques http://www.circumcisioncentre.co.uk/circumcision-methods-techniques.html?Itemid=55 Accessed 20 July 2010

Dunsmuir WD, Gordon EM (1999) The history of circumcision (Winkelman) BJU International, vol 83(1), pp 1–12 http://www.cirp.org/library/history/dunsmuir1/ Accessed 19 July 2010

Fetishism (2010) Encyclopedia of mental disorders http://www.minddisorders.com/Del-Fi/Fetishism.html Accessed 22 July 2010

Gluckman G et al (1995) Newborn penile amputation during circumcision and successful reattachment, vol 153. BJU, South Carolina, 778–779

Grossman E (1982) The evolution of circumcision technique. In: Circumcision: a pictorial atlas of its history, instrument development and operating techniques. Todd & Honeywell, Great Neck, pp 17–34

Lagarde E, Taljaard D, Puren A, Auvert B (2009) High rate of adverse events following circumcision of young male adults with the Tara KLamp technique: a randomized trial in South Africa. S Afr Med J 99(3):163–169

Lowenstein VH (1997) Circumcision. In: Varney H (ed) Varney's midwifery, 3rd edn. Mass: Jones and Bartlett, Sudbury

Mandela N (1995) Long walk to freedom. Little Brown & Co (unabridged editions only), pp 30–36

Morris B (2010) Circumcision—what caused many cultures to ritually remove the foreskin? http://www.circinfo.net/what_caused_many_cultures_to_remove_it.html) Accessed 17 July 2010

Paediatric Death Review Committee (2007) Office of the chief coroner of Ontario. Circumcision: a minor procedure? paed child health, vol 12(4) http://www.pulsus.com/Paeds/12_04/Pdf/zwol_ed.pdf Accessed 20 July 2010

Plank RM et al (2013) A randomized trial of mogen clamp versus plastibell for neonatal male circumcision in botswana. JAIDS vol 62(5), pp e131–137 http://journals.lww.com/jaids/Fulltext/2013/04150/A_Randomized_Trial_of_Mogen_Clamp_Versus.14.aspx Accessed 3 April 2013

Rathmann WG (1959) Female circumcision: indications and a new technique, vol XX. GP, pp 115–120

Reuters (2001) US warns of circumcision clamp injury risk. Reuters Health

Samad A, Khanzada TW, Kumar B (2010) Plastibell circumcision: a minor surgical of major importance. J Ped Urol 6:28–31

Simpson A (2010) Woman with objects fetish marries Eiffel Tower. The Telegraph, London, England http://www.telegraph.co.uk/news/newstopics/howaboutthat/2074301/Woman-with-objects-fetish-marries-Eiffel-Tower.html Accessed 22 July 2010

Sunathrone BM Technologies Sdn. Bhd. Sunathrone (2010) Disposable circumcision device http://www.sunathrone.com/home.htm Accessed 22 July 2010

Taylor JP, Lockwood AP, Taylor AJ (1996) The prepuce: specialized mucosa of the penis and its loss to circumcision, vol 77. BJU, South Carolina, pp 211–295 http://www.cirp.org/library/anatomy/taylor/ Accessed 20 July 2010

Tomlinson D, Shelton L, Caldamone A (2009) An improved device for male circumcision: a modified Yellen style (Gomco) circumcision clamp (poster presentation) 5th IAS conference on AIDS pathogenesis, treatment and prevention, pp 19–22 http://www.ias2009.org/pag/Abstracts.aspx?AID=1397 Accessed 24 July 2010

Tomlinson D, Shelton L, Caldamone A (2009) An improved device for male circumcision: a modified Ross style (Plastibell) tourniquet shielding ring. 5th IAS Conference on AIDS Pathenogenesis, treatment and prevention, 2009 (poster presentation) (accessed July 20 2010 at http://www.ias2009.org/pag/Abstracts.aspx?AID=1398)

Wan J (2002) GOMCO circumcision clamp; an enduring and unexpected success. Urology 59(5):790–794

Weihai Zhenxi Medical Equipment Corporation (2010) Introduction to company and product http://zhenxi-korea.com/index_en_intr.htm Accessed 22 July 2010

Wiss JR (ed) (1948) A Story of Shears and Scissors. J Wiss & Sons, p 16 http://jwissandsons.com/shears-scissors.pdf Accessed 3 April 2012

Yitzchak BY (2010) What does halacha say? http://www.brityy.org/content.asp?dept=1017& article=617) Accessed 8 July 2010

Author Biography

Hugh Young BSc, is a retired broadcaster and editor with a science background. He has published two dictionaries, of Solomon Islands Pijin and New Zealand Maori place name pronunciation (oral, now online at http://nga-ingoa.notlong.com). He has presented three papers at Genital Integrity Symposia, on the rise and fall of circumcision in New Zealand (with Ken McGrath), on circumcision as a memeplex, and on the foreskin and circumcision in popular media, subsequently published. For more than 14 years he has maintained the Intactivism Pages, www.circumstitions.com, a pro-intact website. Pukerua Bay, New Zealand.

Chapter 6
Penile Wounding: Complications of Routine Male Circumcision in a Typical American Family Practice

Christopher Fletcher

Abstract Men 18 years and older seeking medical care in a private, full-service, well-established family practice in New Mexico were offered evaluation as to circumcision status and examined with regards to documentable surgical damage from circumcision. Despite the fact that every circumcised man had visible and definable obvious and undesired surgical side-effects, ranging from minor scarring to extreme twisting and bending, only a tiny fraction of these men, including gay men, were aware of any penile abnormalities, and almost all believed their own penises were "normal". The vast majority of the circumcisions had occurred in the newborn period and had been done for standard non-medical reasons. Contrary to assumptions by parents and physicians, most, if not all, newborn circumcisions leave the victim of the surgery in an obvious physically damaged state, which is universally ignored by the patient, his parents, and the physicians performing the surgery or caring for the male child or adult male victim of circumcision.

Keywords Male circumcision • Genital mutilation • Measurements • Length • Circumference • Skin bridges • Tunnels • Cysts • Deformity • Scar tissue • Meatus • Meatal stenosis

6.1 Introduction

By definition, newborn male circumcision (male genital mutilation or MGM) removes a significant amount of genital tissue from a presumably normal penis, leaving the victim of this brutal and unnecessary surgery damaged and diminished (Goldman 2011; Williams and Kapila 1993). Most American parents, physicians, and adult men are so oblivious to this reality that only a very few circumcised men ever realize that they have had penile reduction "surgery" and are therefore not normal.

C. Fletcher (✉)
School of Medicine, University of New Mexico, Santa Fe, NM, USA
e-mail: docfrodo@earthlink.net

G. C. Denniston et al. (eds.), *Genital Cutting: Protecting Children from Medical, Cultural, and Religious Infringements*, DOI: 10.1007/978-94-007-6407-1_6,

During my 30 years of practice it has become increasingly and painfully obvious that essentially all circumcised boys and men have visible, definable, and measurable penile and genital damage, (Williams and Kapila 1993; Weiss et al. 2010; Baskin et al. 1996) and that there is probably no such thing as a "normal circumcision" and certainly no such thing as a "normal" penis after circumcision. Because almost none of these circumcisions are medically necessary essentially every circumcised male is therefore, by definition, a victim of an unnecessary and botched operation. Most of these iatrogenic penile injuries are never recognized by the patient, his parents and, worse yet, by the examining and/or circumcising physician (Goldman 2011; Williams and Kapila 1993). The more horrendous surgical sequelae are almost always dismissed, minimized (Weiss et al. 2010; Baskin et al. 1996) or covered up, and of course, only rarely acknowledged by the physicians involved (Goldman 2011).

From the boy who is taught by his parents to "poke his penis" in the other side of his underwear to "help it grow back straight" to the physicians who spend only a few seconds, if that, on a genital exam, see nothing, and miss everything, to the circumcisers who believe in their own arrogant fashion that they "do perfect work," we encounter an endless line of wounded men mostly unaware of their deformities.

It is from a gradually developed awareness of the scope of the damage that I decided to do a comparative study of circumcised versus intact men. Prior studies have demonstrated the different types of damage (Williams and Kapila 1993; Weiss et al. 2010; Baskin et al. 1996; Osifo and Oriaifo 2009) but none have placed this within the context of a medical practice. What I witnessed should be no different than what all primary care physicians taking care of circumcised boys and men see regularly, and should easily recognize and therefore document.

6.2 Background

Men who agreed to participate in this observational study were stratified by the demographics of age, height, weight, nationality, race, and religious persuasion. Other than having to be at least 18 years of age and healthy enough to participate, there were no exclusionary criteria. Patients were offered no inducement to participate, were recruited only because they were adult males, and were in the office during an annual exam or non-sick visit. The only incentive to participate was to further personal and scientific knowledge. Confidentially and anonymity were preserved as there were no office or chart records. No treatment was offered or provided. Six circumcised and two intact men who were asked to participate declined.

A convenience sample of 108 men (53 genitally intact and 55 circumcised) was evaluated in the spring of 2010. All but two of the circumcised men had had circumcisions as infants, with one of the other two men circumcised at age 4 and one at age 45 following a zipper accident. The genital status of the participants was unknown to me until their exam, and several of the participants were unsure whether they were intact or circumcised.

6.3 Observations and Measurements

Participating men were examined with respect to (1) length of their flaccid penis, (2) circumference of the distal shaft, (3) sideways leaning of the penis to the right or left, (4) curvature or angular twisting of the penile shaft, (5) presence of a bent shaft, (6) measurement of the vertical and horizontal dimensions of the external urethral orifice (meatus), and (7) presence of surgical mishaps or damage such as skin bridges, tunnels, retention cysts, glans deformity, scar tissue on the shaft or glans, evidence of de-shafting, extraneous surgical scars, and excessive shaft skin removed. Anatomical measurements allowed for calculation of penile volume and meatal percentage and area, a factor which impacts urinary flow. Participants were asked about additional or secondary genital surgery, whether they were aware of any personal genital abnormalities, whether they were bothered by their appearance or abnormalities, and whether they had asked for and/or been prescribed erectile dysfunction medications.

6.4 Demographics

6.4.1 Age, Height, and Weight

The mean (average) age of the participants was 49.69 years old for the circumcised men and 51.64 years old for the intact men. The median ages were 49 and 53 years old respectively. Mean (average) heights and weights were 69.76 and 69.5 inches tall, and 228.03 and 191.59 lbs for circumcised and intact men. Median heights and weights were 69 and 69.25 inches and 185 and 191 lbs respectively.

The circumcised men had been mostly circumcised in the US and a few internationally, with none, to my knowledge, having been circumcised by currently practicing physicians in New Mexico. It was impossible to determine whether the circumcising physicians were pediatricians, obstetrician-gynecologists, family physicians, urologists, or other specialists since none of the circumcisers could be identified by the participants. The two Jewish men in the study had been circumcised ritually.

6.4.2 Nationality and Race

Among the 55 circumcised men, 52 were American by birth, 2 were African, and 1 was a Pakistani with dual citizenship. 35 identified themselves as Caucasian, including 10 Hispanics, 2 were black, 1 was European, and 14 identified themselves as primarily Hispanic. Among the intact men, 43 were born in the U.S., 7 were born in Mexico, 1 in El Salvador, 1 in Brazil, and 1 was British. 12 identified themselves as primarily Caucasian, 40 as Hispanic, including 1 Native American, and 1 as black.

6.4.3 Religious Persuasion

Among the circumcised men, there were 25 Catholics, 4 "Christians", 3 Episcopalians, 1 Mennonite, 1 Methodist, 1 Baptist, 3 "Protestants", 1 Greek Orthodox, 2 Jews, 1 Muslim, 3 agnostics, and 10 had no religious affiliation. Among the intact men, there were 34 Catholics, 2 Protestants, 1 Presbyterian, 2 Episcopalians, 1 Jehovah's Witness, 7 "Christians", and 6 had no religious affiliation.

6.5 Findings

6.5.1 Penile Length

The penile length was measured from base to the tip of the glans (Khan et al. 2012; Richters et al. 1995). Circumcised men had an average or mean length of 4.343 inches with a median length of 4.25 inches and with a standard deviation of 0.49955 and variance of 0.24955. Intact men measured significantly longer with a mean or average length of 4.575 inches, a median length of 4.5 inches, and with a standard deviation of 0.54725 and variance of 0.29948 (difference 0.266 inches, $t = 2.24$, $p = 0.0275$).

6.5.2 Penile Leaning

All 55 circumcised men leaned to one side or the other while only 9 intact men did. The mean (average) angle of lean in the circumcised group was 12.113 with a median of 11° and a range of 2–38°. Of the 9 intact men who had measurable leaning the mean (average) was 4.333° with a median of 4° and a range of 1–10°. Only 1 intact man, however, leaned more than 4°. The difference in angle of leaning was 11.426 ($t = 11.16$, $p < 0.0001$).

6.5.3 Right- Versus Left-Leaning

The majority of circumcised men (44/55 = 80 %) leaned to the left consistent with the presumed majority of circumcising physicians being right-handed (70–95 % of people in the world are right-handed), while 20 % (11/55) leaned to the right consistent with left-handed circumcisers (5–30 % of all people worldwide are left-handed). Asymmetric circumferential cutting leading to leaning and curvature presumably devolves from the location of the standing surgeon relative to the restrained baby boy.

6.5.4 Shaft Circumference

Measurements of the distal penile shaft just proximal to the corona revealed expected differences between circumcised and intact men based on the surgical removal of the foreskin and resultant neurovascular insult to the shaft and glans. The mean (average) circumcised distal shaft was 9.817 cm with a median of 10 cm while the intact men measured on average 10 cm with a median of 10 cm (difference 0.426, $t = 2.66$, $p = 0.0093$).

6.5.5 Shaft Curvature

Men who have been circumcised are frequently noted to have obvious penile curvature, a condition that has led to innumerable jokes, stories, and urban myths, as well as complaints to physicians from female partners and the patients themselves about painful intercourse as well as difficulty aiming their urinary stream. In this study, 28 of 55 (51 %) circumcised men were found to have a twisted shaft with a mean (average) twist angle of 6.964° and median of 5.5°, while none of the 53 intact men had any measurable penile twist ($p < 0.0001$).

6.5.6 External Urethral Meatus Measurements

Previous studies dating back to the 19th century have demonstrated a significant difference in urethral meatal caliber from circumcision-caused contraction of the external urethral meatus. (Berry and Cross 1956; Martin 1881; Morton 1963) In circumcised males, the mean (average) length and width of the external urethra was 6.782 and 1.067 mm with median length and widths of 6.00 and 1.00 mm. In the intact population, the mean (average) length and width were 9.283 and 1.642 mm with a median of 9.00 and 2.00 mm (length: difference 2.339, $t = 5.66$, $p < 0.0001$; width: difference 0.457, $t = 3.87$, $p = 0.0002$) (Figs. 6.1 and 6.2).

6.6 Damages from the Surgery

6.6.1 The Circumcised Men

It seems counter-intuitive but only circumcised men had evidence of *unnecessary* surgical damage to their genitals. Of the 55 circumcised men in the study, 1 (1.8 %) had a bent shaft (Fig. 6.3),

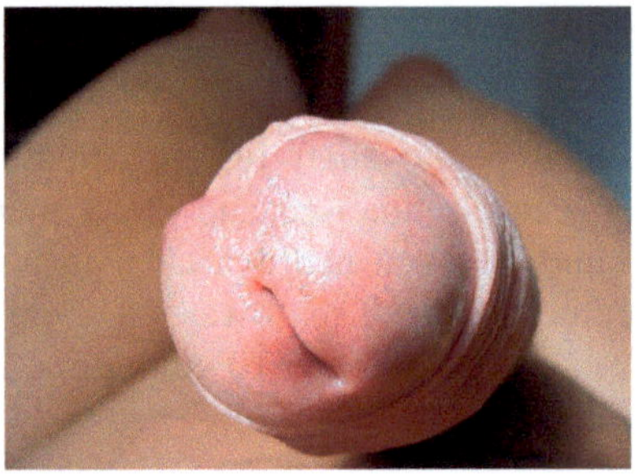

Fig. 6.1 Normal glans penis

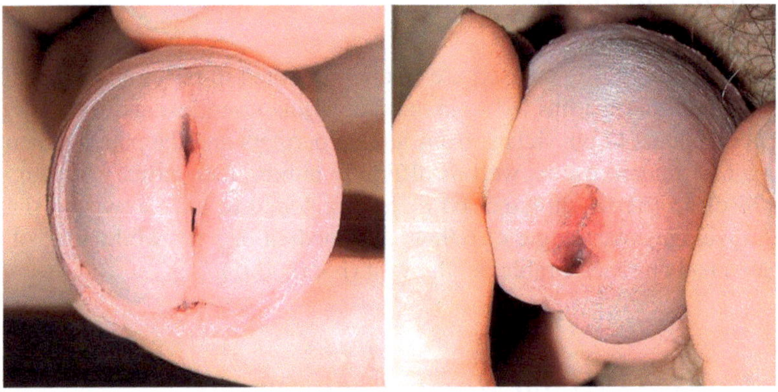

Fig. 6.2 Normal male urethal opening

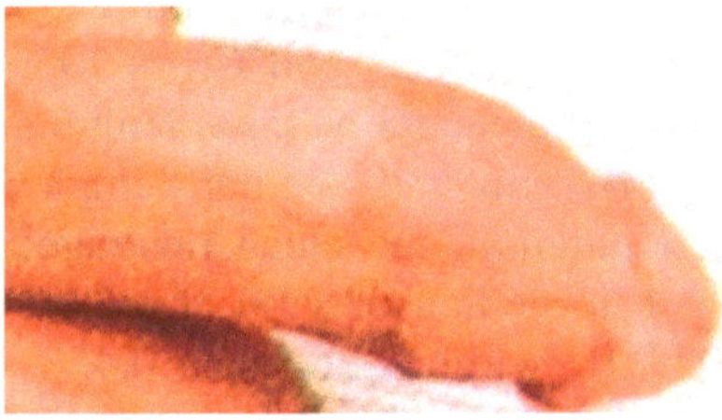

Fig. 6.3 Bent shaft

7 had skin bridges (12.7 %) (Figs. 6.4, 6.5, 6.6, 6.7)

I knew that he had required additional surgery (1.8 %), and fortuitously none had been de-shafted.

Two of the 55 circumcised men (and none of the intact men) complained of a bifid or split urinary stream and had very small urinary orifices on examination consistent with post-circumcision meatal stenosis (Joudi et al. 2010; Van Howe 2006) and scarring. One noted that he had to twist his penis 90° to aim his split stream at the toilet in

Fig. 6.4 Skin bridge

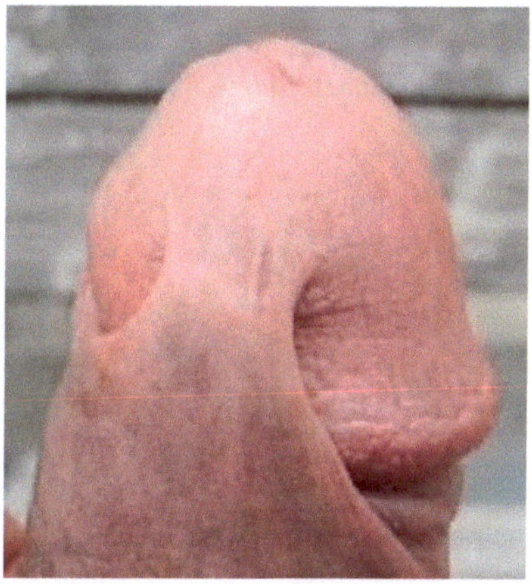

Fig. 6.5 Skin bridge

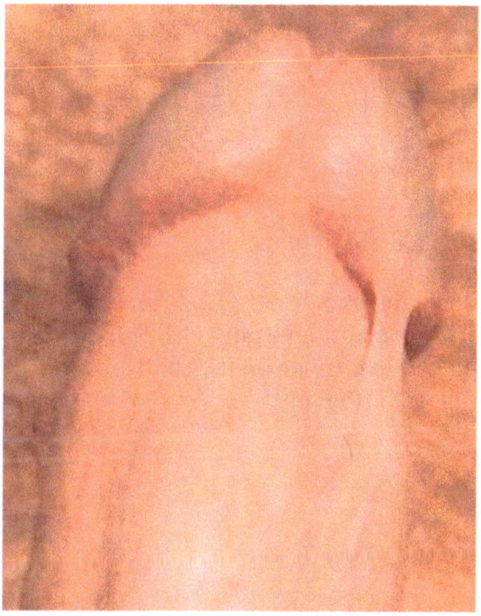

Fig. 6.6 Skin bridges

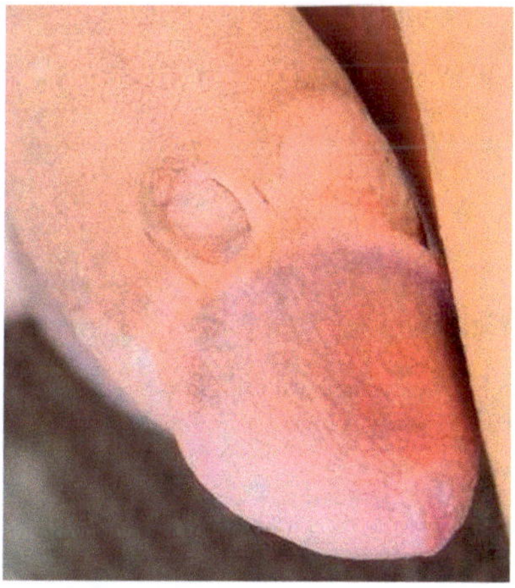

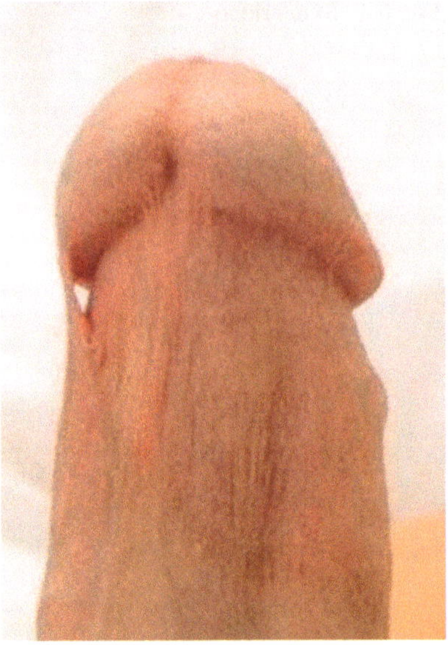

Fig. 6.7 Skin bridge

2 had skin tunnels (3.6 %) (Fig. 6.8)

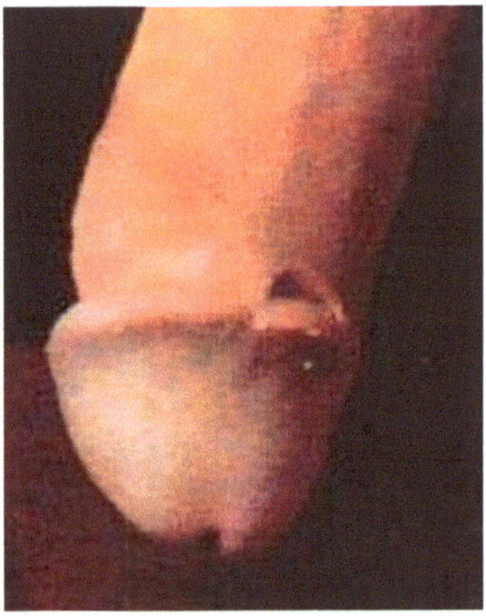

Fig. 6.8 Skin tunnel

7 had retention cysts (12.7 %), 1 had a glans deformity (1.8 %), 25 had scar tissue on the shaft (44.4 %) (Fig. 6.9)

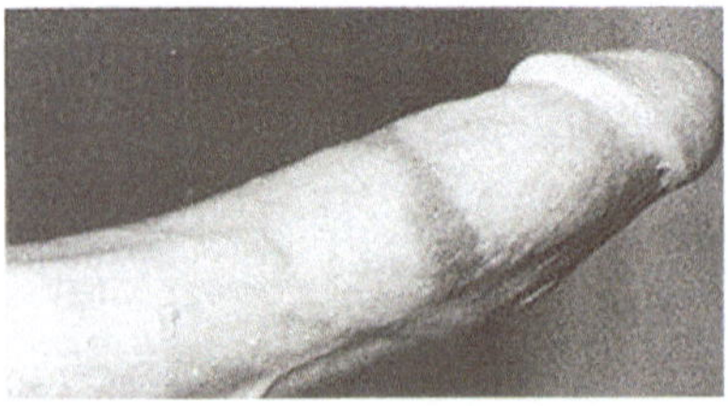

Fig. 6.9

5 had scar tissue on the glans (9.1 %) (Fig. 6.10)

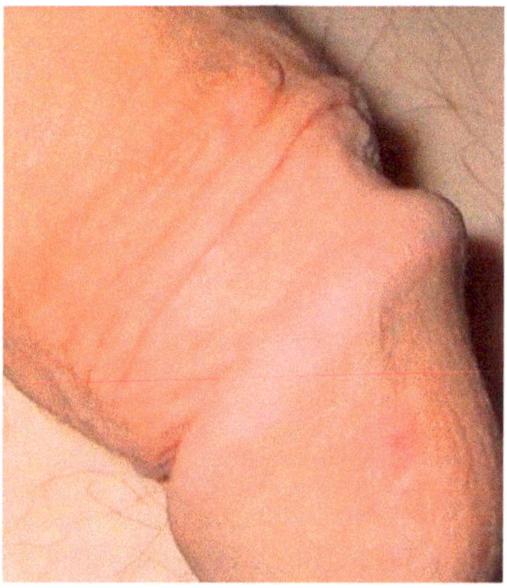

Fig. 6.10 Glans scar

11 had excessive shaft skin removed (20 %) including 1 who had 5 different colored bands of scarified shaft skin (Figs. 6.11, 6.12, 6.13, 6.14)

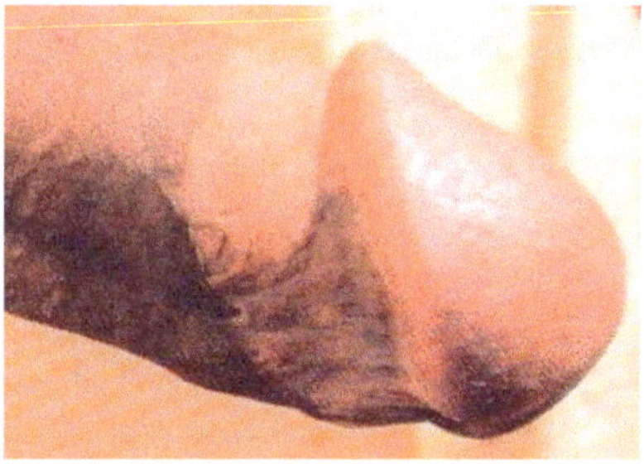

Fig. 6.11 Excessive skin removal with resultant scar

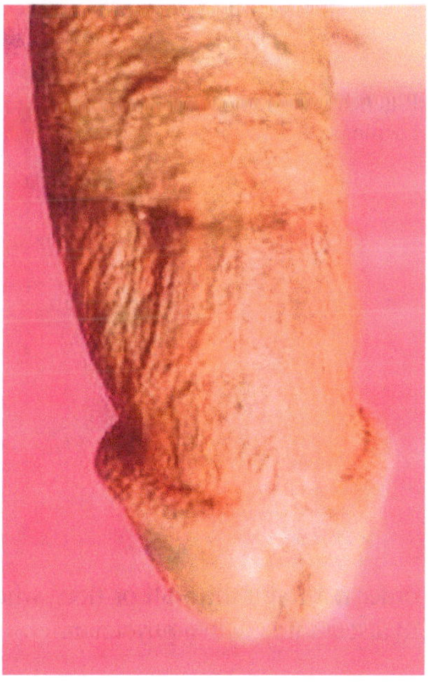

Fig. 6.12 Excessive skin removal

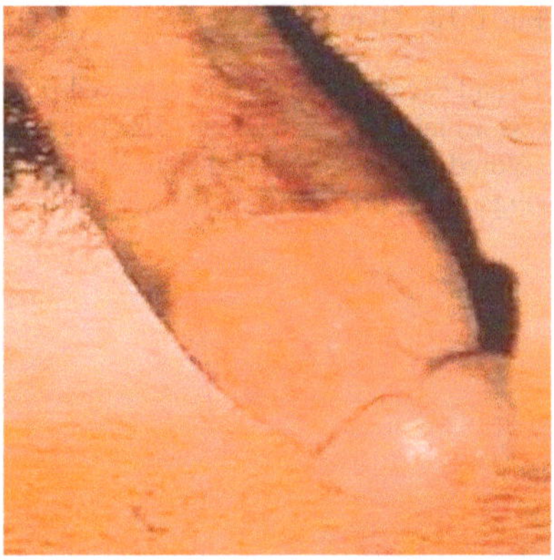

Fig. 6.13 Excessive skin removal

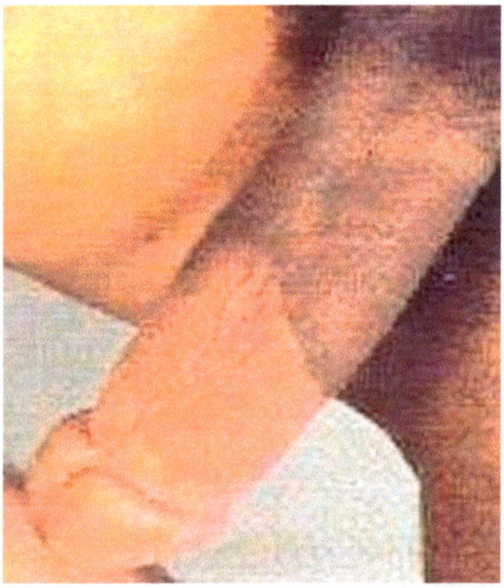

Fig. 6.14 Excessive skin removal

2 had meatal stenosis and scarring causing bifid urinary streams (Figs. 6.15 and 6.16)

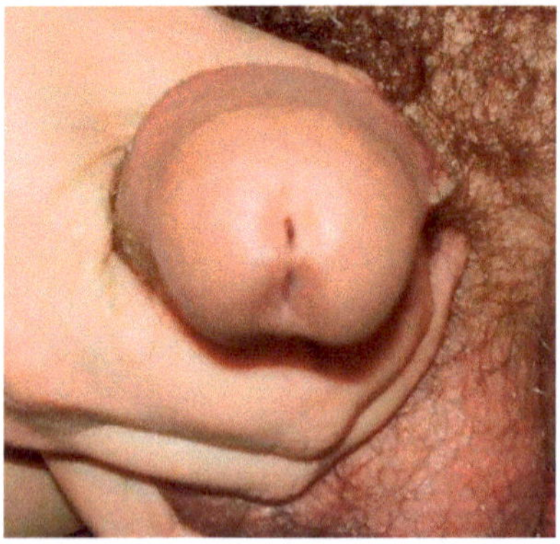

Fig. 6.15 Two meatal openings

order not to hit the wall or floor when urinating. Both men had been too embarrassed to discuss this with a physician.

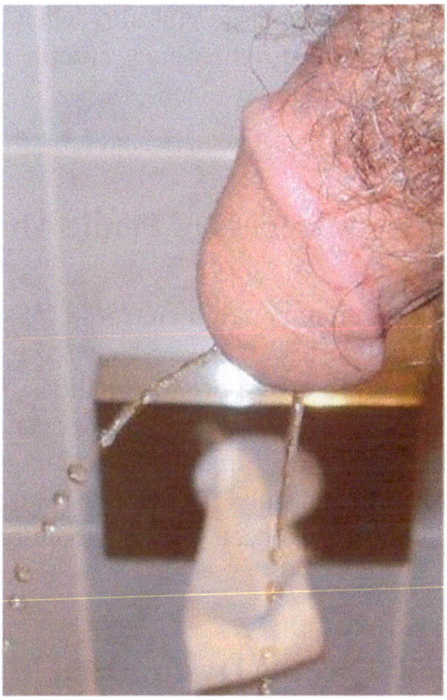

Fig. 6.16 Bifid urinary streams

One patient presented with a 2½ inch long curvilinear scar with suture marks on the ventral shaft and had never noticed it—an obvious Z-plasty plastic surgery repair of a "filleting" his parents (and of course he) were never told about. One complained that his circumcised penis bothered him during competitive cycling because of the significant curvature, two told stories about their tailors cutting one pant leg differently to accommodate a leaning/twisting penis, and one was so upset by his poorly done circumcision (he left his own son intact) that he had switched from Episcopalian to agnostic assuming that somehow his family's religion had been connected to his circumcision damages. One fractured his twisted penis during intercourse requiring emergency surgery (he and his brother had had side-by-side tonsillectomies and coincidental circumcisions by the neighborhood Jewish doctor during the Depression), and another one had 3 side-by-side linear scars with suture marks extending the length of his ventral shaft, also never noticed until his exam.

6.6.2 *The Intact Men*

Of the 53 intact men, one elderly male had developed balanitis xerotica obliterans (BXO) and required surgery, which was partially successful and which left him with scar tissue on his shaft. He was the only intact male to have had any penile surgery. One intact male was told that he was circumcised when he was clearly intact (what a surprise!), one tore his frenulum as an adult in an accident, and one very tall and large male was told by his short girlfriend that he "was too small" (she owned a large vibrator) when he was in fact quite normally sized. He had suffered from psychological erectile dysfunction for several years believing that he was inadequately sized.

6.7 Awareness of Penile Abnormalities

Of the circumcised men, 25/55 (45.4 %) were aware of any penile abnormalities and only 4/55 (7.2 %) were bothered by their abnormalities. The 20/25 (80 %) circumcised men aware of abnormalities during and after the study were still not bothered by their problems. On the other hand, only 3/53 (5.4 %) of intact men were aware of any penile abnormalities, including two men who were concerned that they leaned slightly and only 1/53 (1.8 %) was bothered by his perceived abnormality (the one man who had been told, and therefore believed, that his penis was "too small").

6.8 Erectile Dysfunction Medication Use

Of the circumcised men (average age 63.45 and median age 65 years old), 11/55 (20 %), and, of the intact men (average age 63.07 and median age 67 years old), 15/55 (27.3 %) had asked for, been prescribed, and used medications for erectile dysfunction. Within the two groups, one circumcised man had had a fractured penis and one had had prostate surgery, while in the intact group two men had diabetic neuropathy and one had renal failure. Within the confines of this study, circumcision status was not a factor in asking for or being prescribed erectile dysfunction medication. For each year older, the rate of asking for medication went up by 11.7 %.

6.9 Analyses of Penile Measurements

Using multivariate analysis with penile length as the dependent variable, including circumcision status and BMI in the model, intact men in this study had a penis 5.18 % longer, 4.33 % bigger around, 14.66 % larger in volume in the flaccid state with a meatus 34.18 % longer, 39.48 % wider, and an opening that is 94.97 % larger (all findings $p < 0 .05$). For circumcision adjusting for BMI, intact men had a circumference that was 0.359 cm larger, and when volume was adjusted for height, intact men have a larger penile volume by 15.284 ml. Volume was calculated in standard fashion, and meatal percent (the length of the meatus divided by the radius) adjusts for the size of the penis and avoids the criticism that the meatus is bigger because the penis is larger.

For meatal measurements, circumcision status was the only statistically significant factor. Meatal area diamond (the width times the length divided by 2), which probably underestimates the area, impacts urine flow, which is a function of the radius to the 4th power. The flow from the intact penis is calculated at 3.8 times higher than that in the circumcised men.

As one would expect, but which is rarely acknowledged in American medicine, routine newborn circumcision results in smaller, skinnier, shorter, and surgically altered and damaged penises with a host of distinct and definable surgical complications most of which are not recognized by the owners of these altered genitals. It is just as unusual for physicians, especially those who perform newborn circumcision, to ever mention or discuss these obvious defects and damages or much less examine their male patients in a forthright and comprehensive manner in order to document them. This willful and seemingly blinded ignorance among the physician perpetrators, the surgical victims, and their families leads to perpetuation of a procedure whose complications can be easily documented (Goldman 2011; Williams and Kapila 1993; Weiss et al. 2010; Baskin et al. 1996) discussed, and rarely remedied.

6.10 Conclusions

This observational study of circumcised and intact men with surprisingly similar demographics shows that circumcised men were generally unaware of any personal penile abnormalities. This is presumable due to growing up in a circumcised country and environment where due to cultural and sexual biases they rarely encounter other than their own wounded, but presumably normal, genitals. Even the few homosexual men in the study were unaware of these problems, including one subject who leaned 38° and twisted 18°. The majority of circumcised men do not apparently suffer in silence because they are surprisingly ignorant of what has been done to them, and of course almost universally ignorant of what is normal. A very small percentage of circumcised men are bothered by the various damages done to them, and most were unaware of the obvious, that removal of 40–50 % of the penile skin, leaves you "smaller" and misshapen.

Circumcision damages have been documented previously (Williams and Kapila 1993; Weiss et al. 2010; Baskin et al. 1996) but none within the context of a general practice, and this study demonstrates that circumcised men have smaller and shorter penises (Khan et al. 2012; Richters et al. 1995) have measurable and obvious penile leaning, curvature, and twisting, have significantly smaller external urethral orifices (Berry and Cross 1956; Martin 1881; Morton 1963; Joudi et al. 2010; Van Howe 2006) sometimes leading to problems with urinary flow, and have a variety of obvious surgical scars (Ponsky et al. 2000) most of which they are unaware of. Circumcised men have adapted to the problems without consulting physicians, mostly out of ignorance of what is normal. A good number of these damages lead to abnormal functioning (Goldman 2011).

Most American physicians have been persistent and complicit in minimizing the risks, complications, and damages of newborn male circumcision because this unnecessary surgery has proven to be a highly lucrative part of practice for a good number of them. This complicity extends to the specialty societies representing them (AAP, AAFP, ACOG, and AUA) which have, unlike their counterparts in other developed countries, backpedaled and waffled repeatedly on educational statements to parents.

It is high time for medical educators to be forthright and honest in teaching medical students and residents in training normal male genital anatomy and function, and for physicians who deal with babies and children to be completely honest and ethical with their patients and the parents of those pediatric patients with regards to what is biologically normal. Physician ignorance and deception is medico-legally and morally unacceptable, and solicitation of routine and medically unnecessary newborn circumcision as an intervention that does nothing more than mutilate normal tissue must end.

Acknowledgments Jennifer Urbina, PA, assisted with data formatting and Robert Van Howe, MD, graciously provided statistical analysis of the study findings. Continuous outcomes were assessed with t-tests, using the Welch-Saitterwaite method, and linear regression. Non-continuous outcomes were assessed using Chi square, Fisher's exact test, and logistic regression. Multivariate analyses used backwards selection. All calculations were performed using SAS version 8.2 (SAS Institute, Cary, North Carolina).

References

Baskin LS, Canning DA, Snyder HM, Duckett JW (1996) Treating complications of circumcision. Pediatr Emerg Care 12(1)

Berry CD Jr, Cross RR Jr (1956) Urethral meatal caliber in circumcised and uncircumcised males. Am J Dis Child 92:152–156

Goldman R (2011) Circumcision: harm and psychological factors ignored. The Bay Citizen, San Francisco

Joudi M, Fathi M, Hiradfar M (2010) Incidence of asymptomatic meatal stenosis in children following neonatal circumcision. J Pediatr Urol. doi:10.1016/j.jpurol.2010.08.005

Khan S, Somani BN, Lam W, Donat R (2012) Establishing a reference range for penile length in Caucasian British men: a prospective study of 609 men. Br J Urol 109(5):740–744

Martin WM (1881) Infantile circumcision: a cause of contraction of the external urethral meatus. Ann Anat Surg 4:123–128

Morton HG (1963) Meatal size in 1,000 circumcised children form 2 weeks to 16 years of age. J Florida Med Assoc 50:137–138

Osifo OD, Oriaifo IA (2009) Circumcision mishaps in Nigerian children. Ann Afr Med 8(4):266–270

Ponsky LE, Ross JH, Knipper N, Kay R (2000) Penile adhesions after neonatal circumcision. J Urol 164(2):495–496

Richters J, Gerofi J, Donovan B (1995) Are Condoms the right size(s)? A method for self-measurement of the erect penis. Venereology 8(2):77–81

Van Howe RS (2006) Incidence of meatal stenosis following neonatal circumcision in a primary care setting. Clin Pediatr (Philadelphia) 45:49–54

Weiss HA, Larke N, Halperin D, Schenker I (2010) Complications of circumcision in male neonates, infants and children: a systematic review. Biomed Central Urol 10:2

Williams N, Kapila L (1993) Complications of circumcision. Br J Surg 80:1231–1236

Author Biography

Christopher Fletcher MD, is a family physician in Santa Fe, NM, USA, who graduated cum laude from Harvard College, has an MD from the University of Texas Southwestern Medical School in Dallas, and Residency training in the University of Massachusetts Medical Center Family Practice Residency Program. He has been in public and private practice in New Mexico since 1981, is an assistant clinical professor of family and community medicine at the University of New Mexico School of Medicine, and has a long-term interest in circumcision issues, having not performed one since 1981 and having left his own sons intact. He takes pride in being a supporter of the nurses who founded Nurses for the Rights of the Child at St. Vincent Hospital. He has delivered over a thousand babies and, with aggressive but supportive and caring education of parents, was able to prevent all but ten of the boys he delivered from being circumcised. Santa Fe, New Mexico, USA.

Chapter 7
Male Circumcision and the Potential for Unexplained Male Adolescent Suicide in Northern Ireland

Linda Massie

Abstract NOCIRC of Northern Ireland has had a preliminary meeting with counselors and psychiatrists on the known emotional effects of male circumcision, particularly in relation to adolescent suicide attempts, and is currently developing a training program in this area. Neonatal circumcision is *not* the norm in Northern Ireland where the majority of children are not circumcised after birth. There were 244 male children circumcised between birth and 18 years of age in 2008/2009, with the majority diagnosed as requiring circumcision due to phimosis and urinary tract infections. We have anecdotal evidence that female children may also be at risk locally because, despite legislation, it has been estimated by Forward that 15,000 female children in the United Kingdom are at risk annually.

Keywords Northern Ireland • Circumcision • Phimosis • Psychology • Psychiatry • Suicide

7.1 Introduction

I first became involved in the international campaign to end circumcision following the attempted suicide of my eldest son in 1996, which resulted in his being detained and committed for 3 months to a psychiatric unit in Northern Ireland. As a family, we feel seriously let down by the medical profession in Northern Ireland, both by their suggestion that circumcision was necessary in the first place and by the lack of support or understanding we encountered when my son became distressed due to the effects of this surgery. The problems were further compounded by the psychiatric professional who thought it was so ridiculous to have a problem with circumcision that he must be schizophrenic, and that the solution was to take him to Amsterdam to see a prostitute.

L. Massie (✉)
NOCIRC of Northern Ireland, Glengormle, County Antrim, Northern Ireland
e-mail: nocircni@yahoo.co.uk

G. C. Denniston et al. (eds.), *Genital Cutting: Protecting Children from Medical, Cultural, and Religious Infringements*, DOI: 10.1007/978-94-007-6407-1_7,

7.2 History

Routine neonatal circumcision is not the norm in Northern Ireland hospitals and it is not something that is viewed as a "decision" that is made by parents at birth. Rather it is viewed both by the medical profession and parents as something that may be necessary on "medical" grounds in childhood and in later life. Until the age of seven, therefore, my son was like the majority of boys in Northern Ireland; he had a foreskin. However, he then developed an infection and was referred to the hospital, where I was told by the consultant that he needed to be circumcised because his foreskin was not retractable, that this was a medical problem defined as "phimosis".

At the time, I was a young mother of 23. However, I had been brought up with a healthy disregard for not believing everything I was told and I did not like the idea of my young son being subjected to an operation of any kind, so I questioned the doctor further. Among the questions I asked were "What would happen if we just left it until he was older?" The consultant appeared to become quite agitated with my questioning of his "professional opinion". He told me, in an abrupt fashion, that "without the surgery" my son "would be unable to have sexual relationships when he was older, that to leave the operation to a later date would make the operation more difficult, and that performing the procedure at that time was in his best interests". Every day, I wish I had said, "Fine. We will wait until he is older," but, I felt pressured into feeling that it was for the best.

The year was 1983. The doctor may have read Douglas Gairdner's paper in the *British Medical Journal* in 1949 regarding preputial development in children up to aged 5 but, unfortunately, was unaware of the work of Oster in 1968 in the *Archives of Disease of Childhood,* demonstrating that "phimosis" was not an abnormality in such a young child and that preputial retraction could continue up until at least age 17. The psychological effects of circumcision in young boys had also already been examined by Gocke Cansever in the *British Journal of Psychology* in 1965. At no point, however, was I told there would be any problems of an emotional nature. I was not given any information regarding any potential surgical complications from the surgery and was told it was a minor day procedure. In effect, I was misinformed regarding this procedure and that is something that my son and I have to live with for the rest of our lives. Due to this surgery, my son has never been able to form a sexual relationship, living a life of relative seclusion, and I have to live every day in the knowledge that I consented to an unnecessary procedure that changed his life and mine forever.

Following the surgery, my son who previously had a sunny nature became agitated and withdrawn and slightly aggressive. I put this down to the effects of anesthesia and of him being in pain. I did not know, until many years later when we discussed it, that he had withdrawn his consent to the doctors in the operating theatre and that they had laughed and told him as they anesthetized him not to worry, everything would be fine.

A few weeks after the surgery, I took a photograph of my son and, for the first time, I saw his emotional pain. He was looking at me with betrayal in his eyes and

I did not know why. What I did not know at that time was that he felt violated, mutilated, and angry with me for having allowed this surgery. I assumed, because he had never had an operation before, that he was still distressed by the pain of the procedure. But, now I know that he felt I had not protected him.

For many years, I was unaware of how distressed he felt. When he reached adolescence, he became withdrawn and refused to go to school because he would have had to participate in games followed by open communal showers, which meant that he would have had to reveal himself as circumcised. He also started to self-harm, cutting his arms with razor blades. All he would say, however, was that he was circumcised, he hated it, and that he wanted to die. I was oblivious to his pain and thought it was just teenage angst. After all, lots of people were circumcised and they were fine. At the time, I did not own a computer and tried ringing various organizations for help, but they all told me they had never heard of anyone having a problem with circumcision. I was unable to understand because all he would say was that he hated being circumcised, that he was not normal, that he was not a human being, that he would never know what it is like to be a complete human being, and that he wished he was dead. He was also self-harming and I realized that he was at risk of killing himself.

As a teenager, my son became so distressed he could not go to school because he was afraid if he participated in games his status would be revealed and he could not bear for anyone to know what had happened to him. He started to self-harm as a teenager and then after many torturous discussions told me that he was not a complete human being and he would die not knowing what it was like to be one.

At the time, I did not understand his distress and took him to the GP, sexual counselors, a psychiatrist, and a plastic surgeon, none of whom were aware of the research in this area. My son eventually attempted suicide at the age of 20, due to this lack of understanding on my part and by the medical profession. I finally learned the truth about male circumcision by making contact with the group NOHARMM in San Francisco, which led me to Marilyn Milos at NOCIRC and NORM-UK, who supported my son by letter when he was detained under the Mental Health Act.

A few months later, I travelled to my first international symposium, and I have continued to present papers and publish on this issue since then. I established NOCIRC of NI to ensure that no other family had to endure the lack of support that faced us and still does in many ways today.

Without the support of NOHARMM, NOCIRC, and NORM-UK, I would have been alone. Often, late at night, the only people I felt understood our pain were on the other end of the phone, prepared to support my family in every way and I thank you all for that.

7.3 Statistics on Genital Mutilation in Northern Ireland

Neonatal circumcision is not the norm in Northern Ireland where the majority of children are not circumcised after birth. There were 244 male children circumcised between birth and 18 years of age in 2008/2009, with the majority diagnosed as requiring circumcision due to phimosis and urinary tract infections. We have anecdotal evidence that female children may also be at risk locally because, despite legislation, it has been estimated by Forward that 15,000 female children in the United Kingdom are at risk annually.

NOCIRC of Northern Ireland has had a preliminary meeting with counselors and psychiatrists about the known emotional effects of male circumcision, particularly in relation to adolescent suicide attempts, and they have agreed to take referrals from us in this area. NOCIRC of NI is currently developing a training program.

Never before has a group of people historically had to fight to protect children from what they have seen happen in their own families. I set up NOCIRC—NI so that no other family had to endure the ignorance and lack of help that our family experienced.

7.4 Statistics on Male Circumcision Over a 10-Year Period

A recent study on circumcision trends in Northern Ireland was conducted to determine the trend in circumcision operations over a 10 year period in the 0–13-year-age group and to compare the number of operations performed by pediatric surgeons compared to those performed by general surgeons over the same period. The data was collected from the Northern Ireland Department of Health and Social Services and Public Safety (The British Association of Paediatric Surgeons 2003). There were 769 circumcisions performed in the year 1991–1992, compared with 264 in the year 2001–2002, representing a 66 % decrease. In the 10-year-study period, the number of circumcisions performed by general surgeons fell by 71 % whilst specialist pediatric surgeons performed 56 % less.

7.5 Conclusions

The decrease in rates of circumcision in boys aged 0–13 years in Northern Ireland (2001) is consistent with trends in the remainder of the United Kingdom (British Association of Paediatric Surgeons 2001). The results also suggest a greater decrease in the proportion of circumcisions being performed by general surgeons in district general hospitals compared to those performed by pediatric surgeons.

In recent times, there has been growing concern that too many circumcisions are carried out unnecessarily in neonates and young boys. Several studies undertaken in England and Scotland have identified a decrease in the number of operations being performed (Rickwood et al. 2000; Quaba and MacKinlay 2004). To date, there has been no review of trends in circumcision rates within Northern Ireland.

The aim of this study is to review the numbers of circumcision procedures performed in boys aged 0–13 years in Northern Ireland over a ten-year period and to analyze the trend in the procedures performed by pediatric surgeons and general surgeons over the same period.

Data were collected from the Department of Health, Social Services and Public Safety in Northern Ireland. The total number of circumcisions performed in Northern Ireland in the 0–13-year age group during periods 1st September 1991–1st September 1992 and 1st September 2001–1st September 2002 was ascertained. Data from the Northern Ireland Census Report 4 were used to calculate the percentage circumcision rates during these years. Figures specific to each hospital in which the circumcisions had been performed were also available, allowing comparison between the number of circumcisions performed by general surgeons and pediatric surgeons over the same period.

A total of 769 circumcisions were performed in the year 1991–1992, representing 5.7 % of boys aged 0–13 years. A total of 264 circumcisions were performed in the year 2001–2002, representing 1.9 % of boys aged 0–13 years. Overall, this signifies a 66 % decrease in the number of circumcisions performed in the 10 year period.

In the year 1991–1992, circumcisions were performed in 11 hospitals throughout Northern Ireland. In total, 257 (33 %) operations were performed by pediatric surgeons and 518 (67 %) by general surgeons during this year.

In the year 2001–2002, circumcisions were performed in nine hospitals. Overall, 113 (43 %) were performed by pediatric surgeons and 151 (57 %) by general surgeons. The number of circumcisions carried out by general surgeons dropped by 71 % in the 10-year-period compared with a 56 % reduction by pediatric surgeons.

7.6 Discussion

The decrease in rates of circumcision seen in this study is consistent with trends noted across the remainder of the UK. Furthermore, circumcision rates in boys within Northern Ireland are currently in line with the target of 2 % suggested by Rickwood et al. (2000). However, there are a number of limitations to this study. The retrospective data were derived from DHSSPS statistics, a potential source of bias. Unfortunately, the indications for circumcision were not available, making it impossible to evaluate the impact of changes in disease prevalence or trends in non-therapeutic circumcision during the study period. What many surgeons considered to be phimosis (and treated by circumcision) in fact was physiological non-retractile foreskin. Therefore, the most probable explanation for the reduction in circumcision rate is the improved understanding of the natural history of physiological non-retractile foreskin and the pathophysiology of phimosis.

This study also indicates that the number of circumcisions in Northern Ireland being performed during childhood by general surgeons has decreased substantially over the study decade. Circumcision and other general pediatric surgical procedures have traditionally fallen within the remit and interests of both general and pediatric surgeons. Recent increases in the workload of consultant pediatric surgeons have been noted by the British Association of Paediatric Surgeons as fewer general surgeons continue to perform general pediatric surgery (The British Association of Paediatric Surgeons. Reconfiguration in Paediatric Surgery 2003). The observed decrease in circumcisions being performed by general surgeons may be due to recent changes in general surgical training, which have reduced opportunities for surgeons in training to acquire experience in pediatric surgery (Groves et al. 2010). This highlights an important and potentially worrying trend in the distribution of general pediatric surgery provision in the Province.

References

British Association of Paediatric Surgeons, Royal College of Nursing, Royal College of Paediatrics and Child Health, Royal College of Surgeons of England and Royal College of Anaesthetists. Statement on male circumcision. London: Royal College of Surgeons of England; (2001). Available online from: http://www.cirp.org/library/statements/RCS2001. Accessed Mar 2010

Groves H, Bailie A, McCallion W (2010) Childhood circumcision in Northern Ireland: a barometer of the current practice of general paediatric surgery. Ulster Med J 79(2):80–81

Northern Ireland Statistics and Research Agency. Northern Ireland Census 2001 output. Belfast: NISRA; (2001). Available online from: http://www.nisranew.nisra.gov.uk/census/Census2001Output/index.html. Accessed Mar 2010

Quaba O, MacKinlay GA (2004) Changing trends in a decade of circumcision in Scotland. J Pediatr Surg 39(7):1037–1039

Rickwood AM, Kenny SE, Donnell SC (2000) Towards evidence based circumcision of English boys: survey of trends in practice. BMJ 321(7264):792–793

The British Association of Paediatric Surgeons. Reconfiguration in Paediatric Surgery. London: BAPS; (2003). Available online from: www.rcsed.ac.uk/fellows/meflett/Library/Statements/reconfigpaed.doc. Accessed Mar 2010, published 7 June 2010, doi:10.1136/bmj.c2987 Cite this as: BMJ 2010;340:c2987, NewsDutch medical alliance moves to change thinking on male circumcision

Author Biography

Linda Massie BSc, PGDip, is currently the director of NOCIRC of Northern Ireland, a voluntary charity that she established following the attempted suicide of her eldest son due to circumcision trauma. In 2009, Linda was awarded funding from UnLtd, the foundation for Social Entrenpeneurs, and is developing an educational outreach project for counselors and psychologists in Northern Ireland on the emotional consequences associated with genital surgeries on children. Linda is currently a member of Business and Professional Women UK, which has co-funded this presentation. Glengormley, County Antrim, Northern Ireland.

Chapter 8
Healing the Harms of Circumcision: A Nursing Case Study

B. Maurene White

Abstract This case study records counseling with a couple on the verge of separation due to sexual dysfunction partially conditioned by adverse sequellae of routine male infant circumcision. Their extended family referred them to me for counseling and to support their efforts at restoring their relationship. The couple's motivation to collaborate during assessment and openness to the contemporary option of foreskin restoration as part of their self-managed treatment mitigated negotiating a dynamic, flexible, long-term plan to resolve their problems. Methodology: data collecting of couple and family history, physical examination, discussion of the issues, outlining and negotiating potential solutions, and collaborative writing up of treatment plan. Follow-up: regular in-person or telephone discussion of progress every 2 weeks for 3 months, then every month up to 2 years; further interventions or referrals as agreed on.

Keywords Counseling • Pain • Sexual dysfunction • Foreskin restoration

8.1 Introduction

A study of counseling and intervention with follow-up program was reported up to July 24, 2010, to the 11th International Symposium on Circumcision, Genital Integrity, and Human Rights in Berkeley, California. Follow-up continued until August 27, 2012 with a final telephone call from the couple reporting on their continuing physical and psychological well-being, drawing the case study to a close.

A husband and wife asked for consultation on December 22, 2009, to assess sexual difficulties caused by the husband's circumcision deformity and explore possible treatment for his painful erections, and the resulting painful vaginal symptoms sustained by the wife. Their sexual problems had created such stress in

B. M. White (✉)
Nursing Consultant, Montreal, Quebec, Canada
e-mail: bmwhite41@hotmail.com

G. C. Denniston et al. (eds.), *Genital Cutting: Protecting Children from Medical, Cultural, and Religious Infringements*, DOI: 10.1007/978-94-007-6407-1_8,

the marriage the couple had decided to separate. The outcome of the intervention would determine whether they would continue their marriage or separate.

8.2 Thesis

Unknown to either man or wife, the long-term adverse effects of infant circumcision causes dysfunction of the penis making sexual intercourse uncomfortable, painful and even injurious to the female partner, depending on the severity of the circumcision deformity. The stressors of sexual dissatisfaction are subsequently projected onto other areas of the marriage.

By gathering, collating, and analyzing histories and physicals, and intervening with an ancient self-help, skin expansion technique, many adverse effects of circumcision may be reversed as the remnant layers of the prepuce are stretched to reform a sheath similar to the original prepuce, restoring near normal appearance and function.

This study has value for significant numbers of men with who similar injuries as shown by Williams and Kapila (1993), speaks to those who perform circumcisions and to parents who submit their sons' to circumcision in lieu of protecting their integrity (Williams and Kapila, 1993).

8.3 Nursing Theory

Virginia Henderson (1897–1996) defined nursing as "assisting individuals to gain independence in relation to the performance of activities contributing to health or its recovery." Henderson was one of the first nurses to point out that nursing does not consist of merely following physicians' orders. She categorized nursing activities into fourteen components based on human needs. She described the nurse's role as substitutive (doing for the person), supplementary (helping the person), complementary (working with the person), with the goal of helping the person become as independent as possible.

Henderson's famous definition of nursing was one of the first to clearly delineate nursing from medicine: "The unique function of the nurse is to assist the individual, sick or well, in the performance of those activities contributing to health or its recovery (or to peaceful death) that he (or she) would perform unaided if he had the necessary strength, will, or knowledge. And to do this in such a way as to help him gain independence as rapidly as possible" (Henderson 1966).

8.4 Methodology

Data collection includes receiving histories from clients and their parents, complete physical examinations, discussion of the findings with the couple, collaborative treatment planning and follow-up. The author and the couple completed the initial stages in Montreal between December 26 and 30, 2009. Close relatives of HM, living in Montreal but on vacation, very generously volunteered their apartment for use as consultation rooms.

8.5 Confidentiality

To maintain confidentiality the clients are identified by their family relationships: H for husband, W for wife, HF for H's father, HM for his mother, WF for W's father, and WM for her mother; their ages and nationalities are closely approximated.

Historical and cultural data was collected from H to W by telephone and in person and from their parents by telephone. As both clients are articulate and insightful, they are closely cited, with explanations and theoretical points included as needed.

All their difficulties were considered in detail and treatment options considered until the couple came to mutual decisions on their preferences. They collaborated on planning immediate and long-term treatment goals, including medical referrals, foreskin restoration schedules, journaling, follow-up, and further interventions and referrals, should they need it.

December 23, 2009
H and W discussed their sexual histories and their perceptions of H's circumcision in detail. We discussed their parents' perceptions of their issues and their cultural influences on concepts and emotions concerning circumcision, which were very helpful for both H and W. We all learned a great deal about the entire family, how cohesive, concerned, and devoted they are to H and W.

I first met H a little more than 30 years ago through his mother, a nursing colleague. He was very bright and energetic, and remains so as he approaches fifty; he remains fit, not due, by his own admission, to his own effort, but 'to the gene pool he comes from.' Both his father's parents were from Northern Europe and settled in the United States and his mother is a Canadian of English Scottish descent. He is proficient in four languages and studied in Canada, the US, and Europe. He is an established professional and author. He is enjoying a fulfilling and financially rewarding career. He travels frequently for business and with his family.

The couple's family is close, their relationships are harmonious; their children's happiness and development is next to their marriage in importance. For everyone's sake he wants his marriage to survive and even thrive.

The entire family attends a reformed church; one grandfather and one grandmother are elders; H and W contribute to their church in various roles.

His health appeared sound apart from slightly elevated blood pressure, which is well followed by his family physician. His nutritional status is good and the family pays close attention to their diet, and shops and cooks together. He is a wine aficionado and drinks moderately. He has never smoked tobacco or other substances or used illicit drugs. He exercises moderately, especially enjoying light outdoor family activities.

His affect was serious, very tense, and anxious. His voice at the first meeting was very tense and strained, he was pale, and his face drawn and fatigued.

He confirmed that uneven circumcision scarring deforms his penis, causing pain, dysfunctional erection, and considerable difficulty with insertion for sexual intercourse. H and W realized they were projecting the frustrations of their sexual problems onto other areas of their marriage, leading to the brink of separation. He stated, "I'm half skeptical, half curious about this bizarre stretching system you're promoting, and how it could possibly resolve anything for us. But I'm desperate enough to consider whatever doesn't cause us more pain, and hopeful that you think I may at least lessen my painful erections."

W is two and a half years older than her husband. She is of Northern European ancestry, like her husband, taller than average, well groomed, warm, and presented with a calm, serious mood, but also looking fatigued and drawn. She is the youngest of four children, with three older brothers all born in Europe. The fathers of H and W are second cousins. W and her family lived in both the United States and Europe during her childhood and adolescence. W speaks four languages as does her husband.

She and H met during family reunions all through childhood and adolescence. They briefly studied at the same university. Both pursued careers and other relationships, then met again while working in the same city. After a brief courtship they married to the keen delight of both families and themselves. Their family constellation has been close, supportive and harmonious throughout their marriage.

Her health has been good to date; although menopausal symptoms have been a nuisance for the past several years and she feels her energy level has dropped somewhat. Her nutritional status is good, her alcohol intake is modest. She has never smoked or consumed other substances. Her blood pressure is slightly low. She walks for 15 min twice per day and occasionally uses the gym facilities at her workplace. She enjoys their family ski holidays. She is an amateur musician, her principal diversion and relaxation from her high stress professional career.

W's personality is more outgoing than H at present, although she was also tense and concerned about their sexual difficulties. She states that both partners perceive that their sexual problems are caused by his mutilation.

W says, "Our sexual lives have never been satisfactory, but now have become impossible. I simply can't live in the same house with the man I love without any possibility of satisfactory sex. The grief and frustration are sheer torture. We would both like to explore the system you've described and hope and pray we can make it work for us."

8.6 HM, (Husband's Mother)

HM is a nursing colleague with whom I conferenced in Montreal over 30 years ago; it is she who suggested the option of foreskin restoration to her son and referred the couple for treatment. HM has considerable insight into her son's and the couple's history and, with their consent, contributed significantly to the intervention.

She is Canadian of English and Scottish descent, a retired nursing teacher, and remains up to date with her profession and colleagues.

HM has been happily married to HF for nearly 60 years, learned her husband's language to communicate with his parents, and made sure their children also learned it.

After hearing my presentation on neonatal circumcision over 30 years ago, citing the few studies then available on the risks and damage caused, HM discussed possible problems it might cause later in her son's life. She said then she was concerned about the problems circumcision scarring had always caused her son. As an infant and toddler, he had frequently cried with erections. As a child and adolescent he was anxious and frequently adjusted either his clothing or his penis to try and avoid pain, burning, and itching, which were a constant problem. He favored the longer part of the remnant and often tried to relieve the pain and itching by pressing his hand around the shorter ragged, edge of the remnant.

Neither HM nor HF had consented to circumcision and in fact had refused to sign the consent form. They view it as radical, harmful, and quite against their cultural norms. They were both devastated when H was simply brought to them by a nurse on the fourth day after his birth with the announcement that the pediatrician had just circumcised him.

They were appalled that the pediatrician they had engaged had disregarded their wishes and felt deeply violated, for themselves and for their son. HM was deeply disturbed by the unresponsive lethargic behavior H exhibited following circumcision, "It was as if he were completely altered. He was unable to nurse for nearly 2 days, was limp and pale, not the same vigorous baby at all." She felt deeply betrayed by the pediatrician's disobedient act and was very concerned for HF, who was so extremely angry she feared he would do something drastic. She wondered if there would be ill effects, and indeed there have been, right up to the present.

HM had been noticing the mounting tension and dissension between her son and his wife with alarm and sensed they could be projecting their disappointment and frustration over sexual difficulties onto other aspects of their marriage: "They are beginning to sound like a soap opera or 'The War of the Roses,'" she said during a telephone conversation, "If it isn't dealt with very soon, their marriage will be over, and it will affect our whole, close family."

I suggested to HM that she read anatomy and physiology articles on the foreskin and visit the various foreskin restoration sites as preliminary reading for the couple and to intervene with them, if they wished.

8.7 HF (Husband's Father)

HF is an articulate man, now in his mid-seventies. He came from Northern Europe to join his older cousin, W's father, in a business venture several years before H was born. He met HM at a restaurant close to their workplaces and they were married within the year. H was born the following year.

HF is the most emotionally expressive of all the grandparents. His concern over his son's damage and impending marriage failure was compelling.

He stated he has always felt angry over not only the injury but the fact that he had been circumcised explicitly against both parents' instructions. They had made it clear to the nursing staff and especially the pediatrician that their culture and religion did not sanction circumcision and that they wished their son to look like the rest of the men in their family. When a nurse had brought their son to his mother on the fourth day, explaining he had just been circumcised, HM had phoned him at work in tears.

He questioned the pediatrician, who evaded his questions and glibly told him it was best for his son to look like his peers. HF then spoke to a hospital administrator, and complained of professional misconduct, received a cursory apology, but never received any explanation for the breach of responsibility and trust, even of his written request; he received no appropriate concern for the disregard and disrespect he felt was shown him and his family and has never had closure on the issue, nor, he feels, has his son.

HF said he and the family felt as if their rights, their culture, their family, and their son's life and privacy had been invaded. HF said he had felt angry about the issue since H's infancy and only now that he was encountering people affording him empathy and concern for his son's injury.

HF consulted many pediatricians, pediatric urologists, and dermatologists for the constant irritation of the scarred surface of his penis that H experienced throughout his childhood, and psychologists, for his irritation and "nervousness," all to no avail. The only advice they received, which appalled him and which he refused, was to even the scar by cutting off the longer foreskin remnant.

He said his son and daughter-in-law must be trapped in some form of hell to be living with an injury that not only prevents sexual satisfaction but causes pain with sex.

HF said he had read the literature on D.O.C. (2010), NOCIRC (2010) and NORM (2010) websites and was particularly encouraged by the accounts of men who had succeeded with foreskin restoration. Although his son had been skeptical initially, he hoped someone could convince him to consider foreskin restoration, help him find some pleasure in his sexual life, and preserve his marriage.

8.8 WF (Wife's Father)

WF is HF's distant cousin and about 10 years his senior. They often met at family gatherings when they were young and both families still lived in Europe. He coached HF in athletics and enjoyed the role of elder cousin. As adults they are close friends and business partners.

WF has four children, three intact sons born in Europe and a daughter, W, born two and a half years before H, his cousin's son and his son-in-law.

WF came to North America first and, when his business was beginning to succeed, helped his cousin emigrate to join his developing enterprise. Together they have built a successful business. When H was born in the United States, and circumcised without authority or knowledge of either parent, WF was as distressed as his cousin. He participated with the investigation of the doctor and the hospital. WF expressed dismay and for years has felt partially responsible for the injury, stating that, if his cousin's son had been born in Europe, there would have been no risk of circumcision or the additional injury. He feels grateful his own sons "were born where boys are considered human beings, not objects, with rights to integrity and uninvaded privacy." That H was circumcised, "Was a complete violation of his rights as a person, and showed total disregard for our culture and heritage." I felt my cousin should have sued the doctor and the hospital at that time; we already had the resources to do so, but he said it might harm his son's self-confidence and also drain energy and finances that could help him more in the long run.

WF also feels great concern for W, his daughter, and has high hopes for the intervention. HF has shared his Internet research with WF; both are enthusiastic and feel that it would be the answer to the problem if H will consider it. Both senior men are urging H to be positive about investigating it. WF brought HF printed accounts reporting women's improved satisfaction when their husbands had restored their foreskins. Both W's parents support this intervention and hope their son-in-law's health and the couple's marriage will be preserved and are willing to support them however, they may.

8.9 Histories and Physical Examinations

December 28, 2009. A complete physical examination situates particular health problems in the context of the person's general health. As H's circumcision problem had caused both partners great stress for over 15 years, screening all systems seemed appropriate. Time to do thorough physical examinations was available and the relaxed pace allowed them both to unwind. Each partner was present during the other's physical examination. The focus on the exams and explanations of each phase of examination distracted them somewhat from the anxiety and distress of their sexual problems. It also provided an opportunity to mention the value of touch for enhancing intimacy by opening "conversation" with the rest of the body (Montague 1978).

8.10 History of Presenting Problem

H denies current health complaints except for slight chest pain at the end of and after sexual intercourse. He denies any chest pain at the moment but agreed to report it immediately should he experience it during the course of this counseling situation and that he would seek medical help immediately should it recur. H has annual health checks from his family MD, ophthalmologist, and urologist. He occasionally finds he has sore eyes, slight headache, and stiff neck, which he attributes to overwork at the computer. He agreed to consult his family MD and request a cardiology examination, and to see his ophthalmologist on return home.

H's nutritional status is good, both he and W pay attention to their diet, purchase mostly organic food, cook together when home, have increased the proportion of vegetable and fruit intake, reduced red meat and increased the amount of fish. They are aware of the need for responsible health behaviors.

H gets most of his exercise by walking, occasionally cycles; he plays golf occasionally with business colleagues. He enjoys skiing with his family.

He required surgery twice in adolescence, an appendectomy and a left open radial/ulnar reduction of a fracture caused by a fall. There were no adverse sequellae from either surgery.

8.11 Circumcision History, Physical and Emotional

H was circumcised without parental consent at 4 days of age. The circumcision scar is very unequal, has caused pain, disfigurement, and embarrassment throughout his life.

H recalls pain and severe stinging and itching from his penis, especially the right lateral side, from a very early age. He knew the circumcision was not planned. He says he is a little wary of most doctors as a consequence.

During his childhood H came to understand that only boys are cut; he wondered why boys are singled out for punishment and envied his sister's escape from trauma. Later he also realized through sauna experience that all his male relatives were intact and felt humiliated, alienated, and wondered why he alone was cut.

At age sixteen, during high school in Europe, he also realized his penis had different functions and sensations from other boys of his age. While he and an intact school friend were dressing after a sporting event, his friend's penis became slightly erect, and remained straight instead of twisting and curving. Also, his friend, although slightly embarrassed, expressed no pain or distress at all, in fact, laughed, addressed the persona of his erection and quipped, "Hey, back to sleep!" They both laughed, but H then perceived he had difficulties his friend did not suffer. H began to feel anxious and as if he alone had been singled out for mistreatment of his penis; he wondered whether he could ever be treated and become normal.

H began to research anatomy and sexuality texts and finally understood how deeply he had been affected. He noted how many American versus European texts consider circumcision routine and normal, even with purported benefits. He felt betrayed and developed a marked disregard for anyone "with medical power over infants and children" as he phrased it.

H said, "I have never felt at home, never comfortable, physically, psychologically, or emotionally in my own body. This injury, which I now, finally, no longer take personally but perceive as criminal, was done to me here in North America, where the majority of men my age are circumcised but don't have the same ill effects from it that I do. I consider circumcision abnormal, mine is exceptionally abnormal. I don't look like other American men. I don't feel normal here in North America. I feel even more abnormal in Europe but, if I had been born in Europe, I would have been allowed to remain normal. The medical profession should not have the power, the license to perform surgery that causes abnormality of any degree of severity (Snyder 2009).

Sexual relations with women before my marriage and now with W, whom I love very deeply, have never been easy or satisfactory. Now I understand how deeply this injury has affected my marriage, too; it has nearly destroyed our intimacy at many levels. I don't feel at home with W and am unable to be a normal husband to her. Sex with me makes her very uncomfortable and distresses her, although she makes a great effort to be cheerful. I can understand why she would want to leave me, but it is terribly disappointing. Our families are so close and happy together. I feel that I, or maybe I should say, my abnormality would be responsible for the wreckage of our marriage should we not be able to resolve my injury.

The only place I feel at home is at work. I have put enormous effort into developing myself to the degree that I excel at work and derive the main satisfaction of my life from it, from my profession, where I am recognized and respected. If it weren't for my faith and my career, to say nothing of my family's devotion to us, I would succumb to meaningless, empty, utter despair.

The NORM success accounts were again pointed out to him and I reminded him he had found the courage to persist for nearly 50 years and, while it is impossible to say to what degree he would be able to recover, he could likely expect slow but steady progress for many months, if not years.

8.12 H Physical Examination December 27, 2009

Significant findings.

HEENT No lesions or abnormalities noted; there is considerable tension in his neck, shoulders and upper back.

Breasts Axillary lymph nodes have no masses, irregularities, or swellings.

Lungs Clear on percussion and auscultation, normal heart sounds, all pulses strong and equal.

Abdominal Sounds are normal, no pain, no obvious masses, no enlarged lymph nodes.

Reflexes All normal, L hand and arm strength greater—L dominant.

No bony abnormalities noted, some stiffness in neck, legs, forward bends to mid lower leg.

Skin Normal hair patterns. A few moles on trunk, arms and legs. One significant lesion, a dark irregular mole approximately 4 mm (1/8 inch) diameter with dark radiating striae on left upper arm about 7 cm (2¾ inch) above his elbow. Recommended follow-up with family doctor.

Genitourinary, denies change in urinary flow; no enlarged lymph nodes, no hernias; penis in flaccid state measures 13.5 cm (5¼ inch), remarkably uneven scar; on his L about 1.5 cm of frenulum remains, about 2.5 cm dermal and mucosal tissue remain to almost midline of the glans, the remnant of the prepuce then goes diagonally to the R side of the corona where about 4 mm (3/16 inch) mucosal tissue is exposed; most of the scar on the top of the glans to midpoint of the lower surface appears 'ragged.'

Light touch with cotton ball on the dermal surface of the left side of the remnant elicits sensation, on the mucosal surface, which is dry, elicits slightly more sensation; light touch with cotton ball on the ragged edges of the scar produces a faint burning stinging sensation reminiscent of the much more severe sensations H experienced throughout childhood into adolescence.

H measures his erect penis (I did not examine him) "from the base, over the top of the glans to the urethra" where it is pulled to the right and downwards, at 22.3 cm (8 3/4″).

H states that when he has erections his whole penis bends to the right and his glans penis "curls." The glans is pulled downwards and to the right, causing pain in the scarred area between the glans and shaft of his penis. The same right lateral area cracks and bleeds. He can feel a lump to the R between his scrotum and the ventral base of his penis during erections (I requested that he assess this to determine if 'trapped penis' was part of his trauma syndrome, which it seems to be).

The appearance is not as if his prepuce was circumcised, (cut around) but was cut almost in half lengthwise (hemi-sected). It is difficult to understand how the pediatrician could have made such a distinctive error.

The distorted shape of his erect penis is not conducive to comfortable vaginal penetration.

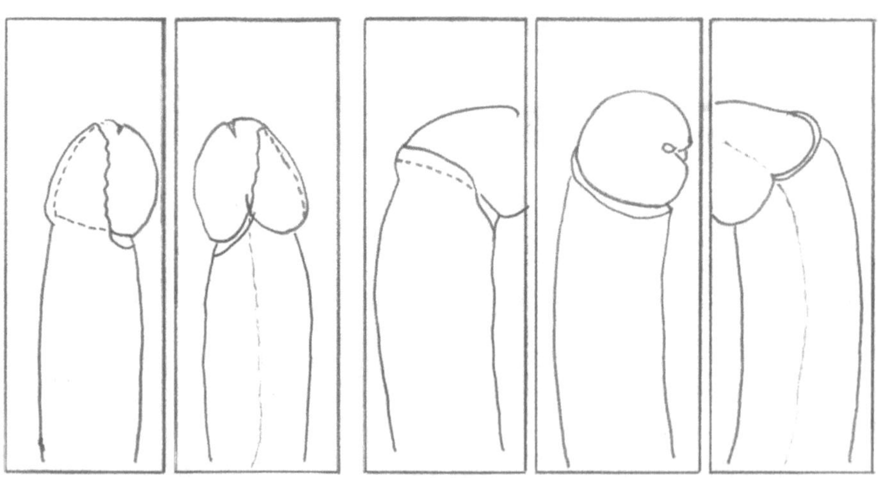

1 Dorsal, Flaccid 28.12.09 2 Ventral, Flaccid 28.12.09 3 Dorsal, Erect 28.12.2009 4 Lateral, Erect 28.12.2009 5 Ventral, Erect 28.12.2009

8.13 W History of Presenting Problem

W denies major health problems but states she has been feeling less energetic lately. She attributes this to the stress of the couple's marriage and sexual situation, professional workload, and menopause.

Menses age 13, had dysmenorrhea due possibly to a retroverted uterus until after the birth of their son; menopause was at age 47, W is now 49.

Para 2, Gravida 2 W was healthy during both pregnancies except for mild gestational diabetes with both. She has had no recurrence of elevated blood sugar since her younger child was born.

Their first child, a boy, was born by normal vaginal delivery after a relatively short labor. H and W had made a firm pre-natal decision their sons would not be circumcised. By insisting on rooming-in, with no exceptions, for the entire 2 days, with doulas in constant attendance, their son made it safely intact through the American Midwestern hospital system. Both parents were appalled that one pediatrician ignored the written refusals and tried to convince them to have their son circumcised. W noted with mixed feelings of pride and sadness, her father-in-law's delight that his grandson is intact.

Their second child, a daughter was born in a birthing center again by vaginal birth and without any untoward events. W stated to me out of H's hearing, that she had less vaginal pain following both births than she sometimes experienced after sex.

W breastfed both their children for 8 months.

Her dysmenorrhea, painful breast cysts with premenstrual tension, have disappeared with menopause.

W notes relatively mild menopausal symptoms apart from decreased vaginal elasticity and lubrication. Sexual relations with other men before marriage to H were satisfactory. W noted she experienced greater comfort and pleasure with her intact lovers and was orgasmic with them, which she very rarely is with H. W has had dyspareunia throughout her marriage to H. Post-coital pain is significant and she has to avoid sex for up to a week until she can recover enough to tolerate it again; she has frequent bouts of cystitis.

At present she is experiencing vaginal pain and sensations of cystitis since intercourse 4 days ago. She frequently has small tears at the introitus to her vagina, more of a problem since menopause.

8.14 Physical Examination

December 27, 09

HEENT Swelling above the suprasternal notch, possibly goiter, for follow-up with her family physician. Slightly dry skin, hair also dry, some falling out.

Lungs clear on percussion and auscultation, slight functional systolic murmur, all pulses strong and equal.

Breasts slightly heavy, no tenderness, no obvious cysts or other masses, normally protruding red/pink even nipples, no discharge, no swellings, redness, heat, pain, or masses in lymph nodes.

Abdomen, some striae, good muscle tone, normal bowel sounds, no pain, no obvious masses no enlarged lymph nodes, slight right upper quadrant tenderness.

Reflexes all present, perhaps slightly slow.

W is flexible, has no joint or muscle pain, had some lower back pain gestationally, none now.

Genitourinary, light excoriation, small crack, 7 o'clock introitus, slight redness exit of urethra, no apparent masses on ovaries or enlargement of uterus (retroverted, difficult to locate/palpate), vaginal tenderness with pelvic exam; 2 × 3 cm bruise, tender to touch at 11 o'clock upper vaginal area; cervical os slightly reddened and excoriated.

Normal secretions. With W's consent, H was shown these perineal and vaginal findings to demonstrate how the injury to his penis, no fault of his own, which he neither consented to nor requested, and from which he suffers considerably, impacts on W and on their marriage (Bensley and Boyle 2001; O'Hara and O'Hara 1999).

8.15 Findings and Discussion

December 29, 2009

Before dealing with the findings relating to the presenting sexual problems, we discussed the other physical findings with the couple, e.g., H's chest pain and the lesion on his arm and his boggy prostate. His chest pain could possibly be angina caused by coronary artery disease. With the significant risk it could be exacerbated by sexual exertion. We realized it was important to defer sex until after the chest pain was assessed and dealt with. H denies chest pain at the moment but agreed to report it immediately should he experience it during the course of counseling and that he would go to emergency immediately. H will also ask the family physician for referrals to assess the mole on his arm and about his prostate.

If H had remained intact, the size increase with erections might still have strained a normal prepuce, but amputation of any part or amount of his prepuce at all would likely have caused erectile distress. The exceptional irregularity of H's partial foreskin amputation imposes additional erectile distress, the consequence of which is severe difficulty with sexual intercourse and brought the couple to the brink of divorce.

One positive aspect of H's situation is that the larger remnant of his foreskin includes the frenulum, which has a significant amount of sensation. Thanks to his father's refusal to allow pediatricians to 'even the circumcision scar' by further amputation, H will have more than usual restored sensation at the end of what is likely to be a lengthy foreskin restoration process.

W will ask their family physician to do a follow-up examination of the swelling in her neck. If it is a goiter, which I think it is, she will require further consultation and likely thyroxin replacement.

I explained how a low thyroxin level could affect her energy level, and sexual response as well as cause digestive slow thinking and other secondary symptoms.

We discussed anatomy and physiology of the penis, prepuce, labia, vagina, and clitoris (O'Connell et al 1998), and evidence of pathological conditions caused by circumcision. Both had already learned some recent information through research at the time of their son's birth, but were very interested in the new physiology (Sorrells et al 2007). They also reviewed the NORM literature for further reassurance on the effectiveness of foreskin restoration and to plan methods and equipment.

We discussed W's vaginal bruising and both partners were clear they will explore ways of achieving sexual satisfaction that avoids any further pain or damage to W, and also to H (Bensley and Boyle 2001; O'Hara and O'Hara 1999; Health Assessment and Physical Examination 2008; Taylor et al. 1996).

8.16 Treatment Plan

December 30, 2009

The first objective was to ensure that the potentially life and health threatening conditions found on preliminary clinical examination received as rapid follow-up as possible.

Next, was finding the most effective, comfortable methods of stretching the short side of H's prepuce until it reached the same length as the longer tissue. We thoroughly reviewed and discussed all the literature on foreskin restoration available, considering each method to see which would be the most appropriate for H's uneven scar.

It seemed evident that he would have to selectively stretch the shorter area and equalize both sides before he could stretch the remnant as a whole. He also wanted to try keeping his glans covered to de-keratinize the surface, and regain some sensitivity. We mapped out a diagram of the areas to receive preliminary attention and planned where and how long to do freehand restoration, t-taping, and x-taping, his methods of choice. He explored the devices available online to consider which he might prefer once he reaches his initial 'equalization' goal.

He chose to begin with freehand restoration during the day as time permitted. This would avoid bringing hair onto the penile shaft and enable the mucosal surface of the glans to be covered by the inner lining of the foreskin, another mucosal surface, as the original foreskin rests on the glans penis. He then decided on devising a modified 'Micropore' X-tape to wear at night. He experimented with the tape samples I had been given by medical supply companies to see which were the most secure, comfortable, and non-irritating to his skin (see Endnote 2).

To encourage non-sexual physical intimacy, something H and W had never explored, I recommended literature on theories and the practices of touch and massage therapy, and that they experiment with full body massage, apart from or included in their sexual experience. They decided that it would be worth a try for both relaxation and stimulation (Inkeles and Todris 1972; Arcand 1986).

Since both H and W had experienced genital pain throughout their sexual lives together, explanation of the concepts of neurogenic pain seemed important. When pain has been a constant, associated with a particular situation for any individual, their mind/body memory of that activity includes the expectation that pain will always occur with it and they actually sense pain even when anatomical and physiological repairs should allow it to lessen or disappear. To overcome this expectation, as pathology that conditioned the pain is being treated, the client may try to replace it with neutral or pleasure sensations and integrate an awareness of pleasure instead. They may try preliminary touch testing and determine whether any pain they perceive is actually physical or more related to expectation, tension and fear. Massage therapy helps alleviate tension and fear and condition expectation of pleasure; it can be a valuable aid in helping clients overcome neurogenic pain, tension and fear of pain (Butler and Moseley 2003; Howes 2004).

We discussed their plans for sex, positions they liked, frequency, varieties, inclusion of 'toys', (I recommended they defer toys until weeks or months after the physical goals are met), fantasy, the comforts of their bedroom, furniture etc. While they had expectations and ideals of conventional 'adult' positions, it was evident to both that it simply had not worked for a long time, in fact, had unfortunately, never worked. And, therefore, major modifications were in order. Both realized it would be wise not to even attempt penetration until H had restored his foreskin enough to reduce the pathological angle (Laumann et al 1997).

W's attaining orgasm had become dependent on trying to maintain a level of excitement while struggling to tolerate the increasing effort and length of time it required for H to ejaculate.

In addition she was experiencing a lot of pain during intercourse, as was evident from the vaginal bruises seen on pelvic examination. Reversal of this problem was equally paramount to finding methods for resolving H's pathological deformity.

We discussed some of the cultural biases for and against sexual positions and styles. I suggested they set aside biases for "sophisticated," 'adult' sexuality for adolescent sexual styles, including manual and oral stimulation, mutual masturbation, and other non penetration modes of sex, until H reduces the pathological angle in his erect penis, which, they were reassured was completely possible with persistence, patience and carefully calculated effort.

We discussed how to make the changes as esthetically pleasing as possible (Beigel 1963; Comfort 1972).

For future reference, when penetration would be possible again, they discussed *a tergo* (from the rear), oral stimulation, side positions, woman on top (Beigel), and a practice shown in a film, *The Decline of the American Empire,* in which lubrication is placed inside a large condom and either H and or W provide the manual stimulation leading to ejaculation (Arcand 1986).

H had developed a masturbation system capitalizing on the longer remnant of his prepuce on which about 75 percent of his natural frenulum on the unaffected side remained. This area has the greatest sensitivity and contributes the most to his orgasmic and ejaculatory capacity so this seemed the best option for his satisfaction; W was aware of this sensitivity and happy to support him. We reviewed their recollections of adolescent avoidance of pregnancy using these methods. They joked about demoting themselves to 'junior high sex' and the prospect of ultimately 'graduating' back to 'adult' sex' after foreskin restoration.

It seemed important to warn H that, when he achieved enough restored foreskin to sense the benefits, he might unexpectedly feel angry that he had missed these pleasures for so much of his life. This and depression are quite common among men who have partially completed foreskin restoration. Some become discouraged at this point and abandon the project, which a sad loss for both partners. This emotional stage of restoration signifies impending success, so it is important that those around them know how to support them when it does occur and help them continue restoring until they should realize the full benefit [NORM (National Organization of Restoring Men 2010) http://norm.org].

Both partners were quite open to all suggestions. Each one's willingness to be as flexible as the other needed, relinquish biases, and plan the healing of their sexual lives was compelling and impressive. They both expressed relief, gratefulness, and no small amazement that H's physical injury and their disappointingly unsatisfactory sexual lives could be overcome and that they would be the ones to do it.

Their discussions about 're'-scheduling their sexual lives was a revelation for them in several ways. H's injury had caused such difficulties that they had both compensated very successfully for their disappointment and frustration by over-developing their careers and working styles to replace their less-than-satisfactory sexuality. This intervention would allow them to return some priority to their sexual lives, but would take considerable change of values and rescheduling.

They bookmarked Internet references for future research. I asked them to read and discuss their Internet findings with each other and then me during follow-up appointments and to ask every question that came to mind, to capitalize on this innovative style of intervention as insightfully and constructively as possible.

For future reference, we planned for the time, whenever H had restored sufficient foreskin, for them to begin sex with penetration again. I suggested they begin with W on top and that she very slowly allow herself to dilate over H's penis. If they wished, from that position they could very carefully change to another, e.g., a side position. I suggested they make all their moves slowly and confirm with each other whether each move and position was good for them both. We planned to review this during bi-weekly, follow-up conference calls.

During conference calls, we would evaluate progress, decide how long or whether to continue particular interventions, and change or add new modalities. I would add encouragement and support when needed, we could have further meetings and examinations if necessary, but we expected and would attain steady progress and eventual success. We again agreed on the priority of follow up on all non-sexual findings, especially deferral of actual intercourse until H's cardiology status cleared, although he would immediately begin freehand and x-tape restoration.

8.17 Follow-up January to December 2010 to August 2012

January 9. H is managing freehand stretching of the short side of his remnant and is managing the X-tape system. Both H and W saw their family doctor last week and consultations with specialists are in progress. H saw his cardiologist later last week, had an angiogram, which revealed three blocked coronary arteries and had angioplasty. There is no evidence of ventricular muscle damage.

The cardiologist recommended avoiding sexual intercourse for a few weeks. H described his foreskin restoration plans to the cardiologist, who has been divorced twice, and who asked for a referral. The cardiologist phoned me before H had time to introduce him, but the surprise call went well. Dr. C is satisfied to work with the website info and literature referrals, and will only call back with questions for which he cannot find answers elsewhere. He states he believes he has the worst type of circumcision.

W has taken some compassionate leave to look after H during his recovery from the angioplasty. Both are glad to have time off and are "working" on massage and getting to know each other in the prescribed new ways (within the cardiologist's recommendations) by resting, reading and absorbing the new information. Although they had been living the difficulties for years, they both say the new information is causing some cognitive dissonance, which they are working to reconcile. I repeated the recommendation they consider yoga as an excellent way of learning relaxation and building up psychological and emotional resources.

January 16. W has been seen by an endocrinologist; the thyroid antibodies study show she has Hashimoto's disease, and that the right upper quadrant pain could be an irritated gall bladder caused by increased acid content of the bile due to low thyroxin levels. The endocrinologist has prescribed a low dose of Synthroid, which she is tolerating well. If the upper quadrant pain, which is not a problem unless she is being examined, is still present in 6 weeks, he will order further tests and refer her to a gastroenterologist. H is working consistently on his stretching program, is beginning to see a slight difference in size and texture of dermal and mucosal layers and feels very optimistic. H states that they will defer adding Yoga to their repertoire, that the "penis yoga" is enough for now! In 2 weeks they will be cleared by the cardiologist to begin experimenting with their new sexual system. Both feel rested and healthier physically and emotionally. W returns to work next week and H the following week

January 30. H states he has grown 2 mm of dermal and mucosal tissue, and is thrilled. He joked, however, that he hopes it will compensate for the skin he will lose from his arm next week! His return to work is delayed due to the dermatology follow-up. A biopsy of the lesion on his left arm showed a significant number of melanocytic cells and he will have a revision of the surrounding area to ensure removal of all malignant cells. He will have the full range of investigations to screen for involvement in any other areas of his body. The dermatologist and cancer surgeon both estimate an excellent chance of no recurrence due to the early stage and grade. Tomorrow he will see the urologist re boggy prostate.

H's urologist is actually a church-mate and one of the several H has consulted over the years. H's father brought him to this man almost 30 years ago. He is the only doctor not to recommend excising the remainder of H's prepuce, but along with other consultants had no further suggestions for resolution of H's injury and erectile dysfunction.

February 13. Foreskin restoration is proceeding well. H feels so much better his voice was actually different and I had to confirm it was him. He was surprised I didn't recognize him and asked if I were feeling well! He says he feels remarkably better. The couple has found time for and much pleasure in their "junior style" sex. H is recovering from the revision of the skin on his left arm and will have physiotherapy with a home program until the end of the month or until the limitation of the range of motion is resolved. W is experiencing greater energy since beginning thyroxin replacement therapy, and is very pleased about it. She reports now, too, that she often had frequency and urgency with pain on urination, but not for the past 6 weeks. She also finds this a considerable relief.

Two weeks ago H's urologist confirmed that his prostate was boggy and had been tending towards bogginess for some time, stating it is not uncommon for some men approaching middle age. H had a routine PSA screening blood test done. H discussed his foreskin restoration process with the urologist who in H's words, "Was amused; for a moment I wondered if he was going to refer me to a psychiatrist! But he simply, rather cynically I thought, said 'Good luck' and opened the door. I'll bring him the *British Journal of Urology* articles and a progress report at the next visit. He may be a little more impressed with academic evidence, when my clinical evidence is there to impress him."

February 27. Foreskin restoration and sex proceeding well. H states that the keratin layers have completely sloughed off his glans penis over the past 10 days and thinks it is because he frequently now keeps the x tape on during the day. Both are surprised and delighted with the look of the new moist, glossy mucosal surface of H's glans penis. H is surprised and pleased with the difference in sensation. He's pleased to have started out with tape that seems to be compatible with his skin, sticks well but isn't difficult to remove. Often he lets it soak off in the hot tub or shower.

March 13. All well, the family is off on March break with their children, both of whom are intelligent and observant and have quickly picked up on their parents' improved mood. Both children were very concerned about H's two surgical procedures and believe that the surgery is responsible for all the benefits they're observing, which W notes, saves inventing other explanations.

March 27. Foreskin restoration and sexual relationship is going very well. H has been researching devices for the time when the remnant is even enough to benefit appropriately from them and has ordered several to try when the time comes. Both parents were surprised at how much happier the school break was this time and credit the relief and relaxation from their previous disappointing, frustrating, sexual struggles with the difference. They feel the whole family is benefiting from their achievement, that it is a fresh start in a positive new direction. H states his relationship with his father is closer, and his father has expressed how extremely happy he is that there is a resolution for the injury and that it is in progress; finding a solution for his son's injury has been a quest for HF throughout his son's life and he feels it is nothing short of a miracle that he has lived to see it fulfilled. H expressed how touched and grateful he is for his father's support and love, and for his mother's background support and concern for both of them, and her relentless ear for new ways, however seemingly unorthodox, for dealing with difficult problems. It was she who referred him for the intervention, which seemed so bizarre he almost deferred even attempting it. Moving testimonies, indeed, to say the very least.

April 24. As per the previous phone call, restoration and relationship are going well. W mentioned that she had a conversation with her mother yesterday similar to that H had with his father a month ago. Her parents are both extremely happy with progress to date, even more that complete resolution, however slow, appears certain. H has had a second visit to the urologist, who seemed surprised and pleased to report that the bogginess has decreased since January. H reported to him again that the counseling and foreskin restoration was affording him the opportunity of giving his prostate more exercise than it had ever had. By H's account the urologist glanced very briefly at H's renewed foreskin segment, pooh-poohed the notion of any change and reserved further comment. H said he was sure that this time he was actually quite curious "but just too 'doctorly' to admit it." H's PSA is normal, a great relief to all. His next visit will be in 6 months. He plans to bring a chart of his progress as well as have significantly more foreskin to demonstrate the value of foreskin restoration. H considers his urologist to be a fine professional and is sure that, once he can see how effective foreskin restoration is, he will understand it as the best option for H's condition, and perhaps prescribe it for others, especially since he was unable to come up with any other clinical resolution for H's significant problem. I asked the couple to begin thinking about intercourse with penetration for our next discussion.

May 12. As per previous phone call, restoration and relationship are going well. We then discussed future intercourse with penetration in preparation for when the angle of H's deformity is sufficiently reduced to permit it; they are doing very well 'junior style" and are gathering ideas for initial positions and position changes, e.g., if they begin with W on top and she very slowly allows herself to dilate over H's penis they might continue in that position for a time, then carefully change to a side or *a tergo* position. They will do preliminary "practice" progressions that are esthically pleasing and physically possible for both. I suggested they not rush the date and assess the possibility according to amounts of remnant stretched and the angle of his glans penis, which should be at least half of the original angle before they attempt penetration. Both H and W seemed to concur.

May 29. H reports that he has stretched the short side of his foreskin remnant 10 mm in the 5 months since he began restoring. He calculates that by the end of July he should have reached 16 mm, almost ¾ of the length of the long side of his foreskin remnant when flaccid. This should reduce the angle of the deformity when erect almost 50 %, according to his further calculation and hope. He and W are very pleased with progress to date. He experiences less pain on erection and estimates that pain with efforts to ejaculate are 25 % of what it was at its worst.

June 26. No new events or particular milestones; all efforts and enjoyment continuing well. Both say they have never had this much physical, emotional, or sexual comfort and relaxation with each other. H has no further doubts that he can succeed, is now confident and perhaps a little too enthusiastic and impatient to reach completion. He has discovered two websites describing faster restoration. One is a surgical intervention, the second a genetic experiment to regenerate foreskin tissues. The surgery is very expensive although that is not a problem, but H has read reports of failures, something he is not willing to risk. The genetic option is not available as therapy, and very much at the experimental stage. He is interested in the genetic system advertising the possibility of recovering the original nerve structures, ridged band, etc., but perceives the notion as farfetched. I suggested he investigate the risks of introducing foreign genetic material into his body, especially onto his penis, adjacent to lymph nodes and other delicate structures where malignancies are known to develop. He has come to the conclusion it will be many years before any significant results of the venture are available, long after his own foreskin is restored and that the slow manual techniques are healthier.

July 17. Foreskin restoration is progressing and the couple's sexual life is continuing well. Both acknowledge feeling anger and depression over H's injury and the loss it caused them for so many years, affecting them so deeply they nearly separated. I reminded them that other restorers have this same experience and cautioned them to expect insights that lead to feelings of anger and depression, to take time to acknowledge the feelings and share them with each other, and then to let them go, not to dwell on them. Since they are both active in their church and are believers, they pray about this aspect of their lives on their own and together, asking for help and comfort, but also giving thanks for the enormous positive changes. They have shared the information with their new pastor who is exploring the benefits for himself and his family. Their pastor has three daughters and they are expecting a son to be born in November. The minister states that H's experience has firmly convinced him that circumcision is completely unnecessary and he has even researched biblical citations to confirm theological beliefs about it, too.

July 27. H measured the angle of his bowing glans penis this morning and reports it is half of what it was at its worst. The couple has cautiously explored careful penetration with no pain, but climax with penetration seemed too difficult so they reverted to manual and oral climax, but they were very encouraged and consider it great progress and a victorious milestone. They plan to continue their manual and oral sex practices until the angle of the deformity is closer to normal, occasionally testing their ability to function with penetration. Both restoration and sexual relationships are going very well. The entire family is travelling together; the tension of H and W's difficulties of last year entirely resolved.

September 25. Both restoration and sexual relationships are going very well. H has added another few millimeters to the mucosal and dermal surfaces of the short side of his foreskin and has begun using a device called constantly applied tension (CAT) designed by an engineer. H, whose first degree is in engineering, considers the device an engineering marvel and believes he will have more rapid results with it. Both H and W have heavy work schedules over the next month, so the next follow-up will be at the end of October.

H reports on behalf of his cardiologist that he seems to be progressing rapidly and that he also has increased both mucosal and dermal layers by 1.75 cm since January 9. Dr. C and his wife are appreciative and send regards and thanks.

October 30. Both restoration and sexual relationships are going very well. H is rapidly reaching the first objective of evening the sides of his foreskin. The angle of his deformity is increasingly reduced, he has an occasional twinge of pain, which he believes is simply neurogenic, and the couple has intercourse with penetration about a third of the time. Both say they still feel a fondness for the "junior" style of sexuality because it was really their first successful, continuing, comfortable sexual experience.

November 23. Both restoration and sexual relationships are going very well. H had a final visit with the urologist mid-month, and the urologist reports the problem of bogginess is resolved and his prostate feels normal. H brought photocopies of *British Journal of Urology* articles by Taylor and Sorrels, which the urologist accepted, and he asked a few polite questions. He had done a little online research himself in the interim and is beginning to admit there may be some value to the method. All other findings from nearly a year ago have been well treated and resolved. The next and probably final follow-up will be in 1 month.

December 22. Anniversary of the referral for intervention. H has expanded both mucous membrane and dermal surfaces to 1–2 mm less on the short side of his prepuce when flaccid. He states the edge is a bit ragged but isn't worried about the appearance, stating it is the functional and sensory aesthetics that interest them both. The angle of the glans with erection is slightly more than 5° off center. The couple is now easily able to have sex with penetration, neither have pain and both are able to climax during regular intercourse. H plans to continue restoring until both sides are equal and he has about 50 % coverage during erection. He joked about a comment he found online by John Erickson "You can never have too much foreskin." This is especially true when you've lived the first 50 years of life with the first foreskin hemi-sected. H will report when he has reached his goal just for the records, but no further follow-up is necessary from either client or nursing standpoint. As a team we declared the intervention successful.

July 7, 2011 W reported that over the July 4th reunion the entire family, especially their children commented on the couple's dramatically changed and harmonious relationship. August 27, 2012 H reported that his sexual fantasies and attitudes towards women have changed to a more peaceful and appreciative nature.

The couple is happy to have the recording of their intervention shared, and feel assurance that many others may profit from their experience.

8.18 Conclusions, Questions, and Directions

Many thousands of individuals and couples have researched and engaged in foreskin restoration independently, have succeeded, and improved their lives and relationships by persisting to completion with it. For others, the injuries and effects on the partner are so severe and their lifestyles so un-conducive to independent research, in Henderson's terms, their *needs* are so great that supportive professional intervention is necessary until they are able to resume autonomous self-care. This nursing intervention, guided by Henderson's theory, accomplished just that. It is the couple's hope, and mine as well, that we have not only achieved their goals but produced a model from which others may profit.

This couple's tragedy was caused needlessly and it is likely that millions more are living the same sexual disappointment and frustration they did, before accomplishing foreskin restoration. Sexual mutilation is a significant public health issue and many people will require intervention through foreskin restoration for many years. There are many who will never be able to complete foreskin restoration and the effects of their frustration and post trauma syndromes will be felt by society for generations. These syndromes are easily preventable by completely eliminating all forms of genital cutting. Future generations need not live these tragedies. The prepuce has been the male "default" sensory organ for over 50,000,000 years and no surgical alteration by the human hand can ever improve it.

It should be obvious to all that it is impossible to know when he is an infant, what size a man's penis will be as an adult or what the proportionate difference between his flaccid size and his erect size will eventually be. H's circumciser cannot be seen as having performed, in his capacity as a physician, of fiduciary responsibility, anything close to a beneficent act, especially by inflicting an exaggeratedly uneven injury. While all circumcision causes sexual dysfunction, more severe injuries make sexual experience impossible throughout a man's entire lifespan. Inflicting injury has no place in medical or nursing practice (Milos and Macris 1992; Mayeroff 1971).

As stories of those who have suffered these iatrogenic injuries are gathered and studies of successful restoration emerge, are entered into the public domain and take hold in collective consciousness, the rate of circumcision can only continue to decline.

Illustrations 1–5

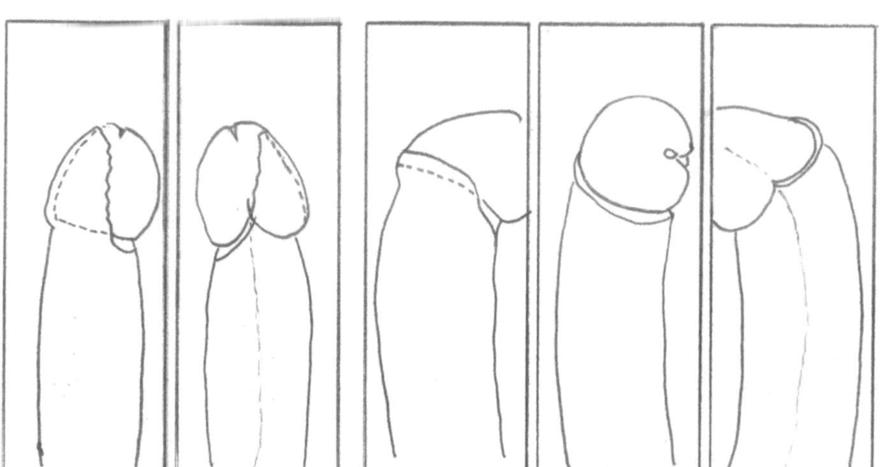

1 Dorsal, Flaccid 28.12.09 2 Ventral, Flaccid 28.12.09 3 Dorsal, Erect 28.12.2009 4 Lateral, Erect 28.12.2009 5 Ventral, Erect 28.12.2009

Illustrations 6–10

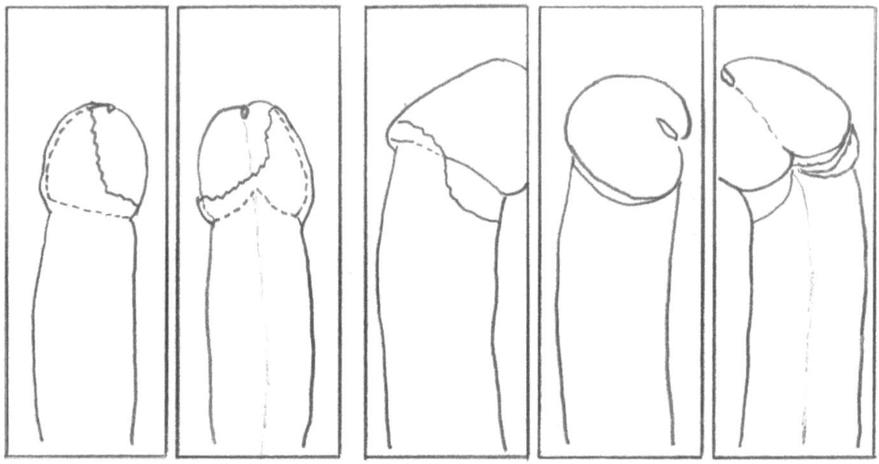

6 Dorsal, Flaccid 24.7.10 7 Ventral, Flaccid 24.7.10 8 Dorsal, Erect 24.7.10 9 Lateral, Erect 24.7.10 10 Ventral, Erect, 24.7.10

Illustrations 11–15

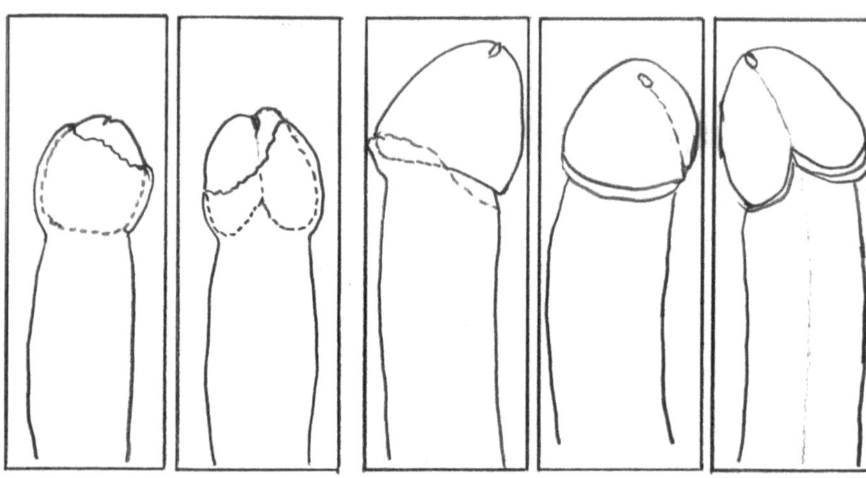

11 Dorsal, Flaccid 22.12.10 12 Ventral Flaccid 22.12.10 13 Dorsal, Erect 22.12.2010 14 Lateral, Erect 22.12.2010 15 Ventral, Erect 22.12.2010

8.19 Notes

1. Dr. W. H. Masters inadvertently contradicted his own findings in his book, Human Sexual Response in an interview in Playboy Magazine (November 1979). He revealed that many circumcised men need to thrust more forcefully than intact men to ejaculate. He stated that the amount of energy required for a

(circumcised) man to climax is about the equivalent of that needed for a fifty-yard dash. While circumcised men and their wives find this statement accurate, intact men state they need a fraction of that amount of energy to climax and their wives state they would find the exaggerated, forceful thrusting distressing and not at all conducive to sexual pleasure (Masters 1979).

2. The freehand method of foreskin restoration is less well known than other methods, yet it is simple and not too time-consuming. There is no need to purchase equipment to do it and it may be done without adhering to any particular schedule. While the method may take longer than some others, it is more relaxed and convenient to do whenever the thought comes to mind, perhaps a few days in a row, with pauses of days, even weeks, then resuming it when convenient again. It may appeal to restorers who are daunted by the variety of methods, number of tasks, and multi-month restoration plan others actually enjoy while restoring their foreskins. Freehand restoration is done simply by encircling the scar with the finger and thumb and gently pulling the mucosal tissue towards the body until it tingles but is not painful. It is useful, perhaps the best way of or if "evening" the scar; for this, tension on the shorter area of the remnant on a daily basis until it is even would be the best preparation for subsequently stretching the remnant as a whole.
3. Over a few months, it is possible to stretch several (2–3) inches of mucosal tissue, (the approximate length of an original mucosal foreskin surface) from the attachment at the coronal sulcus to the scar site.
4. Freehand restoration has several more advantages. It avoids pulling skin with hair from the base of the penis onto the shaft skin. It lengthens the underneath, mucosal surface of the foreskin so that it remains in direct contact with the glans penis, which is also mucosa. Mucosa is more delicate and suited to contact with another mucosal surface than skin is. A useful analogy is that of the inner eyelid (mucosa) as the most appropriate protection and covering for the surface of the eyeball, which is also mucosa.
5. The increasing amount of stretched tissue initially bunches behind the corona then, with further stretching, continues to grow until it comes up over the corona and eventually covers it, then covers the whole glans. Most people are amazed and delighted to watch the growth, enjoy the new sensations, or see their partner enjoying new sensation, where there was previously none. They are also fascinated to see the changes in color and texture of the new surface of the glans penis as it becomes moist mucous membrane again and its color brightens.

Acknowledgments The support and encouragement of Rita F. Cameron, RN, Graduate of the Montreal General Hospital School of Nursing 1931, Supervisor in Obstetrics at Montreal General Hospital 1960–1972 is acknowledged and this study is dedicated to her memory.

References

Arcand D (1986) The decline of the American empire. National Film Board of Canada, Canada

Beigel HG (1963) The meaning of coital postures. In: DiMartino MF (ed) Sexual behavior and personality characteristics. The Citadel Press, New York

Bensley GA, Boyle GJ (2001) Physical, sexual, and psychological effects of male infant circumcision: an exploratory survey. In: Denniston GC, Hodges FM, Milos MF (eds) Understanding circumcision: a multi-disciplinary approach to a multi-dimensional problem. New York, Kluwer Academic/Plenum Publishers, p 207–239

Butler DS, Moseley GL (2003) Explain pain. Noigroup Publishers, Adelaide

Comfort Alex (1972) The joy of sex. Mitchell Beazley, London

DOC (Doctors Opposing Circumcision) (2010) http://doctorsopposingcircumcision.org

Health Assessment and Physical Examination (2008) First Canadian Edition, by Mary Ellen Zatore Estes and Madeleine Buck. Thomson Nelson, Toronto

Henderson (1966) The nature of nursing: a definition and its implication for practice, research and education. MacMillan Pub Co, New York

Howes D (2004) Sensory healing. University of Western Ontario, London, 18 Nov 2004

Inkeles Gordon, Todris Murray (1972) The art of sensual massage. Simon and Schuster, New York

Laumann EO, Masi CM, Zuckerman EW (1997) Circumcision in the United States, prevalence, prophylactic effects, and sexual practice. J Am Med Assoc 277(13):1052–1057

Mayeroff Milton (1971) On caring. Perennial Library Harper and Row, New York

Milos MF, Macris D (1992) Circumcision: a medical or human rights issue? J Nurse Midwifery 37(2):87–96

Montague A (1978) Touching: the human significance of the skin, 2nd edn. Harper & Row, New York

NOCIRC (National Organization of Circumcision Information Resource Centers) (2010) http://nocirc.org

NORM (National Organization of Restoring Men) (2010) http://norm.org

O'Connell HE et al (1998) Anatomical relationship between urethra and clitoris. J Urol 159:1892–1897

O'Hara K, O'Hara J (1999) The effect of male circumcision on the sexual enjoyment of the female partner. BJU Int 83(1):79–84

Snyder JL (2009) "The normal, natural penis and the effects of circumcision" in circumcision and human rights. Springer, New York

Taylor JR, Lockwood AP, and Taylor AJ (1996) The prepuce: specialized mucosa of the penis and its loss to circumcision. Br J Urol 77:291–295

Sorrells ML, Snyder JL, Reiss MD, Eden C, Milos MF, Wilcox, N, Van Howe RS (2007) Fine-touch pressure thresholds in the adult penis. BJU Int 99:864–869

William H. Masters (1979) Playboy interview: masters and johnson—a candid conversation. Playboy Magazine 26:87–121

Williams, Kapila (1993) Complications of circumcision. Br J Surg 80:1231–1236

Author Biography

B. Maurene White RN, graduated from Montreal General Hospital School of Nursing in 1962 and received a Bth in 1988, a DipEd in 1991, and a BA (Medical Anthropology) in 1997 from McGill University. She has worked in different areas of nursing, with special interest in perinatality, and outpost work as a nurse practitioner in northern Canada. She currently develops smartphone applications: iCoOrdiMed for General Health tracking, www.coordimed.com and i4SkinHealth for tracking foreskin restoration progress, www.farreach.org and consults on both projects. Montreal, Quebec, Canada.

Chapter 9
Ten Years of Training: Family Medicine Residents as Conscientious Objectors to Circumcision

Michelle Storms

Abstract Many family medicine residents are opposed to the performance of neonatal circumcision. I will discuss my experiences and insights over the last 10 years providing support for the residents who wish to remain conscientious objectors.

Keywords Residency programs • Circumcision • Child abuse • Torture • Solicitation • Ethical standards • Religion • Conscientious objectors

Family medicine residency programs have the expectation that residents will perform procedures, including neonatal circumcisions. Residents, in general, love learning procedures. However, one-quarter to one-third of residents in the Marquette Family Medicine Residency Program (in Marquette, Michigan, USA) have made a conscious decision to not perform circumcisions. They cite ethical and religious concerns, similar to those given by healthcare providers concerning provision of abortions, abortion counseling, vasectomies, and female contraception.

Employment contracts mandate that physicians provide *medical* care, not *cultural* care. Neonatal circumcision is often performed by non-medical personnel for non-medical reasons, and therefore, qualifies as *cultural* care. Many physicians and healthcare personnel consider circumcision to be child abuse and torture, which is certainly not part of the job description. Nor is the solicitation or arranging for such a procedure part of the employment contract or job description.

Marquette General Hospital has over a 95 % neonatal circumcision rate. The belief held by many in the community and among the medical staff is that parents have the right to request circumcision of their newborn son, and physicians and hospital staff are expected to comply.

The Marquette Residency Program has allowed residents to refuse to perform any procedure, or provide clinical care in any area, that the resident believes violates their ethical standards. For the most part, this has not created any problems.

M. Storms (✉)
Assistant Director and Research Director for the Marquette Family Medicine Residency Program, Marquette, Michigan, USA
e-mail: stormsmd@att.net

G. C. Denniston et al. (eds.), *Genital Cutting: Protecting Children from Medical, Cultural, and Religious Infringements*, DOI: 10.1007/978-94-007-6407-1_9,

However, the refusal to perform neonatal circumcision has generated controversy and division particularly on the hospital birthing unit, and sometimes among the residents. Often, there is no physician available in-hospital to perform circumcisions because the family medicine physician attending, pediatrician attending, obstetrician attending, and the residents available all refuse to perform them.

Many healthcare providers have been forced to call themselves Conscientious Objectors (CO) in order to justify their refusal to participate in the performance of neonatal circumcisions. A recent article by a prominent ethicist questions the need for providers to call themselves *Conscientious Objectors* since any "ethical doctor will object to conducting a clinically unnecessary operation on a child who cannot consent" (Shaw 2009).

Conscientious Objector status originated to allow persons opposed to war from having to take up arms. It then was reframed to allow medical providers and healthcare personnel the opportunity to decline participation in medical care that violated their ethical principles. It is defined by the UN Commission on Human Rights as:

> An individual who has claimed the right to refuse to perform (military service) on the grounds of freedom of thought, conscience, or religion. Conscientious objection in medicine is the notion that a healthcare provider can abstain from offering certain types of medical care with which he/she does not personally agree. This includes care that would otherwise be considered medically appropriate.

The state of Michigan developed the *Michigan Conscientious Objector Policy Act* of 2004, which protects healthcare providers from retribution if those providers, who invoke their conscience, refuse to provide medical care. It "allows providers to decline offering care if that care compromises the provider's beliefs, except in the event of an emergency."

In furtherance of this policy, the "*Medical Conscience Rule*" was passed in December, 2008 by the Department of Health and Human Services. It protects entities or individuals from reprisal if they chose not to provide certain medical services that violate their conscience (notably in the area of abortion services). It was intended to protect providers, educate about protections afforded by federal laws and hear grievances. The goal of the new law was to "prohibit recipients of certain federal funds from coercing individuals in the health care field into participating in actions they find religiously or morally objectionable" and to "prohibit discrimination on the basis of one's objection to, participation in, or refusal to participate in, specific medical procedures, including abortion and sterilization."

DHHS' Secretary Leavitt specifically stated that "healthcare providers should not be forced to choose between good professional standing and violating their conscience." Any healthcare entity found to be in violation of the new law would be subject to a termination of federal support and repayment of funds already received.

Conscientious Objector rulings, as noted in the above paragraphs, address the issue of providing emergency care to adults, but do not discuss how to address the issue of performing procedures on minors for non-therapeutic reasons.

None of the existing conscientious objector laws specifically address the issue of neonatal circumcision, which is unique in that it is an elective procedure performed on non-consenting patients to remove healthy tissue. Many physicians and nurses find neonatal circumcision troublesome for these reasons. They also find it troublesome to be pressured into facilitating the performance of circumcision by finding someone else to do it or someone else to assist in a circumcision. This would clearly not be required of a provider opposed to abortion, or of a Jehovah Witness opposed to hanging blood products on a patient.

Ten years ago, the Marquette residency program was primarily composed of US-trained male residents of primarily the Catholic or Protestant religious faiths. Few residents refused to perform circumcisions while in training, even if privately they expressed opposition to the procedure.

Over the last 10 years, the composition of the residency program has changed to include more females, many foreign medical school graduates from eastern Indian and European countries, where circumcision is not routinely performed, and a diversity of religious beliefs. Some of the male residents are intact and understand the value of the foreskin/prepuce. Many of the residents from foreign countries belong to religions that specifically advise against circumcision (Hindus, Sikhs, etc). There are Catholic priests who are opposed to circumcision, and the New Testament expresses opposition to circumcision. *The Book of Mormon* advises against circumcision. All these factors have created a much higher percentage of residents declining participation in this procedure.

There is also greater awareness of the violation of the infants' human rights by circumcision. Many of the female residents are particularly averse to performing a procedure they consider harmful to the well being of the child. Females, and intact males, understand that circumcision disrupts the mother–child bond.

Residents are also more vocal and assertive than in the past. Previously, residents deferred to authority figures and followed a strict hierarchy, which did not allow for much dissension among the ranks. Residents raised in the U.S. tend to be particularly outspoken in recent years, most likely as a result of their socialization here. Foreign medical graduates are less comfortable challenging the system, but will do so if they believe it violates their religious or cultural beliefs.

Residents who circumcise have tried to coerce other residents into circumcising by emphasizing that they are increasing the workload for other residents, making it inconvenient for others, and that they are not respecting the rights of parents.

Challenging the status quo on the birthing unit has created a strong and concerted kickback. The nursing staff reacted by repeatedly harassing and attempting to intimidate the resident physicians, and even harassing attending physicians and parents, who refuse to circumcise. Nurses state that they are "just being an advocate for their patients." However, clearly they are not advocating for the male infant who has no say whatsoever. One mother stated that she was repeatedly "harassed by nurses until I was crying" over her decision to leave her son intact.

Some physicians have been threatened with the filing of incident reports, and a nurse actually did write up an incident report on a pediatrician who refused to arrange for a circumcision on his patient. Nurses have discussed the "ethical beliefs" of physicians opposed to circumcision with parents. The nurses avoid direct, rational discussions and do not seem to accept that others find circumcision unnecessary, unethical, and a violation of human rights.

The chief medical officer (CMO) of the hospital was contacted about the repeated instances of harassment, intimidation, and unethical/unprofessional behaviors exhibited by nursing personnel on the birthing unit. It was explained to the CMO that such behavior was a violation of federal and state law, and that it no longer would be tolerated. He agreed to discuss the issue with the nursing staff and put an end to it. It was suggested that the nursing staff receive education regarding circumcision, the value of the foreskin/prepuce removed, the complications, and the ethics. This suggestion was not put in place, although attempts have been made at departmental meetings to promote education.

Based on the obvious lack of knowledge, a lecture on circumcision was presented to the family medicine residents in October 2009. Readings were provided in advance of the presentation for the residents to review. These readings included a discussion of the normal structure and functions of the male foreskin and prepuce, the history of circumcision, the ethics and controversies surrounding circumcision, and a full informed consent for circumcision, including all the complications. Interestingly, the room was packed for this discussion. From the questions asked, it was clear the residents had no knowledge of the anatomy and functions of the tissue they were removing by circumcision. Nor did they know any of the history and few of the complications. How can it be that physicians are graduating from accredited medical schools lacking such basic information and education regarding one of the most commonly performed procedures in the US? Clearly, our medical institutions are failing medical students, nursing students, and thus patients, by not providing such basic information needed to provide adequate informed consent. For no other procedure would this be acceptable.

The AAFP conference in October 2009 brought further revelations regarding this issue. Many of the attendees stated they had not circumcised their own children, but continued to circumcise newborns at parental request. They were uncomfortable declining to circumcise despite their obvious negative feelings about it. Such GroupThink is no different than what occurred during World War II with the experimentation on Jews in concentration camps. As Voltaire stated, "Familiarity accommodates any barbarity."

One Michigan family medicine resident at the AAFP conference, originally from Nepal, stated that she was being forced to perform circumcisions and she was afraid to say "No" for fear of being fired. A discussion with the Michigan State University family medicine program directors in December 2009 demonstrated a lack of insight and knowledge on their part regarding the history and ethics of circumcision. However, they did agree to allow residents to decline participation in the procedure. It was emphasized to them that resident physicians need to be informed of the option to forgo performing circumcisions, or any other ethically objectionable procedure.

Neonatal circumcision is a volatile, emotionally charged issue, which is difficult for many to discuss rationally. This alone is a tip-off that something is just not right about the circumcision of non-consenting infants who, as our patients, deserve protection from harm. However, this procedure is culturally embedded in the psyche of our nation. It will require a conscious effort to confront the issues involved. Furthering the goals of being a conscientious objector and eliminating circumcision will require direct open communication with extensive education. It will require an epiphany for many to realize the damage that occurs with neonatal circumcision. It is clear that having a vocal faculty physician and attending physicians presenting the concerns about circumcision to medical students and residents in training has made a difference in Marquette, Michigan.

Reference

Shaw D (2009) Cutting through red tape: non-therapeutic circumcision and unethical guidelines. Clin Ethics 4:181–186

Author Biography

Michelle R. Storms MD, is an Assistant Director and the Research Director for the Marquette Family Medicine Residency Program in Marquette, Michigan. She is an assistant clinical professor at Michigan State University College of Human Medicine. After graduating from Saint Louis University School of Medicine, Dr. Storms completed her Family Medicine residency training at St. Mary's Hospital in Milwaukee, Wisconsin. While a resident physician, she developed an aversion to neonatal circumcision, which led her to challenge the status quo by refusing to perform circumcision post-residency. For ten years, she has provided support to the resident physicians in her program who are conscientious objectors to circumcision. Dr. Storms has published on the topic of circumcision individually and in collaboration with Robert Van Howe, MD. She is on the Health Professionals Board of Intact America. Marquette, Michigan, USA.

Chapter 10
Intersex Surgeries, Circumcision, and the Making of "Normal"

Elizabeth Reis

Abstract So-called "normalizing" surgeries for babies born with various intersex conditions (atypical sex development) as well as infant male circumcision have come under scrutiny in recent years by philosophers, ethicists, and medical professionals. This chapter draws from my recent book, *Bodies in Doubt: An American History of Intersex* (Reis 2009) and argues that, historically, doctors have performed surgeries on infants and children for non-medical reasons. In the case of intersex, surgery was performed so that the baby's external genitalia would align with the gender in which the baby would be reared, supposing (but without substantive evidence) that the child would develop more normally if its gender and physical appearance cohered. Social factors, such as the potential for marriage and the fear of homosexuality, in particular, have motivated these surgeries since the early nineteenth century. Similarly, male circumcision has been motivated by social rather than medical concerns, the incidence increasing and coinciding with the fear of masturbation in nineteenth-century America. As one contemporary doctor has noted, perceptively, circumcision has been a "surgery in search of a disease." My chapter will look at both kinds of genital surgeries, suggesting that irreparable procedures should not be done on infants, with of course the exception of life-saving operations. As intersex children grow older, they can make such decisions for themselves, as can intact boys or men

Keywords Intersex • External genitalia • Gender • Ambiguous genitalia • Disorders of sex development • Chromosomes • Hormones • Genetics • Ethics • Circumcision

E. Reis (✉)
Women's and Gender Studies, University of Oregon, Eugene, OR, USA
e-mail: lzreis@uoregon.edu

G. C. Denniston et al. (eds.), *Genital Cutting: Protecting Children from Medical, Cultural, and Religious Infringements*, DOI: 10.1007/978-94-007-6407-1_10,

10.1 Introduction

My recent book, *Bodies in Doubt*, is the history of the medical management of intersex. Intersex, also known as disorders of sex development or DSD, is a congenital incongruence between internal reproductive anatomy, chromosomes, hormones, and genitals. Not many parents have to face the difficult decisions regarding infant genital surgeries for babies born with intersex. The incidence of infants presenting with ambiguous genitalia is relatively small (about 1/2000 newborns have an intersex condition, though it's not always apparent at birth), and in many hospitals there will be teams of pediatricians, urologists, social workers, geneticists, and ethicists discussing every surgical and social option.[1]

But parents of half of all babies born in the United States typically do confront a largely unspoken ethical dilemma: that of routine male circumcision. Most people don't think of this as a big decision. In fact, male circumcision is not listed in the index of *The Cambridge Medical Ethics Workbook*, one of the prominent collections of case studies, commentaries, and activities used for teaching students major contemporary ethical issues. Yet, it is generally the first ethical decision that parents will make about their baby's life; it has also been the most frequently performed surgery in this country (Gollaher 2000).

"Normalizing" surgery for babies born with various intersex conditions as well as infant male circumcision have both come under scrutiny in recent years by philosophers, ethicists, and medical professionals. Historically, the medical protocol for dealing with intersex conditions is surgical refashioning of the genitals. Typically, so-called corrective surgery has not been done for the baby's physical health but rather for his or her psychological well-being. The supposition (without substantive evidence) is that children will develop more normally if their external genitalia align with their gender of rearing. Social factors, such as the potential for marriage and the threat of homosexuality, in particular, have also motivated these surgeries throughout American history and even today (Reis 2009).

Male circumcision has also been motivated by social rather than medical concerns, the incidence increasing and coinciding with worries about hygiene and the fear of masturbation in nineteenth century America. Today the justification for the

[1] The figures on the incidence of intersex range widely, depending on which conditions one includes in the calculation. One incident in 2,000 births represents a moderately inclusive estimate. Estimators who are more selective in determining what characteristics qualify as intersex put the figure at 2 in 10,000. Researchers at Brown University recently stated that the frequency of people receiving "corrective" genital surgery is between 1 and 2 per 1,000 live births. The Chicago Consensus Conference put the figure at 1in 4,500. See I. A. Hughes, "Consensus Statement on Management of Intersex Disorders," *Archives of Disease in Childhood* 91 (2005): 554–63; Anne Fausto-Sterling, *Sexing the Body, Gender Politics and the Construction of Sexuality* (New York: Basic Books, 2000), 76; Melanie Blackless et al., "How Sexually Dimorphic Are We? Review and Synthesis," *American Journal of Human Biology* 12 (2005): 151–66; and Alice Domurat Dreger, *Hermaphrodites and the Medical Invention of Sex,* (Cambridge: Harvard University Press, 1998), 40–43.

procedure focuses on limiting the spread of certain cancers in America and HIV in Africa. Here, I will look at both kinds of genital surgeries from a historical perspective, suggesting that irreparable procedures should not be done on infants, with, of course, the exception of life-saving operations. As intersex children grow older, they can decide on the appearance of their genitals for themselves, as can boys and men.

10.2 Intersex

Physicians have had a long, fraught relationship with those born with intersex conditions, or atypical sex development. Two recent controversies have brought some of their professional discomfort to public scrutiny. These issues have focused unusual attention on matters usually concealed, and they give us an opportunity to examine our prejudices toward heterosexuality, "normal" bodies, and medicalization. The first storm erupted when a New York doctor was exposed recommending dexamethasone, a Class-C steroid that the FDA has not approved for this use, to pregnant women at risk of bearing babies with congenital adrenal hyperplasia (CAH) (Dreger et al. 2010). CAH girls are often born with a large clitoris, and prenatal dex, as it is called, can mitigate this condition, precluding the "need" (more on this later) for surgery to reduce the clitoris. It has also been suggested that dexamethasone could alter fetal exposure to an excess of androgens. Why is this important? Some speculate that it might reduce a female's inclination toward lesbianism or bisexuality (Meyer-Bahlburg et al. 2008).

The second controversy also involves sexual anatomy, specifically a certain physician's medical management of clitoral reduction surgery. The surgery alone is disturbing, for it relieves no illness. Making matters worse, the doctor in question used a vibrator-like tool to assess the extent of nerve damage on girls and young women on whom he had performed the surgery, crossing the line, even if unintentionally, into sexually inappropriate contact (Dreger and Feder 2010).

It is useful to view these recent controversies over clitoral size and homosexuality in the broader historical context of attitudes toward the intersexed. In *Bodies in Doubt*, I argue that physicians are and have long been influenced by our larger social anxieties, especially concerning marriage and sexual desire. Medical management is fundamentally a cultural, not simply a scientific, endeavor.

In early America, for example, physicians feared that a woman with a large clitoris would act like a man, that she might be tempted to initiate forbidden sexual relationships with other women. Medical writers argued that such women could give sexual pleasure to other women by means of their unusual endowment. One doctor described the clitoris in 1597 as "that part with which imprudent and lustful women, aroused by a more than brutal passion, abuse one another with vigorous rubbings" (Park 1997). The author of an early popular midwifery manual declared in distaste, "some lewd women have endeavoured to use it as men do theirs" (Sharp 1999). Occasionally, writers combined medical writings on hermaphrodites (as they were then called) with quasi-pornographic tales of women with large clitorises having sex with each other, merging, even in the early period, hermaphroditism with same-sex sexual relations (Handy 1808).

In the nineteenth century, when the idea of "sexual inversion" emerged as a scientific explanation of homosexuality, hermaphrodites were considered potential homosexuals or "inverts." If some people's bodies were both male and female, then would such individuals couple with both sexes, or with the "wrong" sex? Physicians as well as lay people have long preferred that one's genitalia matched one's apparent gender and that one exhibited conventional opposite sex desire. When physical ambiguity appeared, many believed that surgery was warranted. They sought to "correct" atypical genitalia, not necessarily for the health, comfort, or pleasure of the patient, but to preclude the undesirable potential for homosexual sex. Even life-long celibacy was preferable to homosexuality. Dr. Samuel Woody wrote in 1896, "So ill-fitted for the generative function and so prone to psychical perversions and moral degradation, such cases should be castrated in early life" (Woody 1896). In the context of surgery and atypical bodies, "morality" meant heterosexual sex if there was to be any sex at all.[2]

There were no easy ways to determine sex in cases of ambiguity, though most physicians remained convinced that the presence of either ovaries or testes (the gonads) would provide the answer. By the first half of the twentieth-century, doctors were able to assess gonads by examining tissue samples under a microscope, and so the sex of living patients could presumably be ascertained. But neither the gonads—or new factors that became accessible: hormonal levels and chromosomes—could (or can, even to this day) tell doctors with absolute certainty the "actual" sex of an individual or whether a particular child would identify as the sex the doctors decided on. Nor were there unmistakable ways to determine a child's eventual sexual preference, no matter what their genitals looked like.

Dealing with intersex adults was complicated because of their established gender identity and sexual desire. Such patients were not always amenable to physicians' suggestions that they alter their anatomy or their intimate habits. How could you convince a person who had lived as a female her whole life that in fact she was a male because she had internal male reproductive anatomy? Physicians attempted this, but their patients often spurned the advice to switch genders. Addressing "the problem" of intersex was simpler with infants or young children, and in the 1950s doctors increasingly focused their attention on childhood intersex. John Money, a psychologist at Johns Hopkins, and his colleagues, Joan and John Hampson, advanced a rationale for choosing gender and performing surgery on infants born with ambiguous genitalia. Their approach came to define intersex management for the next fifty years and, despite some resistance, it lingers. Intersex involves chromosomes

[2] Contemporary intersex activists have written extensively on doctors' commitments to cultural norms. See especially Cheryl Chase (Chase 2002). See also Nancy Ehrenreich and Mark Barr (Ehrenreich and Barr 2005; Walcutt 1999).

and hormones in addition to anatomy, but following Money, external genital morphology became the single most important criterion in the evaluation and treatment of people with intersex conditions. Money and his followers firmly believed that possessing conventional-looking genitals guaranteed healthy psychological development.

Until very recently, doctors surgically sculpted indeterminate genitals to match the gender that an infant was assigned at birth (assignments would be made according to a variety of factors, including hormone levels, chromosomes, and predominant genital shape). On the face of it, it may seem a sensible practice to ensure coherence between one's gender and one's anatomy. Unfortunately, little evidence backed Money's theories, and many intersex people have spoken out about the harm done to their bodies (and their psyches) through these radical interventionist surgeries. Often such procedures were performed to make parents, as opposed to children, feel better. Some girls born with short or absent vaginas have suffered surgical reconstruction to build penetrable vaginas, serviceable for conventional sexual activity. The procedure requires daily dilation to keep the newly built vagina open. This is a painful, scarring process. Intersex activists and ethicists have asked why a small child would need such bodily alteration. Is the "cure" worse than the "affliction?"

For a generation, parents were encouraged to consent to their baby's surgeries so that "normality" could be enforced. And, as we saw earlier, physicians uncritically accepted and acted on their own heterosexual norms, often elevating marriage as a goal to parents considering genital surgery for their children. Heidi Walcutt, in an autobiographical essay, recalled that, in the 1970s, a doctor at the Buffalo Children's Hospital told her that, at age fourteen or fifteen, she would need surgery to increase the depth of her vagina "if you ever want to have normal sex with your husband" (Walcutt 1999).

Similarly, surgeries to repair hypospadias (when the urinary opening is underneath the penis instead of at the tip) are not always medically necessary. By allowing a boy to stand while urinating, such surgery satisfies social, not strictly medical, imperatives. Surgeries to reduce an enlarged clitoris are also cosmetic, not therapeutic (though in some cases surgery is medically warranted to repair confluence between the vagina and urethra). Increasingly, tolerant voices argue that these surgeries should be delayed until adulthood, performed then only with the consent of the person whose body is to be cut.

Intersex activists are currently challenging Money's presumptions and protocols. Beginning in the 1990s, intersex adults and feminists have been working to improve the medical and social attitudes toward people with intersex, focusing in particular on ending the optimum gender of rearing model (the notion that everything has to match in order for parents to raise well-adjusted children) (Karkazis 2008). They argue that the so-called normalizing genital surgery that most infants born with unusual genitals endure does not cure the intersex condition and is often simply aesthetic. Sometimes, as intersex scholar Morgan Holmes has pointed out, surgery to alleviate genital ambiguity might actually have the opposite effect: when boys with micropenises are fashioned into girls they are "actually *made into* intersex persons." "In fact," she argued, "it seems that such a child, in a female assignment, is actually more intersexed following surgery than at the point of diagnosis." [3]

Must bodies and sexual desire be "normalized?" The recent medical interventions mentioned above—prenatal dexamethasone and clitoral reduction surgery—are based on the premise that intersex is a condition that needs to be corrected, even at the expense of a person's basic well-being. Such tampering with hormones or radically altering anatomy can be dangerous to individual health. Prenatal dex, for example, has been linked to cognitive and memory problems, and clitoral reduction surgery reduces sexual sensation. Both treatments have been contrived solely to conform people to our narrow ideals of "normal." Though many doctors and hospitals throughout the country have heeded the cautionary words of intersex activists about the harms of medical interventions, particularly on infant patients, efforts to make the genitals look "normal" and to prevent homosexuality still exist. We continue to be profoundly unsettled by any body that falls outside the parameters of "normal," particularly in terms of sex anatomy, and despite our growing openness to same-sex desire, we remain deeply troubled by that potential as well.

The controversy over whether surgery is necessary at all, and at what age it should be performed, continues to this day. Some critics point out that corrective surgery may do more harm than good by causing incontinence and permanent loss of sexual sensation. As Alice Dreger, an academic historian and past chair of the board of directors of the former Intersex Society of North America (ISNA), put it, "Why perform irreversible surgeries that risk sensation, fertility, continence, comfort, and life without a medical reason?" ISNA's (and now Accord Alliance's) efforts are making headway, but they have not yet been universally accepted. At a 2004 meeting of the Section on Urology of the American Academy of Pediatrics, several leaders in the field cautioned against invasive genital cosmetic surgeries, while others continued to advocate early aggressive operations (Alice Dreger's Blog 2004). Several physicians in Australia recently published a study arguing that despite the controversy, early surgical intervention leads to more positive outcomes in both genital appearance and gender identity (Crawford et al. 2009).

Some physicians and hospital teams have recognized that many intersex conditions require no medical attention; there is nothing medically "wrong" other than that the development of the sex organs diverged from the typical path. Intersex activists have recently tried to persuade doctors to postpone genital surgeries until the intersex person is able to participate in the decision. At a 2005 conference [hosted by the Lawson Wilkins Pediatric Endocrine Society and the European Society for Paediatric Endocrinology and hereafter called the Chicago Consensus Conference], participants agreed on the need for more open communication between doctors, patients, and families, and a more conservative approach to surgery. Perhaps most importantly, the consensus statement acknowledged that there

[3] On the history of the intersex rights movement see Karkazis (Karkazis 2008; Holmes 2002, 2008; Dreger and Herndon 2009; Kessler 1990; Fausto-Sterling 2000).

is little evidence that infant genital surgery does what it has been assumed to do: improve attachment between child and parents, ease parental distress about atypical genitals, ensure gender identity development in accordance with the assigned gender, or eliminate the intersex condition.

Since the 2005 conference that advocated changing the standard of care for DSD, several important changes have been institutionalized in hospitals around the country. Many are now employing a team approach in dealing with intersex patients. Parents are referred not only to the appropriate pediatric subspecialists (endocrinologists, urologists, geneticists) but also to social workers, psychologists, and therapists who have experience with parents and infants with special needs. The team approach, according to Katrina Karkazis in an article that suggests "best practices," should include the parents and the child, if the latter is old enough to understand. "Shared decision-making" is surely a step in the right direction (Karkazis 2010).

10.3 Circumcision

Routine male neonatal circumcision also prioritizes social reasons for genital surgery, at the expense of compelling medical reasons. Most people do not react with horror at hearing about circumcision because the results do not usually involve scarring, incontinence, and loss of sexual sensation—frequent outcomes of intersex genital surgeries. We are accustomed to think that circumcision is a minor procedure that (ironically) makes the baby boy's penis "normal." But what is "normal" about genital surgery on a newborn? What really needs fixing and why? What is the medical justification for intervention?

Infant male circumcision has been characterized as a solution in search of a problem (Wallerstein 1980). Doctors who advocated infant male circumcision in the nineteenth century listed curing "nervous symptoms" as one of the top reasons for the surgery. First thought to thwart disease, it was later promoted to inhibit masturbation, to encourage hygiene, and now again to prevent disease. But, we must ask ourselves if public health anxiety about the spread of HIV and other sexually-transmitted diseases trumps a male's right to his own bodily integrity? Does it make more sense to circumcise infants or let grown men make this decision for themselves?

By the late nineteenth century, worries about masturbation merged with concerns about hygiene and disease. Dr. George M. Beard wrote in 1882 that circumcision may be "needed" in several diseases, including "general neurasthenia (especially sexual exhaustion), epilepsy, and certain paralyses of children" (Beard 1882). In 1891, an article in the *New York Medical Journal* announced, "It is well authenticated that the foreskin is a fruitful cause of the habit of masturbation in children… [T]he foreskin is detrimental to health, and… circumcision is a wise measure of hygiene" (Crossland 1891). At a Royal Academy of Medicine meeting in Ireland that year, physicians debated the procedure and also linked it to masturbation, claiming that circumcision was "a real help to the weakest spot in the human character." "Circumcision is an excellent thing to do," Dr. L. Solomons asserted at the meeting: "It helps to prevent hernia due to straining, and later it helps in preventing masturbation. The ordinary schoolboy is not taught to keep himself clean and, if he is taught, he thinks too much about the matter" (NA 1920).

By 1910, over one-third of male infants in the U.S. were circumcised; by 1940 that number had risen to sixty percent, and by 1980 the rate peaked at eighty-five percent (Glick 2005). It has been falling since; the most recent statistics put the rate at fifty-five percent overall, with regional variations (25 percent in the western states, for example) (Roni Caryn Rabin 2010).

Even into the 1970s, physicians were still mentioning masturbation as a reason for removing the foreskin, though by then avoiding urinary tract infections and cancer also became compelling motivation. In the 1980s, reducing the incidence of sexually transmitted diseases, including HIV, became more persuasive than stemming masturbation, and several studies claimed that researchers could link HIV with circumcision. Today these studies hold an enormous grip on our collective psyche; circumcision advocates wonder how anyone would resist such a minor procedure in the face of a devastating, worldwide epidemic. A recent study published in the *Journal of the American Medical Association* found, for example, that circumcised men had a lower incidence of syphilis and HIV. Last year the World Health Organization said circumcision reduced the risk of HIV transmission from women to men among heterosexual men in Africa by up to 60 %. Just recently, the government of Botswana (a country with one of the world's highest HIV infection rates), decided to circumcise nearly half a million men over the next five years to stem the spread of HIV (NA 2009).

For their part, anti-circumcision advocates (also known as intactivists) question the validity of some of the studies and debate whether it makes sense to prioritize public health at the expense of personal bodily integrity. Consent must be considered. In fact, the 2007 UN Report maintained that the best interests of the child must be respected. It said, "Parents considering circumcision of an infant boy should be provided with all the facts so they can determine the best interest of the child. Because the HIV-related benefits of circumcision only arise in the context of sexual activity, and because male circumcision is an irreversible procedure, parents may consider that the child should be given the option to decide for himself when he has the capacity to do so" (UNAIDS 2008). The report rightly questioned the wisdom and necessity of surgically modifying the healthy bodies of newborns as a possible preventive for sexually transmitted diseases that might be contracted as adults. Any surgery has its immediate risks, and the potential benefits of circumcision won't appear for years. It is conceivable that a vaccine for HIV will be available before these boys are old enough to have sex. Similarly, effective drugs might be available in the next fifteen years. Just recently, *The New York Times* announced that taking antiretroviral drugs can prevent HIV in uninfected people (McNeil DG Jr 2011). Widespread education programs about the need for ubiquitous safe sex and limiting concurrent partners might also be fruitful as alternative methods for limiting the spread of the virus, which, after all, is contracted through risky behavior, not by the presence of an intact penis.

Circumcision has never been strictly a medical issue. Mandated by Jews and Muslims, it is intimately connected to religion, ethnicity, and tradition and thus fuels strong opinions on both sides of the debate. Today's declining rate of newborn circumcision in the United States can be attributed, in part, to the increased immigration and population of ethnic groups, such as Latinos, who customarily have not circumcised their boys (Parikh 2011).

In this country, the American Academy of Pediatrics said in 1999 that the benefits of circumcision are NOT significant enough for the AAP to recommend surgery as a routine procedure (American Academy of Pediatrics 1999). The policy concluded, however, that it is legitimate for parents to take into account cultural, religious, and ethnic traditions, in addition to medical factors, when making this decision. It stated that, to make an informed choice, parents of all male infants should be given accurate information and provided the opportunity to discuss this decision with their pediatrician. But, now even the AAP is considering changing its position. It might argue that circumcision has health benefits—most notably HIV prevention, but also prevention of urinary tract infections, both of which can be avoided in other ways. It should also note that circumcision can itself cause problems: for example, MRSA (drug-resistant bacterial infections, scarring, pain, infection, and hemorrhaging). The AAP hasn't changed its policy yet but, at the very least, it's likely they'll encourage parents to be informed of all the benefits and risks.

Routine male circumcision is largely done for social reasons, not medical reasons, just like the genital surgeries we've seen for intersex infants in the past (and even, sadly, to this day). I think that neonatal male circumcision deserves the same discussion that healthcare providers are now finally encouraging about intersex surgeries. The non-therapeutic removal of healthy body parts from nonconsenting children is a human rights violation and medically unethical, just as it is medically unethical to surgically modify intersex bodies in order to make them conform to typical male and female bodies. It is time we reconsider the cultural imperative to "normalize" children's bodies and to give them the opportunity to make these decisions for themselves.

References

Alice Dreger's Blog (2004) "Urologists: agonize over whether to cut, then cut the way i'm telling you," Oct 14, 2004, Alice Dreger's Blog, Intersex Society of North America, www.isna.org. See also Dreger, Intersex in the Age of Ethics

American Academy of Pediatrics (1999) Circumcision policy statement. Pediatrics 103(3):686–693 (March)

Beard GM (1882) Circumcision as a cure of nervous symptoms. Med Bull Med Surg 248–249

Chase C (2002) Cultural practice or 'reconstructive surgery'? U.S. genital cutting, the intersex movement, and medical double standards. In: James SM, Robertson CC (ed) Genital cutting and transnational sisterhood, University of Illinois Press, Urbana, pp 126–151

Crawford JM et al (2009) Results from a pediatric surgical centre justify early intervention in disorders of sex development. J Pediatr Surg 44:413–416

Crossland JC (1891) The hygiene of circumcision. N Y Med J 53:484–485
Dreger A, Feder EK (2010) Bad vibrations. Bioethics Forum. http://www.thehastingscenter.org/Bioethicsforum/Post.aspx?id=4730&blogid=140. Accessed June 16
Dreger AD, Herndon A (2009) Progress and politics in the intersex rights movement: feminist theory in action. A J Lesbian Gay Stud (GLQ)
Dreger A, Feder EK, Tamar-Mattis A (2010) Preventing homosexuality (and uppity women) in the womb? Bioethics Forum. http://www.thehastingscenter.org/Bioethicsforum/Post.aspx?id=4754&blogid=140. Accessed June 29
Ehrenreich N, Barr M (2005) intersex surgery, female genital cutting, and the selective condemnation of 'cultural practices. Harvard Civ Rights–Civ Liberties Law Rev 40:71–140
Fausto-Sterling A (2000) Sexing the body: gender politics and the construction of human sexuality. Basic Books, New York
Glick LB (2005) Marked in your flesh: circumcision from ancient Judea to modern America. Oxford University Press, New York, pp 181–312 (8)
Gollaher D (2000) Circumcision: a history of the world's most controversial surgery. Basic Books, New York
Handy W (1808) Account of an hermaphrodite. Medical Repository of Original Essays and Intelligence 12, pp 86–87 (May–July)
Holmes M (2002) Rethinking the meaning and management of intersexuality. Sexualities 5(2):159–80 (quotation on 174)
Holmes M (2008) Intersex: a perilous difference. Susquehanna University Press, Selinsgrove
Karkazis K(2008) Fixing sex: intersex, medical authority, and lived experience. Duke University Press, Durham
Karkazis K (2010) Ethics for the pediatrician: disorders of sex development: optimizing care. Pediatr Rev 31(11):e82–e85
Park K (1997) The rediscovery of the clitoris. In: Hillman D, Mazzio C (ed) The body in parts: fantasies of corporeality in early modern Europe. Routledge, New York, pp 178
Kessler SJ (1990) The medical construction of gender: case management of intersexed infants. Signs 16:3–26 (Suzanne Kessler's 1990 pioneering article)
McNeil DG Jr (2011) Two studies show pills can prevent H.I.V. Infection. The New York Times (July 13)
Meyer-Bahlburg HF, Dolezal C, Baker SW, New MI (2008) Sexual orientation in women with classical or non-classical congenital adrenal hyperplasia as a function of degree of prenatal androgen excess. Arch Sexual Behav 37(1):85–99
NA (1920) For and against circumcision. Br Med J 768
NA (2009) Botswana circumcision drive will prevent 70,000 HIV infections: report. The Telegraph, London (May)
Parikh R(2011) Is russell crowe right about circumcision? Salon.com. http://www.salon.com/life/poprx/index.html?story=/mwt/feature/2011/06/27/circumcision_debate_poprx.Accessed June 27
Reis E (2009) Bodies in doubt: an american history of intersex. Johns Hopkins University Press, Baltimore
Roni CR (2010) Steep drop seen in circumcisions in U.S. The New York Times (August 16, 2010). At a recent AIDS conference, a researcher from the Centers for Disease Control and Prevention, Charbel E. El Bcheraoui, reported a severe drop, from 56 percent in 2007 to 32.5 percent in 2009. Though this dramatic figure has not been confirmed, experts agree that numbers of infant circumcisions have been declining
Sharp J (1999) The midwives book: or, the whole art of midwifery discovered. In: Hobby E (ed) The midwives book: or, the whole art of midwifery discovered. Oxford University Press, New York
UNAIDS (2008) "Safe, voluntary, and informed circumcision and comprehensive HIV prevention programming: guidance for decision-makers on Human Rights, Ethical, and legal considerations," UNAIDS, Joint United Nations Programme on HIV/AIDS, p 17 (June 2008)

Walcutt H (1999) Time for a change. In Dreger A (ed) Intersex in the age of ethics, pp 197–200 (quotation on 198)
Wallerstein E (1980) Circumcision: an american fallacy. Springer Publishing Company, New York, p 197
Woody SE (1896) An hermaphrodite. Louisville Medical Monthly 2 pp 418–19 (quotation on 419)

Author Biography

Elizabeth Reis PhD, is professor of Women's and Gender Studies and History at the University of Oregon. She is the author of *Bodies in Doubt: An American History of Intersex* (Johns Hopkins University Press, 2009) and *Damned Women: Sinners and Witches in Puritan New England* (Cornell, 1997). She received her PhD in History from the University of California, Berkeley. Eugene, Oregon, USA

Chapter 11
Intersex Genital Autonomy: A Rights-Based Framework for Medical Intervention with Intersex Infants

Paul Mason

Abstract Children are children first and girls and boys second. If genital surgery on an intersex child is not necessary for preservation of life or treatment or prevention of likely serious illness, the decision whether and how to operate can be deferred until the child is old enough to express an informed view about the options and in a forum that addresses conflicts of interest. That age depends on the intervention and risks. The decision is not a simple clinical one to be taken by doctors, nor by frightened parents following clinical advice, or the dictates of culture or religion. All these criteria are genuinely promoted "in the best interests of the child", which emerges as distinct from "the rights of the child". Such surgery falls outside the range of lawful authority of parents to give a valid consent and requires other authorization. If the child patient and the parent are both unable to give valid consent, it falls outside the ethical and legal authority of the surgeon. Professional associations and ethics committees should be informing their members that, without court or other tribunal authority, doctors perform this kind of surgery at their professional peril.

Keywords Intersex • Circumcision • Female genital mutilation • Best-interest • Chromosomes • Hormones • Rights of the child

---

Apologium In this chapter I have unashamedly relied on the views of adult intersex people as equally valid as those of doctors, lawyers, and judges. I am not intersex myself and have no grounds to challenge the experience of those who are. Some regard them as "activists", as if applying that label somehow affects the validity of their opinions. Nor am I a doctor. I regard both groups as knowing a lot more than I do. Nor am I the parent of an intersex child, and I acknowledge the parents' expertise and the agony of their ongoing decisions and doubts where I have been spared them. All I can hope to comfort them with is that when searching for non-blue and non-pink clothing size 00 for our own baby in 1992 I did find a lot of yellow, green, and purple. I hope the range has improved.

P. Mason (✉)
Former Tasmanian Commission of Children, Family Law Attorney, Brisbane, QLD, Australia
e-mail: pmmason@bigpond.net.au

G. C. Denniston et al. (eds.), *Genital Cutting: Protecting Children from Medical, Cultural, and Religious Infringements*, DOI: 10.1007/978-94-007-6407-1_11,

11.1 Introduction

The difference between the question of medically unnecessary surgery on the genitals of boys (circumcision) and of girls (FGM) on the one hand and surgery on the genitals of intersex babies on the other is the elastic meaning of the word "unnecessary".

The essential thesis of this chapter is that children are children first and girls and boys second. This principle applies equally to girls, boys, and intersex babies and children.

Unlike circumcision and female genital cutting, all players agree on the line between "medically necessary" and "medically unnecessary", however, the emphasis on modern procedures is a tacit acknowledgement that in the past "wrong decisions" have been made.

The decision is not a purely clinical one to be taken by a medical expert, nor one to be taken by frightened parents following that expert's advice, nor by the dictates of culture or a parent's religion. All three of these criteria are earnestly–and genuinely–argued and believed to be "in the best interests of the child".

It is argued that, following *Marion's Case*,[1] this category of surgery falls outside the range of the lawful authority of parent to give a valid consent and requires authorization of a Court exercising the authority of the community–in the English monarchical system the parens patriae power of the Crown. If the child patient and the parent are both unable to give a valid consent, it equally falls outside the ethical and legal authority of the surgeon.

The missing piece of the puzzle is strong advocacy for the rights of a child.

11.2 Clinical and Best Interests-Based Solutions

11.2.1 Intersex

The term *intersex* first emerged in the 1920s (Marañón Gregorio 1929). Its existence used to be identified by external genital appearance in babies and in later childhood by apparent gender role behavior, and in non-industrial societies it still is. In some cases, the degree of difference is so slight that it remains undetected until an adult presents to a doctor complaining that she can't seem to get pregnant.

In the words of Chris Somers XXY, an Australian Executive Member of Organisation International Intersexués:

---

[1] Secretary of the Department of Health and Community Services v JWB and SMB (1992) 15 Fam LR 392 ("Marion's Case").

> Sex is not purely male or female based and neither is it necessarily based on the assumption that a male = 46,XY or a female is 46,XX in fact the reverse may be true (M = 46,XX and F = 46,XY) where their phenotype (body) may be the opposite to that which was assumed and still be fertile or not as the case may be just as the former may be too (fertile or not). Aside of this there are some 47,XXY people who are female in every respect and others mixed and others who may or may not be more predominantly male in all or some respects. And this is only the tip of the iceberg of all the different genetic variations that exist. Whatever it is life is an infinite puzzle of possibilities and none should have to feel that they cannot have a place in society or feel or are from which they are metaphorically or deemed or to be excluded from normal participation with the fundamental rights given to the rest of the human rights, more so in a supposedly sophisticated society such as we have in Australia...[2]

Nowadays, identifying the precise nature of an intersex condition is determined by a complex analysis of chromosome analysis, anatomical shape, and endocrine function. The battery of tools available is impressive.

The Lawson Wilkins Paediatric Endocrine Society and the European Society for Paediatric Endocrinology considered it timely to review the management of intersex disorders from a broad perspective, review data on longer-term outcome, and formulate proposals for future studies. The methodology comprised establishing a number of working groups, the membership of which was drawn from 50 international experts in the field. The groups prepared previous written responses to a defined set of questions resulting from evidence-based review of the literature. At a subsequent gathering of participants, a framework for a consensus document was agreed.

The outcome was the Consensus Statement on Management of Intersex Disorders published in *Pediatrics* 2006.

> First-line testing in newborns includes karyotyping with X- and Y-specific probe detection (even when prenatal karyotype is available), imaging (abdominopelvic ultrasound), measurement of 17-hydroxyprogesterone, testosterone, gonadotropins, anti-Müllerian Hormone, and serum electrolytes, and urinalysis. The results of these investigations are generally available within 48 h and will be sufficient for making a working diagnosis.
>
> Decision-making algorithms are available to guide additional investigation.[3] These assessments include human chorionic gonadotropin–and adreno-corticotropic stimulation tests to assess testicular and adrenal steroid biosynthesis, urinary steroid analysis by gas chromatography mass spectroscopy, imaging studies, and biopsies of gonadal material. Some gene analyses are performed in clinical service laboratories. However, current molecular diagnosis is limited by cost, accessibility, and quality control.[4] Research laboratories provide genetic testing, including functional analysis, but may face restrictions on communicating results.[5]

---

[2] Personal email to author, 23 June 2010.

[3] Secretary of the Department of Health and Community Services v JWB and SMB (1992) 15 Fam LR 392 at 443.

[4] Secretary of the Department of Health and Community Services v JWB and SMB (1992) 15 Fam LR 392 at 444.

[5] Per Deane J. Secretary of the Department of Health and Community Services v JWB and SMB (1992) 15 Fam LR 392 at 449.

Knowing how a human organism is working and why, however, does not tell you whether baby is a boy or a girl or will grow up to be a woman or a man. Parents want to know, and this second line process is called Gender Assignment, not to be confused with gender re-assignment. The process includes the above diagnosis, genital appearance, surgical options, need for lifelong hormone replacement therapy, potential for fertility, views of the family, and, sometimes, circumstances relating to cultural practices.

The most common intersex condition is Congenital Adrenal Hyperplasia (CAH), where an overactive adrenal gland in utero creates an unusually large "hyperplastic" clitoris, resembling a penis. The baby has an uterus and a pair of functioning ovaries and can grow up to have babies of her own. If you reduce the androgen, the hyperplasia is controlled as long as you keep up the medication.

A less common condition, Complete Androgen Insensitivity Syndrome (CAIS), appears in babies with 46,XY chromosomes and has an almost opposite effect: a short penis, and an incomplete closure of the urethra-vaginal sinus, or a condition called hypospadias where the urethra exits anywhere along the shaft of the penis but at the end where most 46,XY babies have it. Of these babies, 90 % identify as females as they grow up but not all.

The baby in the opening description is part of this group and it is on this group, Warne says, that "the controversy is centered". As recently as the 1970s in the West, it was routine to operate on such babies to approximate the female, give them a girl's name, and dress them in frocks. Long-term outcome studies clearly show that a significant number of patients developed severe gender identity problems and some requested surgical reconstruction to affirm the opposite gender to that engineered in babyhood.

> It is easier to turn an artificial penis back into an artificial vagina than vice versa if the patient chooses that in adolescence or adulthood, and for that reason he explains "there is now a strong trend in the opposite direction…regardless of the size of the phallus, because this operation best preserves choice for the individual and because a male gender identity is more likely than a female one.

Babies deficient in 5_reductase (5_RD2) appear female in infancy and are often named and brought up as little girls but "virilize" at puberty. Sixty percent of them go on to live the rest of their lives as males (and all assigned male live as males). Among patients with partial androgen insensitivity syndrome (PAIS), androgen biosynthetic defects, and incomplete gonadal dysgenesis, there is dissatisfaction with the sex of rearing in 25 % of individuals whether raised male or female.

Among patients with partial androgen insensitivity syndrome (PAIS), androgen biosynthetic defects, and incomplete gonadal dysgenesis, there is dissatisfaction with the sex of rearing in 25 % of individuals whether raised male or female.

Professor Gary Warne is the senior endocrinologist at the Royal Children's Hospital, Melbourne, Professorial Associate at University of Melbourne, and Honorary Fellow at the Murdoch Children's Research Institute. Professor Warne was also one of the participants in an International Consensus Conference, convened in 2005 to develop a modern model of best practice for selecting the safest and most effective modality of management of intersex conditions.

At the 5th World Congress on Family Law and Children's Rights in 2009, Professor Warne delivered a brief but informative paper[6] to show that modern medicine and ethical practice–including importantly a multi-disciplinary team not just a primary doctor advising the parents–was quite capable of producing "right decision" for children born with ambiguous gender without recourse to an external arbiter such as a Court or other Tribunal. He concedes there is a role for the independent arbiter in the rare event of the parents disagreeing with "the doctors".

Professor Warne gives the example of a baby with Mixed Gonadal Dysgenesis (MGD), as his diagnosis is gonadal dysgenesis caused by a chromosomal mix-up that occurred when the egg was fertilized. The palpable gonad is likely to be a poorly formed testis. The other one is likely to be as he describes at the opening of his chapter:

> No one in the room is able to say whether the baby is a boy or a girl. The phallus looks too small to be a penis and too big to be a clitoris. There is only one opening, and it is at the base of the phallus. Exploration of the lower urinary passage in the medical imaging department shows that it branches into two, one passage leading to the bladder and the other into a vagina, concealed behind a layer of skin. Ultrasound shows a uterus. One gonad, which feels like a testis, can be felt but the other cannot. Further testing reveals that the chromosomes are a mosaic, with one cell line containing 45 Y chromosomes and one X, and the other containing the 46,XY pattern. Hormonal studies show that some testosterone is being produced but there is evidence of testicular malfunction.
>
> The diagnosis is gonadal dysgenesis caused by a chromosomal mix-up that occurred when the egg was fertilised. The palpable gonad is likely to be a poorly formed testis. The other one is likely to be a streak of connective tissue containing few germ cells, inside the pelvis.

From this sample, the reader will readily identify that the balance of any percentage of a cohort did not have that outcome, or the outcome is unknown.

Hormone replacement therapy is effective in many (not all) children with hypogonadism, or defects in sex-steroid synthesis or resistance to androgen that is normally introduced around puberty.

Babies with micropenis seem to be happy with their assigned gender, male or female, but again there are exceptions, with or without any growth hormone therapy or surgery. Psychosexual therapy for both parents and family is usually enough.

11.2.2 Surgery

There are two types of surgical intervention. One is to remove gonads (testes, ovaries and ovo-testes) that, combined with the genetic origin of the relevant condition, present a future risk of malignant tumor that of course can become life

[6] Warne G. Special medical procedures in relation to children with disorders of sex development and adolescents with transexualism, 5th World Congress on Family Law and Children's Rights, Halifax 2009.

threatening. Once again, malignancy is usually associated with the onset of puberty and, in some cases where the probability of malignancy is low, there may never be any need for surgery if regular biopsies are taken to track the health of the person's gonads. "Streak" or vestigial gonads are particularly susceptible to malignancy.

Malignancy depends not whether one is intersex but how: the highest tumor risk is found in testis specific protein Y encoded (TSPY) positive gonadal dysgenesis and PAIS with intra-abdominal gonads, whereas the lowest risk (5 %) is found in ovotestis85 and CAIS. So there is some good sense in removing the gonads of the highest risk groups, leaving those of the lowest and tracking the health of the in-between ones with biopsy. This table summarizes how the Consensus Statement assesses to most appropriate response base on the evidence that is available at present. Of course, the worst that gonadectomy can do is to render a potentially fertile baby infertile, a subject to which I shall return (Table 11.1).

The other type of surgery is reconstruction, which may be cosmetic (e.g., for ordinary 46,XX babies with unusually large clitoris or labia), curative (e.g., to relocate an urethra to the tip of a penis or open a sealed vaginal opening), or to assign a gender to a baby or child where the anatomy is completely ambiguous or where it is decided to align the babies' genital appearance with the gender in which their parents eventually intend to raise them.

Table 11.1 Risk of germ cell malignancy according to diagnosis

Risk group	Disorder	Malignancy risk (%)	Recommended action	Patients, *n*	Studies, *n*
High	GD[a] (+γ)[b] intraabdominal	15–35	Gonadectomy[c]	12	>350
	PAI5 nonscrotal	50	Gonadectomy[c]	2	24
	Frasier	60	Gonadectomy[c]	1	15
	Denys-Drash (+γ)	40	Gonadectomy[c]	1	5
Intermediate	Turner (+γ)	12	Gonadectomy[c]	11	43
	17β-hydroxysteroid	28	Watchful waiting	2	7
	GD (+γ)[b] scrotal	Unknown	Biopsy[d] and irradiation?	0	0
	PAI5 scrotal gonad	Unknown	Biopsy[d] and irradiation?	0	0
Low	CAI5	2	Biopsy[d] and ???	2	55
	Ovotesticular D5D	3	Testicular tissue removal	3	426
	Turner (−γ)	1	None	11	557
No (?)	5αRD2	0	Unresolved	1	3
	Leydig cell hypoplasia	0	Unresolved	1	2

[a]Gonactal dysgenesis (including not further specified, 46,XY, 46,X, 46,XY, mbead, partial, and complete)
[b]GBY region positive, including the TSPY (fastis-specific protein Y enclosed) gene
[c]At time of diagnosis
[d]At puberty, allowing investigation of at least 30 seminiferous tubules, preferentially diagnosis on the basis of OCT3/4 immunohistochemistry

It all sounds so easy.

The two great medical areas of controversy are prophylactic gonadectomy to prevent malignancy and, of course, deciding to make a baby look like a girl or a boy. The other controversy is existential. If you are safe from malignancy or safe enough to survive with routine biopsies, why should you be a boy or a girl?

> This baby is at risk for a number of things:
>
> A 20–30 % lifetime risk of cancer developing in the gonads
>
> Short stature, which is often associated with this chromosome pattern and which might need growth hormone treatment
>
> Gender dysphoria (unhappiness with one's own gender identity) or worse still, gender identity disorder–a gender identity that is incongruous with the genital or assigned sex.
>
> Other psychosocial problems, related to how well or how badly the parents adapt to the shock of having a baby with ambiguous genitalia and how they raise the child.
>
> Problems with urination. There can be partial obstruction to the outflow of urine caused by narrowing of the outlet, or back-flow of urine into the vagina, setting the scene for recurrent urinary tract infections
>
> Babies with a 46,XY chromosome count and ambiguous genitalia may develop cancer of the kidney and/or renal failure due to a genetic mutation.

Warne's paper describes the three options available:

> Option 1 is to give the child a boy's name and have surgery done that will bring the urinary opening to the tip of the penis, then explore the location and nature of the internal gonad, removing it if it cannot be brought down to the scrotum. The uterus and vagina would be removed at some stage.
>
> Option 2 is to give the baby a girl's name, reduce the size of the phallus to that of a clitoris, reconstruct the opening of the vagina so that it is separated from the urinary opening, and remove both gonads.
>
> Option 3 is to assign the baby as either a boy or a girl, giving a name, and deal with the internal gonad as in option 1, but postpone any surgery to alter the appearance of the external genitalia until the child or adolescent is old enough to decide about their gender identity and about surgery for themselves. Which of these options would be best for the individual? How should we decide?
>
> For Warne it is "rare" for anyone to consent to raising such a child as a boy just because they have a large clitoris and, for him, "the only debate is about when the surgery should be carried out."
>
> At our hospital, we operate at 6–8 weeks and do a one-stage clitoral reduction and genitoplasty. Lesser degrees of clitoral enlargement are left unchanged. Our long-term outcome data indicate excellent results.

2006 Consensus Statement on Management of Intersex Disorders

This chapter arose for a similar process and desire for consistency as the CAH Consensus Statement four years earlier. The instruction describes the rationale and process.

The very next heading is about "Nomenclature" and explains that the authors chose the word "disorders" because other expressions such as "intersex" itself were "particularly controversial", "potentially pejorative", and "confusing". No matter that the word "disorder" is the antonym of "order": that calling something closely associated with the identity of a human being as "disordered" may create a perception both of and by that person that they themselves are somehow "wrongly ordered". Most remarkably, the statement ends that discussion by explaining that "disordered" is defined by conditions that are "atypical."

Why did they not simply use "atypical" as in "conditions of Atypical Sex Development or ASD"? That part of the controversy would not have arisen and the medical profession not have been seen to distance those with ASD as somehow defective instead of as different people. Whilst the authors of the statement protest publicly that they cleared the term with "intersex people" (surely they mean people with disordered sexual development), the controversy that has persisted about the use of the term belies it, non-American groups accusing Intersex Society of North America (ISNA) of perpetuating classic American Imperialism. Not only did the international intersex movement actually split over the issue, ISNA holding fast to DSD and other splinter groups who do not, e.g., Intersex Initiative in Portland.

At the heart of the issue is whether you can consider me intersex and "normal". It is legitimate for the case to be put, for the baby within the debate, that it is ok to be and remain intersex if it is medically safe and to focus on the parents' preparedness for the psychosocial outcomes.

Beyond Science

Chris Somers, an Australian board member of *Organisation Internationale des Intersexués*, the largest intersex body in the world observed, "I do not dislike Gary Warne, though I think he has a lot to learn about what it means to be an intersex person other than seeing us as scientific curios…to be fair to him I think he tries much harder than he used to be, to be more accommodating. Unfortunately, together with others within his profession bar a few, he has a long way to go".

I spoke after Professor Warne at the 2009 Congress and had the opportunity to suggest that the nature of "the controversy" was different from what Warne believed.

The fact is that many ambiguous gender babies–even those without CAH-do grow up to be happy and well adjusted and go on to have babies. Many of them do not think they are in need of surgery. The fact is that the risk of streak gonads becoming malignant is between 20–25 % and they can be tracked with biopsy–especially at puberty–and removed by laparotomy if malignant. Thus, for well over 75 % of people with streak gonads that did not become malignant, the risk was not "high". The argument is familiar to this audience, that a reported 60 % population reduction in HIV transmission to women in some African countries following an otherwise unnecessary surgical procedure does not equate to a 60 % reduction of the risk of a baby in suburban Hobart, Manchester, or San Francisco contracting or transmitting HIV in adulthood, regardless of his longevity, his sexuality, or other precautions he takes. The logic does not work.

Normal

It is a phenomenological fact that each person experiences their own body as "normal" until and unless they are taught otherwise. The prominent early researcher of intersex, Milton Diamond, stressed the importance of care in selection of language that applies to not only intersex but all areas of human difference (Diamond and Sigmundson 2009):

> Foremost, we advocate use of the terms "typical," "usual," or "most frequent" where it is more common to use the term "normal." When possible avoid expressions like maldeveloped or undeveloped, errors of development, defective genitals, abnormal, or mistakes of nature. Emphasize that all of these conditions are biologically understandable while they are statistically uncommon.

A key issue is whether "intersex" is an abnormal medical condition or a normal but rare genetic variation. Following moves by the Intersex Society of North America, (ISNA) in the late 1990s some intersex activists, medical experts, and parents have moved to eliminate the term "intersex" in medical usage, replacing it with disorders of sex development (DSD) in order to avoid conflating anatomy with identity.

L'Organisation International des Intersexués (OII) is the world's largest intersex organization, constituting predominantly intersex individuals. OII recognizes some of the underlying diagnoses that can lead to intersex CAH, Androgen Insensitivity Syndrome (AIS), Kleinfelter syndrome (K. S.), mixed gonadal dysgenesis, Turners Syndrome and more. There are well over 30 diagnoses in the literature that can underlie "intersex" and most of the diagnoses are not amenable to surgery.

The person is not the diagnosis. Not all diagnoses that may lead to intersex result in intersex. We have seen that CAH is one of the most common diagnoses, but it rarely results in intersex for individuals with XY chromosomes and only occasionally for those with XX chromosomes; and not all intersex results in the sex binary expectations of the diagnosis. Many of those with Kleinfelter Syndrome (XXY) are male and live as men, some are female and live as women, and some are neither.

As far as external ambiguities are concerned, the Prader Scale is often referred to as providing some objective scale of reference, 1 to 2 being "mild" megaloclitoris. The scale of external genital appearance identifies 5 points along an unbroken continuum of external anatomical difference from one end of the male/female binary spectrum to the other.

The key concept here in this chapter is that of "normal" or "ordered" as opposed to "abnormal" or "disordered".

> The term 'intersex' has been used in the scientific community for a long time to describe plants and animals that are not either the typically chromosomal and reproductively dimorphic XX-female or XY-male. The term may be used for an individual within an otherwise usually dimorphic species, or for an entire class of beings within a species, such as a non-reproductive class of worker bees, or a population of fish, or XY female rodents.
>
> …Thus all forms of intersex, or atypical sex differentiation and/or behavior, including non-reproductive and neuter classes, transsexed behavior, same-sex acts, and same-sex

pair-bonding, genetic sex-reversal (XY females, XX males), and actual spontaneous sex-changing are important and healthy/necessary parts of life on Earth (Goswami 2009).

If intersex is normal, then the sexual expression of the intersex person will be as diverse, and for the same diverse and largely unknown reasons, as non-intersex people. This idea underlies the argument of intersex people against the expression "Disorders of Sexual Development" or DSD.

OII UK explains its rejection of the "disorder" tag that prompted the separation in the late 1990s and the 2000s of activist groups of intersex people from groups formed to address clinical management issues (OII International 2009).

> OII is not of the opinion that people who are born with intersex variations do not have health needs. Quite the contrary. What we are saying is that being intersex, or of intermediate or atypical sex, is itself not a disorder which requires medical treatment. The term "Disorders of Sex Development" comprises all the different variations which could result in being intersex and makes our SEX (intersex) itself the disorder. It is obvious that people born of intermediate or atypical sex have health problems. That is what OII wants to be treated, our actual health problems, not gender or other cosmetic changes to make us meet norms for male and female.

Whether people are boys or girls, women or men, simply should not matter when deciding what to do at birth and in early infancy. What should matter is medical need.

OII Australia made the following submissions[7] to the 2009 Human Rights Consultation referring to UNCROC Article 37 and raised aspects of personal rights not often considered by others:

> The right to be free from cruel and degrading treatment:
>
> From birth to death intersex can be subjected to an array of cruel and degrading treatments. Intersex people can be assigned a sex and then subjected to surgeries to affirm that assignment. Such surgeries are rarely without complications and usually require extensive follow up surgery as the child grows. Some surgeries where neo-vaginas are created or vaginal modifications are preformed require daily vaginal dilation–this is performed on children as young as two years of age. The surgery is cosmetic and performed to satisfy societal and parental expectations of genital appearance. The child has no part in the irreversible decisions being made. Surgery is followed by extensive gender reinforcement where the child is encouraged to behave in ways appropriate to the assignment and discouraged away from gender behaviour that is at, apparent, odds with the assignment.
>
> The child may be photographed and medically inspected, then written up and displayed in medical journals. Many intersexIntersex who have received these treatments have vivid memories of them, were humiliated by them, and suffer long-term trauma as a result. The surgeries are largely experimental in that surgeons try to incorporate advances with every new case and no two intersexIntersex people are identical in any event.
>
> There are no long term follow ups of intersexIntersex surgery, no medical researcher has spoken to any significant number of intersexIntersex adults, and when they are spoken about they are rarely beyond the age of twenty.

[7] http://oiiaustralia.com/files/submissions/national-human-rights-consultation/ for copy of the Submission; site accessed 5 August 2009.

Genders and Sexes–How Many?

The questions raised reinforce a concept dear to the Intersex Rights Movement: that gender is not a binary phenomenon, nor even a trinary one, but an expression of genetics and flesh largely unrelated to sexuality.

This division of gender from sexuality is anathema to cultures–and parents in those cultures–that are structured on the binary model and often generates fears of a connection between intersex and homosexuality: after all, if a teenager's genitals look "male" why should they exhibit sexual attraction to other males? The modern answer is that they may feel they are male and feel homosexually attracted or they may feel female and feel heterosexually attracted, just like other people at the distal points of the Prader Scale. OII Australia explains on their website (2009):

> Intersex includes people who are sexually diverse in the sense that most are in apparently standard heterosexual relationships as well as GLB relationships, some are in no relationship and some are in relationships that do not fit any current codification.
>
> Intersex includes gender diversity in so far as many intersexIntersex are men or women, some are transsexual or transgender, others are Hijra, twin spirited, no-gendered, pan gendered, multi-gendered and gendered in ways that do not fit current codification possibilities.
>
> If gender is not a binary system but a continuum, then logically there can be no finite number of "sexes" between "very male" and "very female" (OII Official Positions 2009):
>
> The creation of a new category to be designated intersex poses several problems. First of all, how do we define intersexuality? OII believes that there will be never a clear definition and at the same time, that it is not necessary to have a legal definition for intersex-Intersex. We have no clear definitions for what a woman is or a man is. We only assume this to be the case.
>
> The creation of a specific category for the intersexed risks even more marginalization of a group which is poorly understood. We base our legal arguments on the right of every person to determine her/his own identity in the binary system in the hope that eventually there would be no attempt to impose legal sex categories on anyone.
>
> The purpose of OII is to work in favour of human rights for the intersexed by helping people to understand that there are not just two pre-existing sexes. There is an infinite combination of possibilities on the spectrum of sex and gender.

The Androgen Insensitivity Syndrome Support Group (AISSG) is another international intersex organization run by and for intersex people especially those with AIS. They have affiliates in the UK, the USA, Canada, Australia, and Europe (France, Germany, and Spain). Their insistence on cultural and phenomenological "normalcy" of the intersex experience matches that of OII.

This rejection of abnormality by persons whose gender identity does not match their anatomical sex appearance, or whose sex appearance and karyotype is ambiguous, lies at the heart of the issue of rights. They testify that the unhappiness experienced by intersex people is not a disability but a handicap: they do not experience a disability, but they do experience a disadvantage imposed on them by society, culture, family, and sometimes surgery. That disadvantage can be accentuated by their parents and doctors having made "the right decision" when they were babies.

These "activist" groups may seem to be asking for a lot, for visibly intersex children to be respected in the locker room, and for their families and parents to accept them for who they really are without reconstruction or hormone alteration.

But this is the same thing as asking all people to be treated as human beings, not as identical but as having equal rights, to be treated no less favorably on account of irrelevant personal attributes.

To my ears, this argument to be regarded as "normal," recalls the arguments of the women's rights movements, and particularly the "first wave" arguments of writers, like Wollstonecraft (1792) introducing to a disbelieving world of men the notion that women were actually capable of voting.

The book, *The Cook and the Carpenter*,[8] is a novel written by "The Carpenter" about life, love, lust, family, and a crisis on an alternative lifestyle commune in the 1970s. It uses no gender-specific pronouns until after the denouement right near the end, when the communards find themselves in police lock-up and segregated by sex. The Preface reads:

> Since the differences between men and women are so obvious to all, so impossible to confuse whether we are speaking of learned behavior or inherent characteristics, ordinary conversation or furious passion, work or intimate relationships, the author understands that it is no longer necessary to distinguish between men and women in this novel. I have therefore used one pronoun for both, trusting the reader to know which is which.

The reader slips into a world where the "big question" really does not matter and the unveiling of the genders of each character at the end is consequently quite unnerving. I strongly recommend the book to anyone trying to come to grips with the notions being advanced by the adult intersex lobby.

"Medically Unnecessary": "Best Interests" and "Therapeutic" as Criteria

There seems to remain a gap between the medical and legal professions about what is "medically necessary". One of the strongest critics of a frameless "best interests" test for cases involving child surgery is Professor Ian Kennedy. In "Patients, Doctors, and Human Rights", (Blackburn and Taylor 1991) he asserted that:

> The best interests formula may be beloved of family lawyers but a moment's reflection will indicate that although it is said to be a test, indeed the legal test for deciding matters relating to children, it is not really a test at all. Instead, it is a somewhat crude conclusion of social policy. It allows lawyers and courts to persuade themselves and others that theirs is a principled approach to law. Meanwhile, they engage in what to others is clearly a form of 'ad hocery.'

A medical person might recognize Professor Kennedy's argument that, "although there are problems at the edges" of the two concepts, "(a)n intervention is therapeutic if treatment (therapy) is intended thereby".[9]

The law, however, grows from the "problems at the edges". Australian cases have striven to grasp something more objective, some framework by which to balance the right of personal integrity with the strong opinions of the medicos and the

[8] By The Carpenter, copyright Arnold, J., Daughters Inc., Vermont, 1973.

[9] Ibid page 102.

even stronger opinions of the parents. The matrix adopted that has emerged reluctantly has been that of "therapeutic" and "non-therapeutic" and like all language it brings its own semantic ambiguities.

In *In Re Jane*,[10] a case in which authority was sought for surgical sterilization of an intellectually disabled teenager, Chief Justice Nicholson relied on a distinction between "therapeutic" and "non-therapeutic" and used the former in the sense of "treatment of some malfunction or disease". Although the distinction has been criticized (e.g., as "totally meaningless and if meaningful quite irrelevant to [the paramountcy principle]") (per Lord Hailsham *In re B* [*A Minor*])[11] that criticism was explored by the majority in *Marion's Case* before they finally settled on adopting the distinction themselves as at least relevant to the application of the welfare principle:[12]

> We hesitate to use the expressions "therapeutic" and "non-therapeutic" because of their uncertainty. But it is necessary to make the distinction, however unclear the dividing line may be.

Brennan J in *Marion's Case*, though in the minority, attempted a definition as follows:[13]

> It is necessary to define what is meant by therapeutic medical treatment. I would define treatment (including surgery) as therapeutic when it is administered for the chief purpose of preventing, removing or ameliorating a cosmetic deformity, a pathological condition or a psychiatric disorder, provided the treatment is appropriate for and proportionate to the purpose for which it is administered. "Non-therapeutic" medical treatment is descriptive of treatment which is inappropriate or disproportionate having regard to the cosmetic deformity, pathological condition or psychiatric disorder for which the treatment is administered and of treatment which is administered chiefly for other purposes.

His Honor found the "therapeutic/non-therapeutic" distinction to be important in applying the welfare principle, as did the majority, where the right of personal integrity of a child is under consideration:

> 18. ...The test of therapeutic medical treatment recognizes the importance of personal integrity and of the maintenance and enhancement of natural attributes to the welfare of the child. By comparison, the best interests approach is useful only to the extent of ensuring that the first and paramount consideration is the interests of the child, not the interests of others. That approach furnishes no general guidance as to the factors which are relevant to the welfare of the child.

And His Honor found the distinction "clearer" when examining the purpose of the treatment:

> 19. Of course, factual difficulties are unavoidable in deciding whether medical treatment is therapeutic or non-therapeutic but, in principle, the distinction is clear and, in particular, the purpose of therapeutic medical treatment can be clearly distinguished from other

[10] (1988) 94 FLR at pp 30–31.

[11] (1988) AC 199, at p 204.

[12] Secretary of the Department of Health and Community Services v JWB and SMB (1992) 15 Fam LR 392 at 409.

[13] Secretary of the Department of Health and Community Services v JWB and SMB (1992) 15 Fam LR 392 at 423.

> purposes. Therapeutic medical treatment is calculated to enhance or maintain as far as practicable the physical or mental attributes which the patient naturally possesses; it is not calculated to impair or destroy those attributes and the capacities they afford. Thus, there is a rationale which justifies the administration of therapeutic medical treatment without the patient's consent when the patient is incapable of consenting or refusing consent. It needs no argument to show that a malignant tumor of the uterus justifies the performance of a hysterectomy or that multiple cysts on an ovary may dictate its surgical removal.

Deane J in *Marion's Case* satisfied himself with a broader distinction.[14]

> 11...the phrases "therapeutic surgery" and "non-therapeutic surgery" have been used to distinguish between surgery for the traditional medical purpose of preserving life or directly treating or preventing physical illness and surgery for other or wider purposes, such as the enhancement or preservation of the quality of life.

Clinical Criteria and "The Pace of Social Change"

Let us examine one, but the most common, example of "intersex", both antenatally and at birth.

The current definitive medical statement about the exact point of surgical intervention in the case of one (the most common) form of intersex, CAH, is the *Consensus Statement on* 21-*Hydroxylase Deficiency* from the Lawson Wilkins Paediatric Endocrine Society and the European Society for Paediatric Endocrinology.[15]

> *Genital surgery.* The decision about surgery should be made by the parents, together with the clinical team, after complete disclosure of all relevant clinical information and all available options have been discussed and after informed consent has been obtained.
>
> The goals of surgery are: 1) genital appearance compatible with gender; 2) unobstructed urinary emptying without incontinence or infections; and 3) good adult sexual and reproductive function.
>
> Once a decision has been made to raise a newborn as female, surgery for those with virilized genitalia caused by CAH is recommended when the patient has a high proximal junction between the vagina and urethra.

Of these criteria, only criterion (2) positively indicates surgery in the interests of the patient. The other two criteria indicate surgery depends either on the

---

[14] *See* footnote 3.

[15] JOINT LWPES/ESPE CAH WORKING GROUP Writing Committee: Peter E. Clayton, Royal Manchester Children's Hospital, Manchester, United Kingdom; Walter L. Miller*, University of California, San Francisco, California; Sharon E. Oberfield, Columbia University, New York, New York; E. Martin Ritze'n, Karolinska Institute, Stockholm, Sweden; Wolfgang G. Sippell*, University, J Clin Endocrinol Metab, September 2002, 87(9):4048–4053, 4049, http://jcem.endojournals.org/cgi/content/full/87/9/4048. Accessed 28 June 2009). To consider the evidence for best practice, to formulate management guidelines, and to consider innovative therapies, The Lawson Wilkins Pediatric Endocrine Society (LWPES) and The European Society for Pediatric Endocrinology (ESPE) convened a meeting in Gloucester, MA, 14–17 March, 2002. The 40 participating physicians, psychologists, scientists, and surgeons from 12 countries on 4 continents agreed with the [following] consensus statement; this statement is concerned exclusively with CAH caused by 21-hydroxylase deficiency and does not address the other, rarer forms of CAH.

capacity of the parents to manage their own emotions and beliefs about gender or what the patient experiences as "good sex", a fact unlikely to be known until adolescence or puberty at the earliest.

The Consensus Statement assumes that the mechanism and the process for making that decision are unproblematic, as if "high proximal junction" is a question of objective fact rather than subjective value-laden judgment affected by the degree of parental stress. It then continues:

> When the degree of virilization is less (minimal clitoromegaly and the junction between the vagina and urethra near the perineum), surgery may not be necessary. In such cases, the decision to operate should be based on appropriate contrast studies of the urinary tract and examination under anesthesia, with cystoscopy. Surgery to reduce clitoral size requires careful consideration. Total removal of the clitoris should never be performed. If clitoral reduction is elected, it is crucial to preserve the neurovascular bundle, the glans, and the preputial skin related to the glans. The early operation should be a one-stage complete repair using the newest techniques of vaginoplasty, clitoral, and labial surgery and should be carried out at a center with experience of at least 3–4 cases/yr. Revision vaginoplasty is often required at adolescence, and the timing should be decided with the patient and family.
>
> It is recognized that 46,XX children with significant virilization may present at a later age. Consideration for sex reassignment must be undertaken only after thorough psychological evaluation of patient and family. Surgery appropriate to gender assignment should be undertaken after a period of endocrine treatment.
>
> *Psychological issues.* Females with CAH show behavioral masculinization, most pronounced in gender role behavior, less so in sexual orientation, and rarely in gender identity… As the pace of societal change, including the flexibility of gender role, increases, more frequent review of management policies and long-term outcomes is important.

Intersex organizations have observed that intersex people were not involved in the development of the Consensus Statement. To that extent, it is a clinical guide, more in the nature of an engineering manual than an ethical treatise.

It can also be observed increasingly in today's context that children, young children and babies or independent advocates of their separate interests, also were not involved in the development of the Consensus Statement. To that extent, it assumes the consent of the parent equates with the consent of the patient up to an uncertain "later age" and focuses on psychological counselling. It does not purport to be an examination of human rights or of the legal validity of the parental consent. In other words, the Consensus Statement itself sits a bit uncomfortably with societal change, recognizing "the pace of societal change, including the flexibility of gender role".

Whilst the Consensus Statement has the appearance of balance and careful deliberation, it still proceeds from a reductionist clinical perspective on how to "fix" a perceived social, psychological, and cultural problem and maintain a strictly binary gender system as the cultural milieu in which the decision is to be made. The distinction between the interests of the "client" parent and the "patient" child becomes blurred.

The complexity of the ethical and rights issues involved is exemplified in the facts of a family reported by van Mil and Hiort in 2008.

> Physical examination showed a Caucasian child with pinkish-brown skin colour who was normally proportioned and had no dysmorphic features. Stretched phallic length was not

measured initially and the urethral opening could not be localised. …Ultrasound examination showed the presence of uterus and ovaries.

The karyotype in combination with an increased 17-hydroxyprogesterone (17OHP) confirmed the likely diagnosis of a 46,XX DSD with androgen excess caused by congenital adrenal hyperplasia (CAH) due to 21-hydroxylase deficiency. The parents were informed of the diagnosis and rearing of a female sex was agreed. Treatment with hydrocortisone was started. …A diagnosis of classical salt losing CAH was confirmed with 129 mmol/l serum sodium. Fluorocortisone and sodium chloride supplements were added to the treatment regimen. …Genetic testing was suggested to absolutely confirm the diagnosis, but this offer was rejected by the parents. The infant was subsequently discharged from hospital…

A vaginoplasty and clitoral reduction was performed at 1 month of age. The family was then lost to follow up until the mother re-presented in her second pregnancy at 14-weeks gestation. Dexamethasone treatment was started immediately, but was stopped at 20-weeks gestation because a prenatal ultrasound performed at another hospital showed a male foetus. It was recommended that dexamethasone treatment be continued until chorionic villus sampling could confirm the male karyotype. However, this advice was not accepted [by the parents] and a healthy male infant was delivered at term.

During the third pregnancy, the parents did not opt for dexamethasone treatment because of potential side effects, and genetic testing was also declined for religious reasons. The infant was delivered at home, but the midwife admitted the child to hospital because of ambiguous genitalia. Subsequent tests confirmed 46,XX DSD due to CAH in a severely virilised child (Prader stage IV). Despite having two girls with CAH, the parents did not choose dexamethasone at the next pregnancy. Home delivery was again chosen and this time genetic testing was undertaken on cord blood. A male infant was born with CAH, as confirmed by a classic mutation in the *CYP21A2* gene.

Discussion…Initially, the parents appeared to be more preoccupied with how to explain the DSD problem to their relatives and family, than what the future held for their child. In certain cultural settings, the religious scholar is invited to join the MDT in discussions with the family. In the present case, the parents were strongly of the opinion that their daughter should have surgery as early as possible. There has been much debate on the timing and extent of surgery in CAH. The age between 2 and 6 months coincides with a period when the tissues in the vaginal wall are oestrogen stimulated from the transient rise in gonadotrophins, which improves wound healing. It is generally accepted that performing surgery at 1 month of age is too early. The emphasis of surgery is now focused more on outcome of sexual function in adulthood, recognizing that the clitoris is highly innervated and can be damaged during clitoroplasty. Clitoral reduction surgery is no longer undertaken for mild clitoromegaly (Prader stages I and II), but there remains no consensus on the timing for any surgery and whether vaginoplasty should be performed early or late.

In this discussion, van Mil and Hiort discuss some of the clinical considerations and improved wound healing at 2–6 months is the indicator identified as the one relevant to the timing of surgery, not whether it should be done at all. They discuss at length the parents' concerns both social and religious, but absent from both the multi-disciplinary team (MDT) and the parents' considerations was any counter view that the endocrine therapy could be continued until the children were older. The outcome was that leaving all decisions to the parents in all four cases produced one surgery earlier than optimum, one outcome better than the clinicians had expected, another ambiguous outcome that could have been minimized if the parents had not refused pre-natal investigation and treatment, and a male child with CAH.

Other Clinical Criteria

Three other criteria that have been adopted are:

1. Whether proposed surgery reduces a risk of cancer in a vestigial gonad.

There are unquantifiable risks to be balanced here: the statistical (not individual) risk of cancer if the gonads are retained, the risk of such cancer commencing before puberty when the child can be engaged in the debate about their body, the risk of the adolescent identifying as a male and resenting their removal, then requiring ongoing testosterone therapy to maintain some equivalence between body and soul; the risk of teenage depression and suicide.

The view of an academic Board Member of OII Australia by the name of "Chris Somers XXY" is a view worth noting, urging a combination of urgency, risk, and the need for continuing care:[16]

> If all women per se had their breasts removed for the simple reason there are roughly 9 % of the total population who have some predisposition towards breast cancer; then everyone should have their breasts removed.

2. Whether the proposed surgery is reversible or irreversible.

This is important for external ambiguities in both CAH and AIS (and other conditions). It may be that, in a given case, the urethra exits within the vagina or at the base of the penis/clitoris and that surgery on a tiny person involves a lesser quantity of surgery than on an 8 years old or a 14 years old. Either way, the surgery is irreversible and, if risks of backflow and UTI can be managed until the child is old enough to take part in the discussion, the question is as ambivalent as the anatomy. In the case of some hypospadias, it is said that the surgery to exit the urethra at the tip of the phallus is reversible. But, all surgery causes pain and leaves scar tissue, and carries risk of complication and usually side-effects. If ordinary function is possible until the child (probably earlier than 8) is able to express a view, who should make this discretionary decision in infancy?

3. Other medical but more avowedly subjective tests.

The Intersex Adult Perspective: OII

OII has a goal and a strategy:[17]

> We campaign against all non-consensual normalization treatments of infants that are not medically necessary and favour the right of all intersexed children to determine their own sex identity once they are capable of communicating it to us. Furthermore we advise parents to respect the sex identity of their children and to do all that is necessary so that their children can live according to their choice.

---

[16] Email to OII Australia, copied to author dated 29 July 2009.

[17] http://www.intersexualite.org/English-Offical-Position.html.

> Once the child has communicated clearly their own sex identity, it is crucial that the child's identity be respected both by the parents, physicians and therapists who are caring for the child. All steps should be taken to respect the child's own sense of self by being given access to all health care necessary to facilitate life in the sex the child considers most appropriate.
>
> Therefore, we are campaigning in favour of changing the current medical paradigm concerning non-consensual normalisation treatments and against the diagnosis of gender dysphoria or GID in intersex individuals who feel they were assigned the wrong sex. OII affirms that the true sex of the child is determined by its own inner psychological perceptions and that the right of individual intersex persons to affirm their own sex without medical or governmental interference should be a basic human right.

11.3 What Are Rights?

Power theory informs much of existing western law, policy, and practice and is linked to why modern socio-legal systems employ the psycho-legal construct of "competence" as the mediator of young people's and children's rights claims.

It is the essence of the "power" or "will" theory of rights that a "right" is the power to exercise control over someone else: e.g., to enforce your right to cast a vote if you qualify under an electoral law or to stop someone injuring you (Hart 1982).

When such "will" or "power" is predicated on the capacity to exercise such choices, then it is often argued that children by virtue of their immaturity–like intellectually disabled people of all ages–only possess such rights as can be exercised vicariously by competent guardians (Richard 1993).

However, even "power"/"will" theorists are driven to recognize that some rights do not require abilities or personal competencies, e.g., housing, food and shelter. A distinction arises between rights for which one has to qualify and those for which one does not, in other words "welfare" rights vs "liberty" rights, or "participation rights" versus "protection rights" (Framilin 1995; Carney 1992). "Liberty rights" (such as rights to enjoy liberty itself and self-determination) still require a child or young person to satisfy a significant array of prerequisites before becoming entitled to the right.

On the other hand, says Bartholomew (2009), "protection rights" might also be termed "interest rights", "those that require the rights holder to have interests that can be served, protected, and promoted".

Bartholomew conducted an interesting study of "competence" as mediator of decisions by 305 randomly selected GPs in Victoria, Australia, to offer requested medical services to 14 years-old girls, namely prescribing oral contraceptives in confidence from the patient's parents.

Bartholomew makes the point that, while few theorists would deny a young person's rights to "welfare" or "protection", power or will theorists still assemble "a significant array of prerequisites" before young people become entitled to "participation" or "liberty" rights. Bartholomew's study showed many GPs unquestioningly refusing the service, some likewise providing it and some in the middle qualifying the provision of the service by reference to their personal perception of "the best interests" of the patient.

But what of pre-verbal infants? Whilst rights theorists posit that these babies have "protection rights" or "interest rights" requiring no competency qualification, the questions begged are "protection from whom?" and "what interest personal to the baby?".

This chapter explores the right of babies and "Gillick incompetent"[18] minors to protection from "unnecessary" genital surgery.

11.4 The Clinical/Legal Interface Identified

11.4.1 David Reimer/Brenda–John Money and the Debate About Brain Sex

During his professional life, Money was respected as an expert on sexual behavior, especially for allegedly demonstrating that gender was learned rather than innate. Many years later, however, it was revealed that his most famous case was the result of fraudulent reporting on the part of Money.

The subject of Money's fraud was his involvement in the sex reassignment of David Reimer. Money reported that he successfully reassigned Reimer as female after a botched 1966 infant circumcision. In 1997, Milton Diamond reported that the reassignment had failed, that Reimer had never identified as female or behaved typically feminine. At age 14, Reimer, who had fought against being forced to see Dr. Money since age 7, refused to see Money again, threatening suicide if he were made to go. Reimer's parents then decided to tell Reimer the truth about his past and his biological sex. Reimer immediately ended the hormone treatments he had been forced to undergo to stimulate female sex traits, and began hormones to bring about the male puberty prevented by the removal of his testes by Dr. Money. He ceased using the name, Brenda, which his parents had chosen for him after he began treatment with Dr. Money, and chose a new name, David, for himself. At 15, with a different medical team, he sought a mastectomy, testosterone therapy, and a phalloplasty. Later, he married a woman who had children from a previous marriage and lived as a man until his suicide in 2004 at age 38 (Diamond and Sigmundson 1997).

Money's theories led to the acceptance in the 1960s of three "givens" in paediatric practice at the time:

> Gender identity and sex differences were solely a matter of social learning rather than biology.
>
> A male with a penis too small to put into a vagina could not find a satisfactory social and sexual place in society.
>
> A functionally "acceptable" vagina could be constructed surgically.

These axioms still have historical influence on modern clinical thinking.

---

[18] Gillick v West Norfolk AHA (1986) AC 112.

11.4.2 Re A [In re A (1993) 16 Fam LR 715]

Professor Warne, in his paper, is guilty of setting up a classic straw man: the closing paragraphs of his paper about misguided and untrusting "activists" refers to a common confusion of transexualism with intersex. He dismisses the Australian Family Court case of Alex as being irrelevant to the issues, as if some imaginary "activists" had suggested it was. The case that is truly relevant is that of A, not Alex:

A was born with Congenital Adrenal Hyperplasia (CAH) resulting in megaloclitoris. His condition was described as "extreme," his clitoris exactly like a penis, and his labia fused over, like an empty scrotum. His older sister was also born with CAH but had no surgery. Genetically, he was 46,XX but at about 12 months he was, on the authority of his parents and the advice of his own medical advisers, genitally reconstructed to give him feminine appearance. He was also given cortisone to suppress the continuing output of excess male hormone. His parent brought him up as a girl, to no avail. In 1993, he presented to the court, at the age of 14, he was feeling like a boy and experienced pain in his surgically reconstructed clitoris when it became erect. Through his parents, he sought authorization for a double mastectomy, radical hysterectomy, and oophorectomy, extension of the clitoris, closing of the labia, and construction of a scrotum with prosthetic testes, and continuing hormone therapy.

The Court agreed, mainly on the basis that, although the processes were irreversible, "the most important matter of concern" was A's psychological and emotional state. He had experienced suicidal thoughts and continuing him as a male in a female body was likely to have devastating consequences if the Court waited until he turned 18 and could make his own choices *sui juris.*

This kid had to go through not one but two major surgical procedures on his most private parts. Whilst Warne and the surgeons would try to characterize this case as one of transexualism, not intersex, it would be disingenuous to deny the possibility that the boy was always a "boy" even when they made the "right decision" and shaped him as a girl. To me, it is a perfect example of what OII describes as him being neither a girl nor a boy but himself.

11.5 "Parental Rights"–Parental Consent as a Mediator of Surgical Assault: Children's Rights Held on Trust

11.5.1 Parental "Rights" and "The Pace of Social Change"

Parental rights were once "more absolute" than they are now. The law is changing and the direction in which it has been changing over the last 20 years has been in favour of the child's "interests" or "protection" rights which do not require him/her to prove any fact in order to assert. It is unsafe to rely on older authority about the balance between parental and children's rights, especially since the late 20th century analysis of rights both conceptually and in terms of international treaty law has increasingly subsumed the human rights culture of the post WWII period.

In *Gillick*, Lord Fraser said this:

> It was, I think, accepted both by Mrs. Gillick and by the D.H.S.S. and in any event I hold, that parental rights to control a child do not exist for the benefit of the parent. They exist for the benefit of the child and they are justified only insofar as they enable the parent to perform his duties towards the child, and towards other children in the family. If necessary, this proposition can be supported by reference to *Blackstone Commentaries*, 17th ed. (1830), Vol. 1, p. 452, where he wrote "The power of parents over their children is derived from…their duty,"

And Lord Scarman said in relation to parental rights:

> But the common law has never treated such rights as sovereign or beyond review and control. Nor has our law ever treated the child as other than a person with capacities and rights recognised by law. The principle of the law, as I shall endeavour to show, is that parental rights are derived from parental duty and exist only so long as they are needed for the protection of the person and property of the child.

In *Marion's Case*,[19] Justice Deane noted the common law pronounced by His Lordship Vice-Chancellor Bacon as recently as 110 years before, "the sacred right of a father over his own children"[20] up until the age of majority–then, of course, 21 years of age:

> Thus, it was said by Sir William Brett, MR, in In re Agar-Ellis; Agar-Ellis v. Lascelles(198) (1883) 24 ChD 317 that a father was merely "insisting upon his right" when he refused to allow a daughter who was nearly seventeen "to live with her mother, and (had) put her into many and various places to live" (at p 324).
>
> The actual decision in In re Agar-Ellis was based on an assertion of almost absolute paternal authority until the age of twenty-one(201) i.e., that it was "the law of England… that the father has the control over the person, education, and conduct of his children until they are twenty-one years of age…The guiding principle was said to be that "when, by birth, a child is subject to a father…the Court should not, except in very extreme cases, interfere with the discretion of the father, but leave to him the responsibility of exercising that power which nature has given him by the birth of the child".

Justice Deane identifies the march of history.

> For one thing the basis of that extreme view [that parental authority persists unabated until a child attains full adulthood] was not merely that the father enjoyed the right of legal guardianship. It was a perception of "the natural rights of a father" which were "greater… than those which a testamentary guardian, or any other guardian, can have" (205) per Brett MR, ibid., at p 327. That perception could not survive, without significant qualification, either the law's recognition, under the impetus of legislative developments, that the position of the father in relation to a child was "not superior to that of the mother" (206) Storie v. Storie [1945] HCA 56; (1945) 80 CLR 597, at p 608, or the law's increasing insistence that, while it is commonly convenient and accurate to speak of parental "authority" and parental "powers," the relationship between parents and a child is, from the parents' point of view, more appropriately expressed in terms of duty (207) See, e.g., J v. Lieschke [1987] HCA 4; (1987) 162 CLR 447, at pp 458, 463; Gillick v. West Norfolk AHA (1986)

[19] Secretary of the Department of Health and Community Services v JWB and SMB (1992) 15 Fam LR 392 at pages 439–440.

[20] Re Plomley; Vidler v. Collyer (1882) 47 LT (N.S.) 283, at p 284.

AC, at p 184; Report by Justice, the British Section of the International Commission of Jurists, Parental Rights and Duties and Custody Suits (1975), pp 6-7; Dingwall, Eekelaar and Murray, The Protection of Children (1983), p 224.

His Honor then identified two broad modern propositions, which although he was in the minority, were inherent to the reasoning of the majority:

> The first of those propositions is that parental authority exists to authorise such surgery *for the purpose, and only for the purpose, of advancing the welfare of the child.* It does not extend to authorizing surgery because of a perception that it is in the interests of those responsible for the care of the child or in the interests of society in general (e.g., for eugenic reasons). That which constitutes the welfare of a child in a particular case falls to be determined by reference to general community standards, but making due allowance for the entitlement of parents, within the limits of what is permissible in accordance with those standards, to entertain divergent views about the moral and secular objectives to be pursued for their children.
>
> The second broad proposition is that, at least in relation to a serious matter such as a major medical procedure, *parental authority can be validly exercised only after due inquiry* about, and adequate consideration of, what truly represents the welfare of the child in all the circumstances of the case.

So the right of the parent no longer qualifies as an "interest" right or "liberty" right, but is rather one for which the parent not the child has to satisfy "a significant array of prerequisites"[21] before he or she becomes entitled to exercise it.

On the other hand, as we have seen, the child's right to protection is a "liberty" or "interest" right that derives from the child's individual human right to nurturance and protection, common to all humans. It requires the rights holder to have only an interest that can be served.

We no longer have an irresistible force and a yielding object. We do not even have an irresistible force and an immovable object. We have a yielding force (the right of the parent) and an immovable object (the right of the child).

11.5.2 Gillick-Competence and the Emergence of a Right of Genital Autonomy

Especially in the intersex arena, the age at which a child can understand the importance of medical options depends as much on the complexity of the condition as the age of the child. There is no point asking a child with vestigial gonads whether a biopsy is a good idea, but there remains every point in waiting till they reach puberty to ask them if they want to remain fertile, or to have genitals shaped like most other boys or most other girls.

The statement of Lord Scarman in *Gillick v West Norfolk Area Health Authority*[22] is the locus classicus of the legal determinant of a child or young per-

[21] Bartholomew, op cit page 6.

[22] Gillick v West Norfolk AHA (1986) AC 122.

son to give or withhold consent to medical treatment. Mrs Gillick sought a declaration that a pamphlet issued by the Health Authority that purported to authorize medical practitioners to give contraceptive advice and prescriptions to children independently of their parents' knowledge and consent was unlawful, on the basis that it was incorrect. His Lordship said:[23]

> Parental rights... do not wholly disappear until the age of majority....But the common law has never treated such rights as sovereign or beyond review and control. Nor has our law ever treated the child as other than a person with capacities and rights recognised by law. The principle of the law...is that parental rights are derived from parental duty and exist only so long as they are needed for the protection of the person and property of the child.
>
> A minor is, according to this principle, capable of giving informed consent when he or she achieves a sufficient understanding and intelligence to enable him or her to understand fully what is proposed.

That was the passage adopted by the majority in Marion's Case when they constructed the now Australia-wide binding principle of common law based on the limits of parental "power" rather than "right".[24]

So modern Australian law is that "parental right" really is a misnomer; the right exists as against third parties but does not automatically exist as against the child's rights; the parent's right is moderated by qualification and is therefore a "welfare" or "participation" right of the parent, rather than a "liberty" or "protection" right as explained at the outset of this chapter. The reverse is true of the child's right in the surgical setting.

It follows that the "right" of the parent and the "right" of the child do not coincide. In other words, the "right" of the parent to give a valid consent to surgery will conflict with the "right" of the child in all but the clearest case, namely where the child's life or immediate protection from harm is threatened.

It is my argument that the distinction is not so clear-cut, and that the decision of what is and is not medically unnecessary for an infant and immediately blurs the distinction considerably, as does the "pace of social change".

The question seems to be emerging not as who had rights over the bodies of children historically, but as who makes the decision nowadays?

11.5.3 What Consent to Surgery is Outside the Ordinary Authority of a Parent...

It must never be forgotten that Gillick was decided in 1986 and *Marion*'s *Case* in 1993. At the time of Gillick, there were no Microsoft Windows, mobile phones, or disposable cameras or Internet, and the hole in the ozone layer had not been

---

[23] Lord Scarman, Gillick v West Norfolk AHA (1986) AC 122 at pages 183–184; see also page 189, 194–195.

[24] Secretary of the Department of Health and Community Services v JWB and SMB (1992) 15 Fam LR 392 at 400.

discovered. In the year of *Marion*'s *Case*, the High Court handed down the *Mabo* decision, but GPS was not invented, nor LED lights, vaccine for Hepatitis A, nor had the human genome been sequenced. The "pace of societal change" has not only continued but has accelerated.

In Australia, the law since *Marion*'s Case is clear that, regardless of the child's Gillick-competence, there is an undefined class of medical treatments that, by their nature, are beyond the authority of parents to authorize. Without the authority of the parents and without the authority of the Court, any treatment that involves the administration of drugs or the touching of the patient lacks valid consent and constitutes an assault.

So, what surgery does fall outside the ordinary authority of a parent to consent to, at least where the child is incapable of understanding the purpose and nature of the procedure, or is incapable of expressing opposition to it?

The Majority in *Marion's Case* set out [25] what has since been taken as the *ratio decidendi* of the case:

> ...sterilisation requires invasive, irreversible and major surgery. But so do, for example, an appendectomy and some cosmetic surgery, both of which, in our opinion, come within the ordinary scope of a parent to consent to. However, other factors exist which have the combined effect of marking out the decision to authorise sterilisation as a special case. *Court authorisation is required, first, because of the significant risk of making the wrong decision, either as to a child's present or future capacity to consent or about what are the best interests of a child who cannot consent, and secondly, because the consequences of a wrong decision are particularly grave* [my emphasis].

What does that value-laden expression "grave" mean? The Majority explained this:[26]

> The gravity of the consequences of wrongly authorising a sterilisation flows both from the resulting inability to reproduce *and from the fact of being acted upon contrary to one's wishes or best interests* [my emphasis]. The fact of violation is likely to have social and psychological implications concerning the person's sense of identity, social place and self-esteem. As the Court said in *In re Grady* (1981) NJ 426 A 2d, at pp 471–472, a decision to sterilise involves serious questions of a person's "social and biological identity"....
>
> The far-reaching consequences of a general rule of law allowing guardians to consent to all kinds of medical treatment, as well as the consequences of a wrong decision in any particular case, are also relevant. As Nicholson C.J. pointed out in *Re Jane* in the passage quoted earlier (1988) 94 FLR, at p 26; 85 ALR, at p 435; 12 Fam LR, at p 685; (1989) FLC, at p 77,256, such a rule may be used to justify other procedures such as a clitoridectomy or the removal of a healthy organ for transplant to another child.

From this passage, many commentators have distilled the following elements of infant surgery that require Court approval:

1. Invasive
2. Irreversible

[25] Secretary of the Department of Health and Community Services v JWB and SMB (1992) 15 Fam LR 392 at 410.

[26] Secretary of the Department of Health and Community Services v JWB and SMB (1992) 15 Fam LR 392 at 411.

3. Major
4. Significant risk of making the wrong decision as to
   a. the child's present or future capacity to consent *or*
   b. the child's present or future "best interests".
5. Particularly grave consequences of a "wrong" decision.

So if "grave" consequences of a wrong decision may flow where the "fact of violation…involves serious questions of a person's social and biological identity", sterilization by those criteria would seem to be no different from genital surgery, other than genital surgery to save a life or cure disease.

11.5.4 …and Who Decides?

Professor Warne correctly identified that the real issue is not what is "the right decision" but who makes it. He says the parents and the doctor. Saying it does not make it correct.

In *Marion's Case,* Justice Deane,[27] was content to leave the decision about *reversible* genital non-urgent surgery entirely to parents, and ventured briefly into the realm of rights, but in this he fell into the minority.

Approaching the validity of the parent's consent from the perspective of the parent results in circularity and internal inconsistency, and it is difficult or impossible in the clinical setting to extricate the distress of the parent from the rights of the child. This emerges from the next but one passage by His Honor:[28]

> Even in the area of surgery for other than conventional medical purposes, there are circumstances in which it plainly lies within the authority of the parents of an incapable child to authorize surgery on the basis of medical advice. Plastic surgery to correct serious disfigurement for purely cosmetic purposes is not "therapeutic" within the accepted meaning of that word "concerned with the treatment of disease, palliative or curative": Butterworth's Medical Dictionary, 2nd ed. (1978), p 1700 and constitutes an obvious example. Male circumcision for perceived hygienic–or even religious–reasons is another. On the other hand, one can think of equally obvious examples where parental authority would not extend to authorize surgery for other than conventional medical purposes even though it was thought by the parents to be for the ultimate welfare of an incapable child. The surgical amputation of the right hand of a child who was an habitual "pickpocket" might conceivably be seen by parents who were fanatical biblical literalists(225). See the Bible, New Testament, Mark 9:43 as being justified as conducive to the child's overall welfare. The authorization of such an operation would be beyond parental authority, however, for the reason that it could not, according to the standards of our society, properly be seen as so justified.

[27] *See* footnote 3.

[28] *See* footnote 4.

Justice Deane approached Marion's conundrum and that of her parents as if the seductively simple act of adopting a "best interests" perspective would itself provide an answer. His solution that a Court decision would be an unnecessary burden where surgery is in the interests of the child "according to general community standards" is circular and leaves he decision with anyone who thinks it is desirable even if not necessary. Judges make Family Law decisions every day that are lambasted in the tabloid press and by "shock jocks", so how does one gauge "community standards", let alone adduce evidence about them?[29]

He did however, hold the view adopted by the majority in relation to the narrow question of sterilization:

> In a case where such surgery is not obviously necessary, the need to protect an incapable child from unjustified surgery involving irreversible sterilization outweighs all other considerations. Notwithstanding the expense, inconvenience and other disadvantages of court proceedings, it appears to me that, in the absence of some special statutory procedure, such proceedings represent the only adequate protection.

This puts even him at odds with Professor Warne in the case of gonadectomy that the doctors think is unarguable.

The matter has clearly become not what is or is not in the best interests of the child, but rather who decides that.

11.6 Rights-Based Solutions

The search for consistency is the search for a stable framework through which to filter these difficult decisions. Clinicians, parents, and the Fourth Estate in "clear-cut" cases will utter an exasperated "pshaw!!" as if there could be any debate. On the other hand, it is hard cases that make hard law, and few clinicians and parents will brazenly declare that they consider themselves impervious to the rule of law. The role of law is to set a rule by which the easy and the hard can both be universally assessed; to draw the line.

Reliance on a "best interests" test alone, without a rights perspective, necessarily imports each individual decider's understanding in each individual case whether that particular procedure is inside or outside "community standards", that is whether or not the general procedure is or is not in the best interests of the individual child, whether that surgery is "normal" or "accepted".

A Rights-based approach has the potential to ensure the decision of the individual procedure, at this point in time, is in the best interests of the child or whether it can be deferred until the child is old enough to understand the procedure or ceases to be a child.

[29] *See* footnote 5.

11.6.1 2004 The Family Court of Australia

By contrast, the reasoning of the majority of the High Court of Austria in *Marion's Case* was not based on an objective assessment of clinical risk dictating "best interest" on the one hand, or nebulous and individualised notions of "best interests" in the sense usually applied in parenting cases of "what decision will produce the "best" outcome for the child?" on the other hand. They eventually settled on a rights analysis[30] but not the "right" one might have expected:

> One more thing should be said about the basis upon which we have concluded that sterilisation is a special case with respect to parental powers. As we have indicated, the conclusion relies on a fundamental right to personal inviolability existing in the common law, a right which underscores the principles of assault, both criminal and civil, as well as on the practical exigencies accompanying this kind of decision which have been discussed. Our conclusion does not, however, rely on a finding which underpins many of the judgments discussed; namely, that there exists in the common law a fundamental right to reproduce which is independent of the right to personal inviolability.

Since *Marion's Case*, the Family Court has implemented a set of court rules known as "Medical Procedure Applications".[31] The Rules are subordinate to the main Legislation the *Family Law Act* 1975 (*as amended*) so the paramountcy principle applies and, provided the Court has jurisdiction,[32] the Rules set out the evidence that must be adduced (Rule 4.09) and provide for urgent priority listing of the application (if possible within 14 days of filing the application) (Rule 4.11).

If there is no Independent Child Lawyer (representing the best interests of the child) one shall be appointed on the first return date of the application at a directions hearing. The Independent Child Lawyer is appointed notwithstanding the incapacity of most subject children to communicate, because the ICL has the role of representing the underlying interests of the child where they diverge from the interests affecting the other parties (usually the parents and the medical team or hospital).[33]

Rule 4.09 prescribes the evidence that must be adduced to satisfy the Court that the proposed procedure is in the best interest of the child. The evidence required–and which is expected to have been gathered before the application is filed for enabling an expedited decision–includes reports dealing with:

- The exact nature and purpose of the proposed procedure;
- The condition for which the procedure is required;
- The long-term physical, social, and psychosocial effects on the child (1) if the procedure is and (2) if it is not carried out;

[30] Per Mason CJ, Dawson, Toohey and Gaudron JJ. Secretary of the Department of Health and Community Services v JWB and SMB (1992) 15 Fam LR 392 at 412.

[31] These Applications are dealt with in Chap. 4 of the Family Law Rules 2004.

[32] Cf Minister for Immigration and Multicultural and Indigenous Affairs v B [2004] HCA 20 and P v P [1994] HCA 20.

[33] See Re K (1994) 17 Fam LR 537; FLC 92–461.

- If alternative and less invasive treatment is available the reasons the proposed procedure is recommended instead of the alternative treatments;
- Whether a child capable of making an informed decision agrees;
- Evidence of how an incapable child is otherwise incapable of making a decision;
- Whether the parents or caregiver agree.

A 1998 pamphlet issued by the Family Court of Australia *A Question of Right Treatment–Special Medical Procedures for Children*, does not have the force of a statute nor even a court rule but is rather a Factsheet for doctors, social workers, parents, and children's representatives. It gives as examples of Special Medical Procedures:

- Irreversible and sensitive procedures (e.g., sterilizations, tissue donation);
- Parents or guardians will not consent to medically necessary life-saving treatment;
- Parents or guardian are in dispute about a significant and medically recommended treatment;
- When a procedure is *ethically contentious* (my emphasis);
- When a child refuses life-saving treatment;
- When a parent or guardian does not want the child to continue with mechanically assisted life support.

"Ethically contentious" was not a phrase used by any of the judges in *Marion's Case*, but recalls Justice Deane's category of "not obviously necessary".

11.6.2 2005 San Francisco Human Rights Commission

In April 2005, the San Francisco Human Rights Commission investigated and reported on "normalization" therapies, including not only surgery but also suppressant therapies like antenatal administration of dexamethasone.

Their report[34] includes an instructive history of the US Intersex Rights Movement by Dr. Alice Dreger and Cheryl Chase, both founding members of the Intersex Society of North America, as it then was. It took evidence from 26 adult individuals who identified as intersex, including Mani Bruce Mitchell, Coordinator of the Intersex Trust of Aotearoa/New Zealand. The Commission made inter alia the following findings:

> 1. Infant genital surgeries and sex hormone treatments that are not performed for the treatment of physical illness, such as improving urinary tract or metabolic functioning, and

---

[34] A Human Rights Investigation into the Medical "Normalization" of Intersex People, Human Rights Commission of the County and City of San Francisco, 28 April 2005, located at www.sfgov.org/humanrights.

have not been shown to alleviate pain or illness (hereafter referred to as "normalizing" interventions) are unnecessary and are not medical or social emergencies.

2. "Normalizing" interventions done without the patient's informed consent are inherent human rights abuses.

3. "Normalizing" interventions deprive intersex people of the opportunity to express their own identity and to experience their own intact physiology.

10. "Normalizing" interventions performed to alleviate a parent's social discomfort about their child's intersex anatomy violate the patient's human rights.

14. "Normalizing" interventions violate most medical standards of informed consent, including the standards put forth by the United Nations' Commission on Human Rights, the American Convention on Human Rights, and the American Academy of Pediatrics' standards.

16. Parents have the right to provide informed consent for medical treatments that are necessary for the physical health of an intersex child, and not for "normalizing" procedures.

11.6.3 2009 Australian Human Rights Commission

The AHRC (formerly the Human Rights and Equal Opportunity Commission HREOC) seems to have taken the view that parents are the final arbiter of genital surgery on their babies.

In 2008–2009 the AHRC conducted an extensive review of the rights of intersex people, focusing on the disadvantages suffered by adult intersex people in relation to names, birth certificates, passports, and the myriad of government forms that ask the citizen to tick one of two boxes. In relation to surgery on intersex infants and human rights, they have published a July 2009 paper, *Surgery on intersex infants and human rights*,[35] which contains the seeds of the argument at the heart of this chapter.

11.7 Best Interests Meets Rights

11.7.1 1999 Constitutional Court of Columbia

Constitutional Court of Colombia in the jointly run matters of *Sentencia No. SU*-337/99 and *Sentencia No.* T-551/99.

The two sets of parents had given consent for infant intersex surgery but the surgeons had refused to accept that consent for fear of malpractice liability. The parents sought declarations and the Constitutional Court held that although it was–in that culture and time–the parents who had authority to give valid consent to

[35] Available at http://www.hreoc.gov.au/genderdiversity/surgery_intersex_infants2009.html. Accessed 5 August 2009.

what was otherwise a grievous assault. This mirrors the judgment of Deane J in *Marion's Case*.

However, the Columbia Constitutional Court decided that in order for that consent to be valid it had to be:

- In writing;
- Complete, that is, including the risks, other modalities of treatment, the effect and benefits of delay and psychological support to the children;
- Given more than once over a period of months.

For present purposes it is noteworthy from a rights perspective that the Court there adopted the view that

- intersex was not a disease;
- intersex did not need a "cure"; and
- the extra steps were dictated by the paramountcy principle of the best interests of the child.

There remains, however, in the judgment, the *non sequitur* that parents have a greater capacity to understand the issues and exercise the requisite authority than judges informed by expert evidence and responding to strong advocacy for the conflicting interests of the child.

11.7.2 2006 Julia Greenberg, Thomas Jefferson School of Law

In a superbly researched work, Julie Greenberg, Professor of Law at Thomas Jefferson School of Law, San Diego, California, [36] came up with what she described as the legal, ethical, and clinical "compromise" solution.

Greenberg identified three positions:

The Dominant Protocol, which is the medical model based on John Money's somewhat discredited work that relies on the wisdom of doctors as uniquely qualified to decide, and advising parents of the benefits of early surgery in order to obtain their consent. This is the model currently adopted by the American Academy of Pediatrics;[37]

The Moratorium Model, advocated for by the Intersex Groups, such as OII, IANZ, and AISSG; and *A Middle Ground Approach*, discussed by Daaboul and Frader (2001) which relies on parents being uniquely qualified to make these life-changing decisions for their babies, based on "true informed consent". In as

---

[36] Greenberg, Julie A. "International Legal Developments Protecting the Autonomy Rights of Sexual Minorities: Who Should Decide the Appropriate Treatment for an Intersex Child?" Ethics and Intersex 87, Sharon Sytsma, ed., Springer, 2006.

[37] "Policy Statement : Evaluation of the Newborn with Developmental Anomalies of the External Genitalia" 14 Pediatrics, 106 (July 2000) at 118.

much as this consent relies on information received (at least in part) from surgeons, this to me is a variant of the Dominant Protocol, but is the one adopted by the British College of Physicians. The source of the parents' authority in this model is notably unspoken, culturally based in what is "acceptable" at the time of the decision to operate. With the emergence of human rights in the 1970s, adults–including quite old adults–perceive through that prism that their rights of choice and personal autonomy were taken away by therapeutically unnecessary surgery when they were babies or elementary school age.[38]

Greenberg's chapter, after analyzing *Marion's Case* and the Australian and other intersex, gender dysphoria, and sex assignment of children cases, concludes that judges are not trained or competent to make the decisions themselves (a view I do not share when appropriate admissible evidence is before them).

Instead, Greenberg's article settles on recommending a formalised variant of an approach taken by the Constitutional Court of Colombia Greenberg suggests a "Middle Way" structure including:

- A permanent Committee (instead of a Court or Tribunal),
- Multidisciplinary with endocrinologists, pediatricians, psychologists, and sociologists as well as intersex adults who have undergone a range of different treatment modalities to advise the parents.
- Functions to provide guidance to the parents, ensure any consent is fully informed, and freely given in a stable psychological frame of mind; gather and present data on different modalities; provide continuing education of parents, intersex adults, and the medical profession.

Like a true lawyer, Greenberg concludes that the compromise is that which will displease everybody: the "knife-happy" will be forced to wait and will miss some surgery because some parents decide to adopt non-surgical approaches and the moratorium advocates will lose some infants to carefully and balanced informed consent by parents.

Like ms and intersex adults, but she still does not include an advocate for the child's interests in so far as they are distinguishable from the parents' interests and the clinicians interests. It needs to be repeated that it is the baby who is the patient, not the parent.

11.7.3 2006 Consensus Statement on Management of Intersex Disorders

Intersex activism and the legal significance of the independent rights of the child in the interpretation of what is "reasonable" and "tolerated by society" are likely to be increasing through the 21st Century, not abating. Professional associations and

---

[38] Refer to testimonials posted on OII, ASNA, AISSG websites.

ethics committees should be informing their members that without court or other tribunal authority doctors perform this kind of surgery at their professional peril.

The Consensus Statement recognizes this as a social force. The greatest advance made by the Consensus Statement is to open up the "right decision" to ideas beyond the immediate and allowing the voice of the child indirectly in the formalization of the need for an inter-disciplinary team:

> The Multidisciplinary Team
>
> Optimal care for children with DSD requires an experienced multidisciplinary team that is generally found in tertiary care centers. Ideally, the team includes pediatric subspecialists in endocrinology, surgery, and/or urology, psychology/psychiatry, gynecology, genetics, neonatology, and, if available, social work, nursing, and medical ethics.22 Core composition will vary according to DSD type, local resources, developmental context, and location. Ongoing communication with the family's primary care physician is essential.23 The team has a responsibility to educate other health care staff in the appropriate initial management of affected newborns and their families. For new patients with DSD, the team should develop a plan for clinical management with respect to diagnosis, gender assignment, and treatment options before making any recommendations. Ideally, discussions with the family are conducted by one professional with appropriate communication skills.24 Transitional care should be organized with the multidisciplinary team operating in an environment that includes specialists with experience in both pediatric and adult practice.

The team approach increases the prospects of parents having space to consider: in the case of CAIS "Parental choice allows deferment until adolescence, recognizing that the earliest reported malignancy in CAIS is at 14 years of age".

11.7.4 2009 5th World Congress on Family Law and Children's Rights, Halifax, Nova Scotia 23–25 August 2009

Resolution 6 of The World Congress followed the protocol of the Murdoch Institute and the Melbourne Royal Children's Hospital almost to the very letter, but with two important differences.

The Congress resolved that it:

A. encourages the adoption of the ethical practices and principles of the Royal Children's Hospital, Melbourne, those principles being:
   - I. Minimize physical risk to child;
   - II. Minimize psycho-social risk to child;
   - III. Preserve potential for fertility;
   - IV. Preserve or increase capacity to have satisfying sexual relations;
   - V. Leave options open for the future; and
   - VI. Consider the wishes and beliefs of the parents.

B. notes the debate as to whether issues of disorders of sexual development should be left to the time when the child attains Gillick competence, even in terms of therapeutic intervention.

The nuances lay in the departure from the Royal's principle VI which reads "respect the wishes and belief of the parents". The word "respect", as one of its connotations, has the meaning "follow". Parents cannot be trusted to make "the right decision" any more than doctors, largely because the parents are shocked to be told that the sex is unclear. Shocked is a classic medical understatement: they will usually be stunned, overwhelmed, terrified for their child, for their grandchildren, for themselves as they try to explain to their own families and friends. In the 6–8 short days Professor Warne gives them to make "the right decision", will they have utterly overcome their alarm, be placid, and rational, or will they do whatever the doctor thinks best?

Does this not mean that the decision of the parents is in reality the decision of the doctor or the professional team assembled to advise them? And, how can the doctor, who sees him or herself as one amongst equals with the rest of the multidisciplinary team, be objectively satisfied that the parents do not regard him or her as the god-head, the principal decider of the team?

11.8 Conclusion

It is the argument of this chapter that sex assigning genital surgery on children is:

- invasive (the clinical perspective),
- irreversible (the welfare perspective),
- serious (the cultural perspective),
- not always medically necessary at the time nominated by the professional team.

Further, doctors have made "wrong" decisions in the past and the best practice Consensus Statement makes it clear that many determining factors remain unknown, uncertain or unknowable. To the same extent that they are still shocked and ignorant, parents are likely to be conflicted between their own fears and shame on the one hand and their obligation to the child to make the "right decision" on the other.

When doctors and parents come to acknowledge that their professional and emotional interests do not coincide with those of the baby, they will be able to accept the role of the community in protecting the rights of those without a voice.

Although a minority judge in *Marion's Case*, Justice McHugh articulated the conflict of inherent interest between the parents and the child using a test of objectivity, but without identifying by whom or how that conflict is to be resolved:[39]

> One other matter needs to be noted. The powers which the parent exercises on behalf of the child are exercised in the course of a fiduciary relationship(299) See the description of a "fiduciary" in Hospital Products Ltd. v. United States Surgical Corporation [1984] HCA 64; (1984) 156 CLR 41, at pp 96–97. At all events, the role of the parent, when acting for

[39] Per McHugh J. Secretary of the Department of Health and Community Services v JWB and SMB (1992) 15 Fam LR 392 at 458.

> the benefit of his or her child, and the role of a fiduciary are sufficiently similar to make at least some of the principles concerning fiduciaries applicable to the parent–child relationship. Thus, in principle, a parent can have no authority to act on behalf of his or her child where a conflict arises between the interests of the parent and the interests of the child.

For a proposed protocol that is rights based yet more balanced by proper medical concern for the infant's immediate and medium term physical and mental health, I turned to another of the intersex lobby groups:

AISSG Australia has published [40] a Preferred Treatment Paradigm For Children With Intersex Conditions:

> The AIS Support Group Australia supports calls for a moratorium on non-urgent medical intervention in children with intersex conditions. This includes gonadectomies on children with AIS and clitoral recession, but does not mean all surgeries should be stopped completely. The preferred treatment paradigm of the AIS Support Group Australia is simple:

1. Obtain an accurate diagnosis from an expert in intersex conditions–preferably an experienced paediatric endocrinologist.
2. Raise the child as a boy or a girl–depending on medical advice and with the complete support of the parents.
3. Give parents complete information about their child's condition. A booklet describing the condition is best so they can refer to it if they have any questions between doctor visits.
4. Offer the parents and any other family members peer support and professional counselling.
5. If surgery is medically required, discuss all treatment options with the parents, including the consequences of not having the surgery. Ensure parents are given the opportunity to ask questions and seek support and counselling. A period of several weeks to consider alternatives is also advised if medically possible.
6. Ideally a child should be educated about their condition in stages as they become old enough to understand certain concepts.
7. When a child with an intersex condition is around 12 years old (or just prior to puberty), they should be given professional counselling and told about options to treat their condition. Counselling should also include an opportunity for the child to openly discuss their gender. This will give those raised in the incorrect gender an opportunity to voice this to the counsellor.
8. From this point on, the child's consent should be given for any further medical intervention, including hormone therapy.
9. If the diagnosis of an intersex condition is made later in life, doctors should still provide their patient with complete disclosure and offer the contact details of the AIS Support Group Australia.

This paradigm still relies on the perceived commonalty of purpose and good intentions of all involved which, as the Bay of Pigs near-disaster showed, could engender erroneous "group-think" blind to conflicts of interest.

To the AISSG list, I would merely add:

10. If irreversible surgery or irreversible endocrine therapy is proposed to commence before the child's 18th birthday, that an application be made for the authority or approval of a suitably informed and expeditious court or tribunal of competent

[40] AISSG Preferred Treatment Paradigm For Children With Intersex Conditions [monogram], 28/3/2003, AISSG Australia Inc., Altona Meadows, Australia.

jurisdiction, including as parties the parents, the child, and an independent representative for the child's separate interests.

The missing element from the Consensus Statement proposal remains the separate interest of the Child. Whilst increasingly recognizing the potential for deferment to include the understanding of the post-verbal child and to preserve options for that later time, it is still based on optimizing clinical outcomes and a hint of protecting professional territory. Even this model still avoids a built-in contradictor, a Devil's advocate embracing the rights of the child, a baby, teenager, and adult.

They do not, for instance, propose that an independent advocate for the separate interests of the child be included in the team or committee, a party, if you like, with a clear brief to argue the counterpoint, in jurisprudential terms a "contradictor".

The prognosis is good, however, that the medical world and the child rights and intersex community will soon be able to reach common ground when this hurdle of understanding is overcome.

References

OII Australia (2009) On Terminology. http://oiiaustralia.com/about/terminology/. Accessed 4 Aug 2009

Bartlomew T (2009) How general practitioners determine young people's rights. Youth Stud Aust. 28(2):5

Blackburn, Taylor (eds) (1991) Human rights for the 1990s. pp 90–91

Carney T (1992) "Reconciling the irreconcilable? A rights or interest based approach to controllability" in children, rights and the law. In: Parker S, Seymour J (eds) Alston P. Clarendon Press, Oxford, pp 119–125

Daaboul, Frader (2001) Ethics and the management of patients with intersex: the middle way. J Pediatr Endocrinol Metab 1575

Diamond M, Sigmundson HK (1997) Sex reassignment at birth: Long-term review and clinical implications. Arch Pediatr Adolesc Med 151(3):298–304

Diamond M, Sigmundson HK (2009) Op.cit cited at http://en.wikipedia.org/wiki/Intersexuality. Accessed 4 Aug 2009

Framilin B (1995) "The case for children's rights: a progress report" in the handbook of children's rights; comparative policy and practice. In: Franklin B (ed) Routledge, New York, pp 3–22

Goswami BA (2009) About the general scientific and medical use of the term "Intersex", OII Australia website, http://oiiaustralia.com/files/articles/term-intersex-term-dsd/. Accessed 4 Aug 2009

Hart H (1982) Essays on Bentham: studies in jurisprudence and political theory. Clarendon Press, Oxford

Marañón Gregorio (1929) Los estados intersexuales en la especie humana. Madrid: Morata

OII International (2009) http://www.intersexualite.org/Organisation_Intersex_International.html. Accessed 4 Aug 2009

OII Official Positions (2009) http://www.intersexualite.org/English-Offical-Position.html. Accessed 4 Aug 2009

Richard D (1993) Children, rights and childhood. Routledge, London

Van Mil E, Hiort O (2008) Three out of four: A case discussion on ambiguous genitalia. Eur J Endocrinol 159(1):S91–S93

Wollstonecraft MA (1792) Vindication of the rights of woman: with strictures on political and moral subjects

Author Biography

Paul Mason was appointed Commissioner for Children for the Australian State of Tasmanian in 2007. The Commissioner is a State appointment independent of the elected Government of the day, responsible for advising Government about all matters concerning the health, welfare, development, education of children and their protection from all forms of abuse and neglect. His other primary function is to raise public awareness about these matters. Before that, he had three decades' experience working in all areas of family law including complex parenting and child protection cases, both as a solicitor and barrister across Australia. He is deeply committed to the human rights of children and a strong believer in their capacity to make valuable contributions to all decisions affecting their welfare and development. Brisbane, Queenslan, Australia.

Chapter 12
The SAR/ROHAN (The Possession): A Response of Somali Women to Pharaonic Circumcision/Infibulation (PhC)

Pia Grassivaro Gallo, Stefania Gazzea and Antonio Iaria

Abstract The Somali rite of possession was interpreted by Lewis (1993) as a reaction of weak and marginalized people to the difficulties of the environment in which they are forced to live. They can be young shepherds isolated with the herds for a long period of time, divorced women neglected by their husbands, women who are still trying to survive or who are struggling to thrive in an urban environment, where they bear the heavy pressure of their family. The rite of possession is an instrument that allows women to attract attention in order to obtain material rewards they cannot normally gain. Our contribution presents the womens prayer to Allah in the *Timàn Adde* camp so that they can be freed from pharaonic circumcision (PhC). The prayer (*Dikrì*) has been included into the PhC Prevention Program prepared by Mana Sultan Abdurahman and has been practiced every Friday since 1977 in the Lower Scebelli. Women pray in a circle, singing, dancing, and eating together. In this way, they become the protagonists during this celebration day, in which they are all equally important and their difficult problems can be shared. In particular, our contribution, after having investigated the *sar* in its sociological, psychological, and anthropological aspects, presents four possession cases that occur during the *dikrì* of the women of Merka. These *sar* are testimonies of the difficult condition of Somali womens traditional life increased by new elements of suffering connected to the contingent situation.

Keywords Possession rite • Sar/Rohan in Somalia • Female genital cutting • Pharaonic circumcision/infibulation • Custom • Sociology • Anthropology • Psychology

12.1 Introduction

In 2007 in Merka (Lower Scebelli), Mana Abdurahman organized a Prevention Program against Pharaonic Circumcision (PhC) aimed to a change in tradition of excissory population: *in primis*, of mothers and grandmothers of the girls at risk,

P. Grassivaro Gallo (✉) · S. Gazzea · A. Iaria
Psychology, University of Padua, Padua, Italia
e-mail: pia.grassivaro@uipd.it

G. C. Denniston et al. (eds.), *Genital Cutting: Protecting Children from Medical, Cultural, and Religious Infringements*, DOI: 10.1007/978-94-007-6407-1_12,

rigid keepers of the tradition, and of all the other components of the extended family, including the male sector, which represents a relatively ambivalent role with regards to the custom.

The program uses a traditionally important moment of Somali women, the "*Mallin Jog*" ("Day of Being Together") (Dirie and Miller 1998, pp. 48–49; Hamed Sceh Nur, personal communication 2007; Sara Hamed Qali, personal communication 2007; Marian Ismail, personal communication 2007), proposed by Mana in the *Timàn Adde* camp. The meeting, held each Friday, assembles women of the close-by villages and the evacuees (IDP-Internal Displaced People) of Mogadish, to discuss their daily problems (Grassivaro Gallo 2009; Grassivaro Gallo and Busatta 2010).

The event in the video-cassette started with the *Dikrì* (Declich 2005, p. 65) a prayer of women to Allah for liberation from PhC. Literally, *dikrì* means "to mention God" but also includes marabouts and their attributes: it is an important liturgical act with Islamic origins that people perform with litanies and body movements. The protagonists are in circles and divided by gender, repeating litanies for hours, accompanied by rhythmic body movements and simultaneous body undulations. When chants and movements join a peak of excitation, some participants fall into a trance and are helped by the others. The rhythm decreases progressively, the excitation of the chants decreases, and the participants fall out of their trance.

The repetitive undulations leave little space for the creativity of the individual; creativity and free body movement are permitted only for those under a trance during the prayer.

In particular, during the *dikrì* of Merka, there were four cases of possession–*Sar/Rohan*–that aroused our interest. These cases were verified within the Prevention Program of PhC that had stimulated us to dig deeper into the possession rite called *Sar/Rohàn*. *Sar* for the better known Somali term and *Rohàn* for the term used by the women of Merka.

12.2 Overview of the Rite: The *Sar*: Definition, Origin, Spread

People believe that a supernatural being becomes reincarnated in the body of a specific person during possession; then other people force the being to leave the possessed body. The reincarnated supernatural being is called the Genius (*Zar* in amaric), the ancient name that was given at times to the celestial sky; in Somalia, it is translated as *Sar.*

The phenomenon of possession in the Somali tribes resulted from special rites, but very often was simply the spontaneous result following a collective state of excitement. Traditionally, the possession occurred during particular conditions of psychic exaltation of the solitary nomad as well as in the crowded reunions during the tribe assembly (Curia 1998/1999, p. 111). In the trance, the final rite is to expel the genius and to restore the individual back into his normal state.

The rhythm is particularly important for the possession. Each dancer is possessed by a specific spirit who has its own rhythm and specific type of dance. Generally, the possessed fall to the ground, become senseless, and start to shake and move slowly; then, gently they rise and start to dance to the rhythm designated by the chant. In this manner, people can liberate themselves gradually from the possession.

The possession rites occur throughout the East African coast, Egypt, North Africa and along the Arabic Peninsula as far as Iran. Although called with different names, its origins come from Ethiopia. Probably it was established simultaneously with the slave trade on the coast of Eastern Africa during the end of 18th and the beginning of the 19th centuries. The phenomenon is generally attributed to women, but has also spread to male immigrants from Somalia, who were frustrated by being treated like second class citizens (Lewis 1993).

12.3 Sociological Aspect of the Rite

The rite can be performed individually or collectively, but also is dynamic and in many ways changeable. It stays faithful to conserve and preserve specific rules that constitute the ritual. People characterize the rite, in fact, through its specific repetition. In the ordinary and banal use of the term, and sometimes with a pejorative tone, a rite is an action that is distinguished, above all by its stereotypical modality.

The rites evolve and regress with time. But, in general, the changes take place in a slow and imperceptible way, unless some religious innovation abruptly dissolves an entire ritual to create another, the latter in turn will keep repeating.

According to Levi Strauss (1966), the rite helps people during moments of crisis and mourning; through the rite, the individual has the possibility of re-elaborating and surpassing acute threatening existential moments, such as catastrophes, wars, earthquakes, and individual mourning. But it offers, an effective way to face the daily crisis of populations or groups that live in precarious situations to them in the hostile world. Each component of each culture knows how a specific rite functions and knows that through its various stages will lead to resolution of the crisis. The drain of anguish through the means of dance and music helps individual reintegration that becomes a collective form: participation from the community gives meaning to the individual and their suffering.

According to Lewis (1983), in the rite, the two functions of expression, through symbols (gestural, verbal, behavioral) and communication are joined together: like true language that transmits meaning. According to the outside observer, one can consider the dual reaction of compassion, that is participation and comprehension, that is the rational explanation.

12.4 Sociological Aspects of the Possession Rite

We could define "autogenic therapy" as all the therapeutic strategies expressed in the possession rites and handed down. One can use these as a source of faith to overcome psycho-physical disturbances and to redeem oneself from a state of marginalization, unease, and isolation that generally affect women during ordinary life (Lewis 1983). As a result, female possession is the most widespread (Eliade 1951; Lewis 1993; Smith 1954).

In Muslim Africa, the female predominance in these social acts can be explained by the restrictions of women in their participation in public and ceremonial life. This would leave an emptiness that could be filled also by the cult of possession.

However, the possession rituals constitute an important occasion of socialization and celebration for the entire population of each village.

The ritual is rich in collective social behaviors, gestures, sounds, dance music, and mythological or symbolic references. It involves all the participants, especially those who are more suffering (and enter more easily into an inner and cultural relationship with the divine or spiritual entities).

We can define the possession as a sort of social trance, an altered state of consciousness of some people that is reflected in the collectivity and that is inserted in its particular context.

In the end, we should underline the duality of the cults of possession, as they have the ability to provide healing and bring social benefits. With the initiation to the rite, the woman can achieve a therapeutic social role recognized by the community (Curia 1998/1999).

In the analyzed video, some cases of the women's possession are shown. They, with the vibrant rhythm of the music and the frenzy of a group dance, fall to the ground and roll, while invoking Allah or the names of the prophets, in a state of rapture. These altered states of consciousness become filled with sacred value, mystical and therapeutic power, which induces a condition of well-being and absolute fulfillment, producing an analgesic and euphoric effect, until rehabilitation (Prince 1993).

In the background there is the involvement of all the other women attending the celebration. They facilitate the trance, accelerating the rhythm of the chant, aiding the possessed on the ground, helping her to resolve her loss of consciousness through particular religious supplications.

12.5 Psychological Aspect of the Possession Rite

A concept by Lewis (1972, p. 90) reveals the relation between anthropology and psychology: "The possession, like a traditional practice, does not attract much interest in the younger generations anymore as it did with the previous generations. This decline seems to coincide with the birth of the modern psychology and of the psychoanalysis: many of the medical symptoms associated with spiritualism in our own past and in traditional society are now examined on the psychoanalyst's couch."

In the possession, the symptoms associated with rite resemble those described by S. Freud in his studies on hysteria (Freud and Breuer 1892). Hysteria was characterized by a confused state, a restriction of consciousness, an absence of spatial and temporal orientation. At the reawakening, the subject does not remenber anything (amnesia). The attack would consist only of motor phenomenona, epileptic seizures, or cataplexy, but the survey conducted in hypnosis provides evidence of an amnesic psychic process. The motor manifestations of the attack are always related to the mental content of the subject and are an expression of his inner torment. The possession rite expresses itself with accentuated and uncontrollable motor movements, a reflection of a manifestation of an oppressed and altered state of consciousness. Hysteria is a neurosis that manifests physical symptoms without a biological cause: it is distinguished from simulation because the subject is not fully conscious of the significance and of the real intentionality of his own behavior. Hysteria is also associated with witchcraft; the same can be said for the possession rite.

There are two mechanisms involved in a hysteric attack: exhibition of the disturbance and use of the symptom. The need is expressed in a distorted way, symbolic (as conflictual), by the "symptom."

The utilization of the symptom is often an explanation of the phenomenon of the *sar* in Somalia by the male population, concerning the manifested behaviors of the women. The wives call it "possession by the *sar*" while the husbands call it " to make oneself ill." They interpret this affliction like a deceptive fabrication used by the women against men. The *sar* spirit that possesses the women demands luxurious clothing, perfume, and delicious food from the men (Lewis 1993). Symptoms may disappear only when these cost demands are satisfied and the costs for the catharctic dance ("strike the *sar*"), directed by an expert shaman, are paid (Curia 1998/1999, p. 114). The male attitudes remain ambivalent: the men believe in the existence of these *sar* spirits, but become sceptical when it happens to their own women and when they must pay the expenses themselves.

In hysteria, the subject can live only by exposing himself to the attention of others, to be perceived is an indispensable condition to exist. This is a convergence point with the practice of the *sar* that acts like a deterrent against the abuses of negligence and deprivation, typical of a sexist culture.

In key ethnopsychiatry, we must add another perspective (Nathan 1990). For example: a woman faints. In western societies that believe in a single method to solve things, the scientist researches the strategies to help the woman regain consciousness from her "disturbance." In the society that does not believe in science as the only solution, the explanation of the same occurrence is different: a spirit has possessed her; to resolve the problem one must know the spirits. The woman becomes the unconscious informer of an invisible world.

The cultures that accept multiple modes of thinking, in regard to solutions, appeal to divination; the western world appeals to scientific diagnosis.

In academic psychopathology, the scientists use the symptoms to classify the illness. The spirits do not exist in a world that follows a one-way solution but only in the worlds with multiple causes and therefore evoke for themselves the existence of such a universe. According to Natan (1990), the only objective of true scientific psychopathology is the more precise description of therapy and of their techniques, never of the sick: "We cannot continue to find mental sicknesses in the sick."

Therefore, the potency of the action and the systemic description of the activity of the specialists, differs according to the culture of reference. In particular, the anthropologist should "realise the glance of psychology and psychiatry", knowing the phenomena of our corresponding society and the syndromes that one examines in comparison to the cultural anthropologist.

In the proposed explanation of the psychologist regarding the bizarre behavior (in terms of unconscious motivation or failure of a defense mechanism), we should not hope to find a definitive explanation that becomes institutionalized and that closes the door to anthropological analysis. We, instead, should manage to classify and render constant a series of similar symptoms that can treat different societies according to a variety of wide institutionalized ways.

The specification of the symptoms, the diagnosis, and cures become a sort of convention implied with the acknowledged effect, but moreover, culturally.

12.6 The Anthropological Aspect of the Possession Rite: J. M. Lewis's Studies in Somalia

J. M. Lewis, in 1978, carried out studies on the shepherd nomads of Somalia, a patriarchal Muslim population (1993). Their religion is dominated almost exclusively by men who occupy the main religious offices of authority and prestige; while the women are considered weak and submissive creatures and are forbidden to access mosques.

The women also have active participation in nomad life, but only with regard to the laborious shepherding of the flocks of sheep and goats and of leading the camels when they transport the material for construction of an *agàl* (their temporary housing in the bushes). However, the right to own camels is denied to women, which is their family wealth; women find a disadvantage regarding the inheritance of all forms of property. In this culture, dominated by males, possession occurs according to Lewis in 4 contexts.

The first context concerns cases of love or unrequited love. If a girl is abandoned by her boyfriend, who had promised in private to marry her, she will begin to show symptoms of apathy or of true physical illness. Her condition will be attributed to possession (indicated by the term "to enter"). This interpretation of the disillusioned girl's condition is in accord with tradition because romantic love is denied to her. Only nowadays, some Somali youth, educated in the western world, describe these cases as a true type of love sickness. In the case of the abandoned girl, there is no other available institutionalized way for her to express her offended feelings. Her private emotions and sentiments are of little interest in the legal world dominated by men. The sickness, which consequently becomes associated with care and attention, offers to the girl some comfort. Deprivation is part of the background of the possession.

The second context regards the entrance of a natural spirit, the anthropomorphic *Jinn*, a capricious entity ready to possess anyone without warning.These spirits are eager for luxurious clothing, frippery, and delicious food (these are the *sars:* either spirits or associated symptoms). The spirits are responsible for the hysterics young camel shepherds sometimes fall into after periods of isolation in the bush with their flock, and they are consequently subject to possession when they return to the community and are in the presence of girls. The remedy involves the percussion dance of the *sar*, which the girls also participate in, to free the spirits from their friends. Even in this case, one can find deprivation, aggravated by states of starvation from the lack of food that afflicts the sherpherds during isolation, and especially during drought.

The third context is the most common and regards women, especially married women. When wives are in difficulty, they get involved in fights for their survival and the survival of their children; alone in a hostile environment and/or neglected by their husband, they are at risk of the jealousy of other wives and are constantly threatened by instability of their marriage that could easily result in repudiation. They often share the house with their mother-in-law and sister-in-law, who constantly observe her.

The fourth type of possession concerns men who are psychologically disturbed and who display special difficulties in dealing with societal pressure. The spirits that possess these unfortunate subjects are considered particularly harmful. The spirits, in these cases, are religious and are also found in the Koran.

In conclusion, according to J. M. Lewis, the possession concerns urban women, but to a lesser degree rural and nomad women. The latter live in the woods, where they usually do not wear veils, herd small flocks, and enjoy considerable freedom and autonomy unlike those living in the city where more women are marked by possession.

In all the cases, the *sar* represents the instrument through which they redeem themselves on a psychological level from an inferior condition. Moreover for the urban woman, it is the occasion to reclaim the possessed property otherwise negated by the husband. In fact, in the state of trance in the presence of many people, the woman speaks for the *sar* spirit that is in her and makes requests for donations, jewelry, and new clothes that she would otherwise not be able to obtain, while the husband is frightened by her performance and cannot escape from these obligations. For this reason, Leiris (1988), a french anthropologist, considers the possession an urban practice associated with an opportunistic character, while resulting more authentically in a rural environment.

12.7 The Possession During the *Dikrì* in the Women of Merka

We have reflected many times on the identities of the Somali women present in the celebrations held every Friday. From the information collected, we come to the conclusion that they are split into two principle types: the women belonging to close villages or from the town of Merka itself, and the evacuees from Mogadish, who all gather in the *Timàn Adde* camp on the edges of *Ayuub* village where there is a nutrition and learning center for IDP children.

Life in the camp was described by Mana in an interview (personal communication, 2005): "…the women are divided in groups. A group constists of 30 units, organized by daily work tasks: at four in the morning, the women collect milk in various villages and return to the camp at nine with a tank of milk on their back. Then, three or four women distribute the milk into containers; another group, formed by about twelve women, delivers and sells the milk to homes. Around five in the afternoon, the women return to the camp with the empty milk containers on their backs. Inside, they have their earnings from the day: from $0.50 to $1.00, a small plastic bag with some sugar, five or six small tomatoes, an onion, one or half a pepper, and a kilo or half a kilo of rice or corn to make polenta with, some oil. A liter of milk was also saved for personal use. Around 5:30 pm, the women start to prepare dinner 'polenta or bread and some sauce' their only meal of the day. At 6:00 pm, the sun sets."

It is in this camp, *Timàn Adde*, that the women come together for the weekly PhC Prevention Program, that started with the *dikrì*.

The women arrived by foot from long distances to share a day of festivity, celebrating according to tradition, with music and chants and a shared meal; they commit themselves to Allah before facing the most important aspect for which they are meeting: to discuss, whether they should continue or lessen the excissory tradition.

It is a day reserved for themselves; they leave their children at home, so that they can be freer. The few men present in charge of the "order of service," are on the outskirts of the meeting.

In the *dikrì,* the women are standing and arranged in circles and move and undulate their bodies with their arms raised in front of them with the hands following the rising rhythm and the obsessive repetition of the litanies in unison; the last elements induce the trance in some subjects. The sequence, with which the event verifies people repeat, is always the same. At the acme of the rhythm that was accelerating progressively, one of the participants is distinguished from the others by placing herself in the middle of a circle and by covering her head with her veil; she is isolated from the others (*uakugelbotài,* literally "go out of head"). She falls to the ground and loses her senses, while her companions continue to sing the litanies. In the case described, and particularly within the video, one catches a glimpse of the feet of the woman in trance; they are decorated with henna tattoos and nearby are her sandals. Some women come to help her and order many times for her to put on her sandals and to rise, knowing that she is in a state of trance (she has the *rohàn*). This phrase, exclaimed clearly many times, has supplied us with key interpretive data. Also the translator that provided us with the Somali translation, had confirmed that this is a case of possession, which she called *sar.* When the woman's companions surround her during her trance, she refuses to put on her sandals to get up. They permit her to follow a special *dikrì* to expel the *sar* and to recover her consciousness. As a result, she agrees to get up, but makes a request to a special mediator to turn to Allah: the *Shek Abdulkàdir Gilàni*, a much venerated marabout in the Somali tradition.

The film is interrupted at this point, leaving us in doubt about whether the *dikrì* will be followed immediately, or if the woman will recover her consciousness immediately after.

12.8 Ending Considerations

The context of possessions, identified by J. M. Lewis, are linked through the common theme of confinement and frustration present in different ways.

The *sar* of the women of Merka seem to fall under the third typology presented, in which the women live in difficulty because of their personal conditions. These conditions are aggravated by traditional and/or contingent factors with which they are confronted on a daily basis today in different ways from the past.

First they face the problem of PhC. The Somali diaspora and the pilgrims who travel to Mecca had brought the woman in contact with other women (non-western, and often Muslim) that transferred the knowledge and conscience of the detriment of the practice to them (Mana, personal communication 2005). On the other hand, when the women return to Somalia, they find a strong popular adhesion to the custom still intact. The women of Merka, reunited by Mana for the weekly celebration, are torn over such incongruity and plead to God; the cases of possession verified are a testimony to their suffering aggravated by this new anxiety.

The women, through the possession, intend to elevate their voice through the only means known in their culture that gives them freedom of expression. They feel legitimate to expose their convictions, opinions, and new hold of conscience through these means, and hope to dissuade their companions with whom they practice the Prevention Program, from continuing the tradition.

The rite of possession could be the starting point for change.

It is for this reason, we believe, that Mana inserted the *dikrì* into the weekly celebration, of the women of Merka against PhC.

We consider the difficult life in the refugee camp of the evacuated women, who were previously mentioned and add to that inner frustration to which the women are forced to submit. Each time a woman looks for or brings food from outside the village, the probability that she will be raped is very high (Declich 2005, p. 72). The woman that is raped often does not expose it, a victim of her own shame. However, she will remember it, keeping the weight of the violence with her. The sense of violation of her intimate confines, the sense of inevitability and vulnerability that such experience transmits to the violated women are not publicly expressed, except through negativity and silence that only contributes toward her frustration and confinement.

The argument was analyzed and traced back to the source in a very extensive way; it is reported here only as a testimony of the difficulty at a global level of evacuated Somali women. These women have little cultural means through which to express themselves; only the ecstatic trance allows them freedom of expression in a male dominated world that is threatening and despotic.

References

Curia M (1998/1999) Itinerari terapeutici in Somaliland. Thesis Dissertation in Psychology, University of Padua pp 111, 114
Declich F (2005) Quando il silenzio è memoria. Cleup, Padova, pp 65, 72
Dirie W, Miller C (1998) Il fiore del deserto Garzanti (ed), Milano, pp 48–49
Eliade M (1951) Le chamanisme et les techniques archaiques de l' extase. Payot, Paris
Freud S, Breuer J (1892) Sulla teoria dell' attacco isterico. Opere 1. Bollati Boringhieri, Torino
Grassivaro Gallo P (2009). Il superamento dell' infibulazione a Merka (Somalia): il "Progetto" e il "Programma" di Mana Sultan Abdurahman Ali Isse (Merka1953–2007), Scienzaonline.com. Accessed on 18/03/2009
Grassivaro Gallo P, Busatta S (2010) Preventing Infibulation: Mana Sultan Abdurahman Ali Isse at Merka, Somalia. In: Denniston GC, Hodges FM, Milos FM (eds) Genital autonomy: protecting personal choice. Springer, dordrecht, pp 125–136
Leiris M (1988) La possessione e i suoi aspetti teatrali tra gli etiopi di Gondar. Ubulibri, Milano
Levi Strauss C (1966) Antropologia strutturale. Il Saggiatore, Milano
Lewis G (1983) Giorno di rosso splendente. Saggio sul rito, Angeli F (ed) Milano
Lewis JM (1972) Le religioni estatiche. Studio antropologico sulla possessione spiritica e sullo sciamanesimo. p 90, Astrolabio. Ubaldini, Roma
Lewis JM (1993) Possessione, Stregoneria e Sciamanesimo. Contesti religiosi nelle società tradizionali. Cap.2: i culti di possessione nel loro contesto, pp 47–82. Cap.6: il potere del passato: "sopravvivenze" africane nell' Islam, pp 137–155 (a cura di Lanternari V.), (Italian translation from english by A. Di Nola), Liguori, Napoli, 1993. Original edition: religion in contest. Cults and charisma. Cambridge University Press, Cambridge 1986
Nathan T (1990) La follia degli altri. Saggio di etnopsichiatria. Ponte delle Grazie, Firenze
Prince R (1993) Sciamani ed endorfine. Fattori esogeni ed endogeni nelle psicoterapie, "Attualità in Psicologia" 8:69–83
Smith M (1954) Baba of Karo. Faber and Faber, London

Author Biography

Pia Grassivaro Gallo Ph.D., Associate Professor of Anthropology, University of Padua's Psychology Faculty, and former teacher of Applied Biology, Human Genetics, and Anthropogenetics, currently retired. Her research on the biology of current human populations has taken place in several developing countries, particularly Somalia (from 1972 to 1985). At the invitation of the Somali Ministry of Public Health (1981), she was invited to take part in a scientific mission to Somaliland. From 1988, she has been responsible for the Padua Working Group on FGM, dealing with African immigrants in Italy. Since 2000, she has studied the expansive forms of the traditional interventions on female genitalia, carrying out field research in Central Africa (Uganda, Malawi, and Congo RDC). She was co-coordinator of the VIII International Symposium on Circumcision and Human Rights. Padua, Italy.

Chapter 13
Genital Stretching Among the Venda Ethnic Group (South Africa)

Erika Dionisio and Franco Viviani

Abstract Different interventions on the body are topics of great interest for anthropologists, as they were historically found in populations lacking the concept of "separateness" from their own body, reducing it to an instrument, a conveyor of symbols. Interventions on genitalia are of particular interest, not only because of their symbolic value, their inter-ethnic impact, and the ethical and moral questions they raise, but by the fact that they are sometimes adopted from surrounding populations as a "founding" cultural trait and maintained over a period of time. In this chapter, we present some data on the genital stretching of women from the Venda group, an ethnic group in South Africa; a practice that became a part of their system of rites and, due to "modernization," is now fast disappearing.

Keywords Genital stretching • Circumcision • Venda • Female genitalia • Labia minora

13.1 Introduction

Lesser studied and lesser interpreted than "mutilating" interventions on female genitalia, genital stretching (GS) is found mostly in the Great Lakes region of Africa. The practice involves the manipulation of the *labia minora* at a young age, which are elongated until they reach some centimeters of length. The populations that practice this custom usually claim that it is used to prepare girls for marriage, as it offers greater sexual satisfaction to their partner. In contrast to infibulation– where the woman is "closed": Lévi Strauss (1970) said that "the woman must be closed upwards because she is open downwards," alluding to the fact that the mouth is the first and most important means of communication and, therefore, must remain closed for women–this practice apparently permits women to have

E. Dionisio · F. Viviani
Anthropology, University of Padua, Padua, Italy

F. Viviani (✉)
FISPPA and Department of Human Movement Studies, University of Padua, Padua, Italy
e-mail: franco.viviani@unipd.it

G. C. Denniston et al. (eds.), *Genital Cutting: Protecting Children from Medical, Cultural, and Religious Infringements*, DOI: 10.1007/978-94-007-6407-1_13,

unlimited sexual communication. However, this is not the case among the populations that have been studied until now, because the risk of uncontrolled sexual forces is restrained by rules and taboos regarding a woman's sex life, social relationships with peers and mates, and sometime the importance of the maintenance of virginity. These rules are often taught in institutions, labeled as "initiation schools" by anthropologists. This is an improper term for women, as the term "initiated" implies to become part of a system of power, but women are not usually part of such systems, as it is the male group that enters into alliance with other groups, thanks to the exchange of women. It, therefore, would be better to use the terms "introduction" or "introductory" schools (IS). However, the fact that the practice of GS is dying out (at present, it is only found in marginal areas of the Venda region) makes it of interest for us to gather, and then report on, data on Venda women. This chapter reports the results of a survey on genital stretching carried out among the women of the Venda population in South Africa by one of the authors (Dionisio) in 2009. Data was collected through interviews, focus groups, and observations. Self-reports of the knowledge and attitudes of the people/women were occasionally used.

13.2 Some Characteristics of the Region and its Inhabitants

The Venda territory constitutes a very small part of the Limpopo area in the Northern Transvaal of South Africa, close to the borders of Zimbabwe and Mozambique. It is located between 22°15′ and 23°45′ South and 29°50′ and 31°30′ East (Benso 1979). The words *Vhavenda* and *Bavenda* are used interchangeably when referring to *Vhavenda* people, along with *Tshivenda and Venda.* However, these last two are specifically used for their language. Linguistically belonging to the Bantu-speaking family, according to Lestrade (1927): "the phonesis and phonology of TshiVenda finds its nearest equivalent in the Karanga group, and it is quite sharply distinguished from the Sotho and Thonga group in this regard. As far as the grammatical structure is concerned, TshiVenda is sharply marked off from the Sotho and Thonga groups, and sharply reminiscent of the Karanga groups to the north-east of the latter, namely, the whole of the East African group of Bantu languages." The Venda language, therefore, is a distinct language, sharing close ties with the Shona (spoken in much of Zimbabwe) and the South African Sotho language. To summarize, the TshiVenda (or LuVenda) emerged as a distinct dialect in the sixteenth century, with the vocabulary being similar to SeSotho, and the grammar similar to the Shona dialect of Zimbabwe. Roughly 875,000 people in South Africa speak TshiVenda, while some people residing in areas such as Zimbabwe use different variants of TshiVenda. Around one million people speak TshiVenda. Its' origin is uncertain, as, over time, the various groups using the language gradually welded into a whole, as it incorporated many diverse peoples belonging to different ethnic groups (Hammond-Tooke 1974). It is assumed (West 1976) that they came from the North (possibly from near Lake Malawi) at the end of the seventeenth century, but their entry into the settlement area could have been earlier.

The Venda settled and built villages in the Zoutpansberg. Over time, they were raided by the Pedi, Zulu, and Tsonga populations. Consequently, they fortified their villages, locating them strategically, and building fences or walls—the Venda knew how to build with stone. Traditional Venda huts were thatched and had walls made with stakes, although nowadays these walls are often plastered and decorated. Cattle did not represent a great source of wealth. They kept goats and sheep, but were mainly agriculturalists. They were skilled in pottery, basketry, woodwork, weaving, skin dressing, and metal-works. They are the object of many stereotypes among their neighboring populations, as they are considered to be mystical, highly secretive, and masters of the occult. Traditionally, they were farmers and hunters living in the mountains, but they recently faced a deep change to their lifestyle as they moved into towns. This move changed many of their traditions, including GS and the surrounding scenarios permitting this practice, such as the IS, where girls are prepared for their future adult life. Nowadays, the practice of IS has almost disappeared, and where it does still exist, it is profoundly modified.

13.3 The Venda Culture

The Vhavenda culture is actually a hybrid of different cultures, with their closest affiliation being the Shona people of Zimbabwe, but the *Lemba, Lobedu,* and *North Sotho* peoples are also similar (Krige and Krige 1943). Other major influences were the *Tsonga, Lobedu, Zulu, Swazi* and others. The Vhavenda share many cultural characteristics of other East African peoples (Benso 1979). These include forbidding the consumption of pork, and extensive male initiation rituals, which begin with the *Thondo,* followed by the *Murundu* initiation school where male circumcision occurs (Junod 1927). This ritual aims to train men in the ways of self-discipline, endurance, and proper tribal customs and conduct. The Vhavenda also engage in female instruction of moral and behavioral rules (IS), which undergoes three phases: the *Vhusha*, the *Tshikanda,* and the *Domba.* This admission process continues throughout the course of the females' lives, up until they get married, the first beginning shortly after their first menstruation and the last two before marriage. IS is meant to prepare women for their roles as wives and mothers. The Venda culture is rooted in mythical and ancestral beliefs best reflected in their closeness to elements of nature, animals, such as crocodiles, and water, together with strong connections with the ancestral spirits. Musical instruments, called *Phala–phala*s, are made from the horns of the kudu or sable antelopes, and produce an array of sounds used to call people together for gatherings. Venda drums are also used, and they come in two forms–a small narrow drum held between the legs and a large round drum often attached to a tree or pole. The drums are collectively named *Ngoma,* and hold sacred status, since the Singo

King was believed to have a drum, known as the *Lungundo or* "drum of the dead," that could protect people from harm.

13.4 Introductory Schools for Girls

13.4.1 Vhusha

In contrast to male circumcision, which was adopted from the Sotho, *Vhusha* rites are probably more genuine Venda customs (Blacking 1964). The most important part of this school is the teaching of *milayo* (formulae). Warmelo (1932) asserted that the practice prepares the girls for later life. Traditionally, the passage from childhood to adolescence was marked by the *Vhusha* ceremony. Before this ritual, a girl was referred to as a *musidzana* (a small girl), and afterwards she was always referred as being a *musidzana vha khomba*. The term *khomba* means 'dangerous,' implying that sexual intercourse could from now on result in pregnancy. Sometimes the term *khomba* was used as an alternative to *Vhusha* in referring to the ceremony. When the first sign of menstruation occurred, the girl had to inform her mother or one of the elder women of the village (*kraal*). Then, the father was informed of the occurrence as well. The *Vhusha* was held in the village of the district chief. The ceremony was usually postponed until there were more girls ready for the rite. Men were excluded from the ritual. *Vhusha* was usually held after sunset in the chief *kraal*. All women living within a reasonable distance came in troupes. A fire was lit in the *khoro*, where the women removed their clothes and danced naked except for their ornaments. The initiates were stripped and had to stand at the back. The women danced close to a fire with the accompaniment of the drums, as well as trilling and singing. The singing and dancing went on all night long. At sunrise, the party broke up and the women went home.

The initiates remained in the *kraal* in the public hut, called *tshivhambo*. The ceremony continued for six days, supervised by two female instructors. Whenever the initiates left the *tshivhambo* they were enveloped in a blanket, and had to walk in a couched position. The instructors were always naked except for the *shedu*. Every morning the initiates went to the river, walking in single file, led by one of the instructors who beat the drum as a warning to males that the party was approaching, and they should keep out of the girls' way. A great deal of time was given to sexual teaching. Girls were warned against becoming deflowered before marriage, and they were taught how to have sexual intercourse without this occurring. An old woman often showed even very young girls how to stretch the *labia minora*. According to Stayt (1968), during the *Vhusha,* a great deal of time was spent on this practice.

To help the dilatation, a bat is killed and cooked, the resulting concoction being rubbed on the parts, so that, as the bat has a curtain across its legs, its essence will facilitate the growth of a similar curtain across the legs of the initiates. Often a stone is tied to the parts to hasten the process. This manipulation results in the formation of a regular apron a few inches in length. Some of the data regarding this is discordant. Interviews conducted during our field research showed that the practice of stretching the *labia minora* is performed prior to *Vhusha.* GS is suspended when menarche occurs. Reference to the use of powdered bat wings is in accordance with previous reports. Warmelo (1932) saw that, before puberty, girls begin to practice the custom of *u kwevha.* This term describes the pulling out and the lengthening of the *labia minora.* Elder women incited the young girls to perform it. When the *Vhusha*-rites of the older girls were taking place, they went to the river to wash. Older girls inspected them to see whether they had protracted *labia minora.* If a girl had not accomplished the manipulation, she could bring shame on the group. According to some students GS is not a practice unique to the Venda, as it is carried out by neighboring populations as well. It is strongly connected to the girls' IS. It comes before *Vhusha.* The procedure and rituals differ from all the modalities previously studied; differences are found even from village to village.

13.4.2 Domba

The *Domba* ceremony occurred at irregular intervals, depending on the local chief. Unlike the *Vhusha ceremony*, boys were also required to join in the dancing. This ceremony, which lasted three months or longer, gave the girls a basic sexual education, information about childbirth, and included a physical examination. Boys and girls had to learn *milayo* and songs, all of them with sexual content. Girls found to be deflowered were traditionally beaten and ridiculed. The initiates learned "the python" dance, in which nearly-naked girls joined in a long sinuous line holding one another closely. Sometimes boys and girls formed alternate lines. They marched slowly in a circle in a rhythmic dance with the accompaniment of drumming and singing. In this vein the simulation of sexual intercourse under a blanket occurred (inciting the disapproval of the missionaries). Thus, the days passed in dancing, education, and manual work. At the end, the participants were washed and shaven and then they could socially re-emerge, after a six-day seclusion. The whole cycle may be seen as a general preparation for marriage. It was important for a woman to have attended a *domba* at some stage of her life, as it established her seniority. If one was not held in her district, the girl could attend one elsewhere.

13.4.3 Hali, Sungwi, or Musevhetho

Musevhetho is the practice of circumcision for girls. This is not a practice originating in Venda customs, but was adopted from the Sotho population. The reason for this rite is the desire of women to be on a par with their circumcised husband. The practice is popular for a small section of the people, especially where the *murundu* (male circumcision) has the strongest influence. Infant daughters are circumcised solely because the parents want them to avoid marital problems in the future.

Sungwi is not a "tribal" institution but is performed locally. To perform it, the chief must be consulted. The function is held in a hut in a small enclosure outside the village. Here *nonyana*, the spirit of *musevetho,* lives and manifests himself to the initiates. This figure is a man disguised in bark and reeds. During the first night of the ceremony, the initiates are greeted by *nonyana,* who is inside his hut. One by one the girls are taken into the hut where the *nonyana,* touched by the initiate, emits a weird noise. Then the initiates dance in the enclosure late into the night. The dancing is repeated for several months (*musevetho* goes on for up to three years). The girls are taught the laws of *musevetho.* The operation is carried out by an old woman, *nonyana.* Girls are taken to a secluded place near the river, where the clitoris is cut. At the same time the girls are branded with a mark on their outer thigh. Today this form of clitoridectomy has been abolished (this was evident in the interviews), and the ritual of branding on the thigh has been kept in rare circumstances only.

13.5 Materials and Methods

During Spring 2009, an intensive qualitative survey was carried out in the Venda region, using semi-structured and open-ended interviews, focus groups, narrative field logs, diaries, and drawing tests. Semi-structured interviews were carried out with six Venda women (four living in rural areas and two in urban locations). Three of them were born in the Vhembe district, the others in different areas. Two focus groups were organized, all of them contained Venda women living in the Vhembe district. In the first ($n = 5$) the average age was 56.2 years (minimum was 42; maximum 86), in the second ($n = 4$) the ages ranged between 60 and 78 years of age (average was 69.2 years). Regarding their marital status, there was an equal number of married, widowed, and divorced participants.

Semi-structured interviews were carried out with four males, whose average age was 55.7 years (minimum was 42, maximum 73), all of them of Venda origin, married, and living in the Vhembe district. Only one of them was born in the Vuvhani district. Twenty-seven pairs of drawings were collected from girls, whose average age was 19.7 years (minimum was 17, maximum 34). Each girl was requested to draw two pictures. In the first, they were asked to represent how they imagined a couple's relationship when a woman was elongated and to make a short comment. In the second drawing, they had to represent the case of a marriage with a non-elongated woman and to make remarks or observations. From the analysis of the first drawing, two clusters emerged. One group depicted the image in a positive light, whereas the other group did not. In this context, only the elements resulting as significant or in its proximity are reported. Seventeen subjects (63 % of the total) depicted the image positively, compared to ten subjects (37 %) who did not. The difference between the two was significant ($X^2 = 27.0$; $df = 1$; $p < 0.001$). Most of the data was coded, analyzed, and interpreted according to Miles and

Huberman's instructions (1994). Their statistical significance was assessed by agglomerative hierarchical cluster analysis using Ward's method (Fabbris 1997), because an examination of the dendrograms was performed, then Chi square test and t test were performed in order to validate the clustering solutions.

13.6 Results

13.6.1 Interviews

The term used by all the women for GS was *u'kwevha*. They mentioned some neighboring populations practicing GS, in particular Shangaana and Sotho. All women claimed that the practice is out-of-date, and is now only an occasional occurrence. According to the women, the discontinuation of the ritual is due to: modernization, "civilization", Christianization, the disappearance of the girls' IS, the opposition of missionaries to the practice, and the fact that it is no longer considered necessary. In detail, 66.7 % described how *u'kwevha* was performed. A synthesis of the various versions could be sketched as follows: the *labia minora* was stretched by the girl with her fingers, first for 15 min and later on from 15 to 30 min. The girl crouched on divaricated legs (or was even sitting). She usually manipulated herself alone, early in the morning, behind the hut. In the afternoon, she manipulated herself again in the bush, but this time in a group. Manipulation was helped with the use of plants, "the ashes of the burned wings of a bat," *murenze* flowers, and leaves of *mahushule*. Then a piece of grass was used to measure the length of the labia.

Girls started the manipulation when they were 8 or 9 years old, depending on the family and the village customs. On average, the length of the labia had to reach four centimeters. *U'kwevha* was performed before menarche (and stopped during), marriage, and pregnancy. During manipulation, the girls were asked not to sing or dance because this could affect the secrecy of the rite, as nobody was supposed to see it. Sometimes, when they were in the bush, they played some instruments: reed and musical bow. *U'kwevha* was considered to be painful only for the first few days, as it was believed that the muscles had to adapt to manipulation. Old women checked the girls at regular intervals.

Those who did not perform *u'kwevha* were not stigmatized linguistically; in fact, there were no particular words to differentiate the girls who performed it and those who did not. However, those who chose not to undertake GS were socially isolated, as they were excluded from playing/socializing with their peers. There was not a specific person to initiate the first manipulation. She was usually an older woman, such as the girl's mother or grandmother, and sometimes the girl's older sister. All the females interviewed believed that GS gave greater sexual satisfaction, and that it prepared the body for marriage as a gift to the partner, in the belief that the elongated labia were better able to hold the penis, thus assuring fertility. Furthermore, it was associated with the concept of beauty and womanliness. The men interviewed stated that they preferred "elongated" women, however, they did not refuse their wife if her body had not been prepared according to the tradition. Both males and females declared that in the past virginity was fundamental. No sexual education was furnished during *u'kwevha* because it was imparted in the initiation schools (*Vhusha*). This is because female sexual education was and still is an exclusively female duty, and fathers are excluded from their daughters' education.

13.6.2 Drawings

From the first drawing (where the women are elongated), there emerged two groups: one (17 subjects, 63 % of the total) depicted the image positively, two (10 subjects 37 %) who did not. The difference between the two was significant ($X^2 = 27.0$; df = 1; $p < 0.001$). Sexual intercourse is considered more positively in the first group, with 76.5 % of the participants (n = 13) considering it to be positive, in respect to 23.5 % that did not (n = 4). In the second group, four subjects (40 % of the cases) refer to sexual intercourse, while six subjects out of the ten (60 %) did not consider this aspect ($X^2 = 3.6$; df = 1; $p = 0.058$). In the first group, 58.8 % of the participants (n = 10) believed that the "man is satisfied," while the subjects in the second group did not mention this aspect: this difference between the groups was evaluated to be significant ($X^2 = 9.3$; df = 1; $p < 0.01$). The relationship of a couple was considered to be "not good" mainly by the second group (60 % of the cases), while none of the subjects of the first group considered this aspect. Clearly, the difference is significant ($X^2 = 13.1$; df = 1; $p < 0.001$). As all the girls that practice manipulation receive a form of sexual education, this aspect was highlighted more in the first group (29.4 %) in respect to the second (0 %), thus the difference between the groups was evaluated as being close to significant ($X^2 = 3.6$; df = 1; $p = 0.057$). The adjective "good" (or any other positive evaluation of GS) is absent in the second group, and used more in the first (29.4 %), with the same results of the latter aspect considered. Regarding the knowledge/absence of knowledge of GS by males, the absence of knowledge is more associated with the second group (40 % of the cases), in respect to the first (5.9 %). The difference is significant ($X^2 = 4.9$; df = 1; $p < 0.05$). As far as the positive evaluation of the second drawing is concerned, 11 subjects gave a positive evaluation, while 16 subjects from the second group (68 %) did not. The sexual act is more associated with the first group (100 % of the cases) compared to 12.5 % from the second: this difference is significant ($X^2 = 17.2$; df = 1; $p < 0.001$). Partner dissatisfaction is more associated with the first group (45 %) than the second (12.5 %) ($X^2 = 3.7$; df = 1; $p = 0.055$). The belief that a non-manipulated woman can induce polygyny is more associated with the first group (54.4 % of the cases), whereas none of the second group held this belief: this difference is also significant ($X^2 = 11.2$; df = 1; $p < 0.001$). The idea that the girls do not receive a sexual education if they do not undertake GS is more associated with the first group (36.4 %) than the second (6.3 %). Here again the difference is significant ($X^2 = 3.9$; df = 1; $p < 0.05$). Male satisfaction is more associated with the second group (31.3 %), in respect to 0 % of the second: the difference is again significant ($X^2 = 4.2$; df = 1; $p < 0.05$).

13.6.3 Drawing Test

The Machover test (1949) was utilized, as it can be used on adults. It is a projective method permitting the personality of a subject to be evaluated in a dynamic sense from his/her graphic productions. Free graphic productions permit the perception about the self of an individual to be inferred. Each subject was asked to produce two drawings: in the first, the subject was asked to depict how they imagined the relationship in a couple where the woman was elongated. In the second, they were asked to depict the couple's relationship when the woman was "straight". In both cases they were also asked to make comments. The following analyses were performed:

- Formal (width of the drawing, position, and so on)
- Graphic (line engraving)
- Content (different body parts and details)
- Comments

To highlight the differences between the first and the second drawing, comparisons were carried out using the McNemar's test (Fabbris 1997). No statistical differences emerged, and only some of the content had any statistical significance at all (Fig. 13.1).

Statistical differences emerged for the hair, the neck (larger and more enhanced in "woman 2"), and the hands (more represented and enhanced in "woman 1"). In the representation, the positioning of the woman at the top of the page is more evident in "Woman 2." (Fig. 13.2)

Statistical differences were found in the representations, as the position of the woman at the top of the page was more commonly found in "men 2." The average

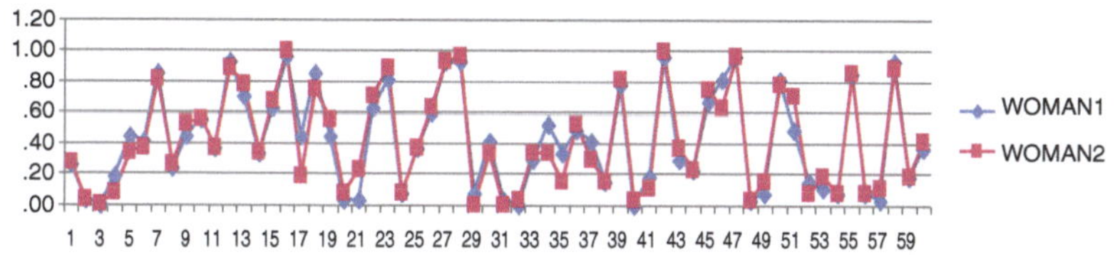

Fig. 13.1 How women were represented

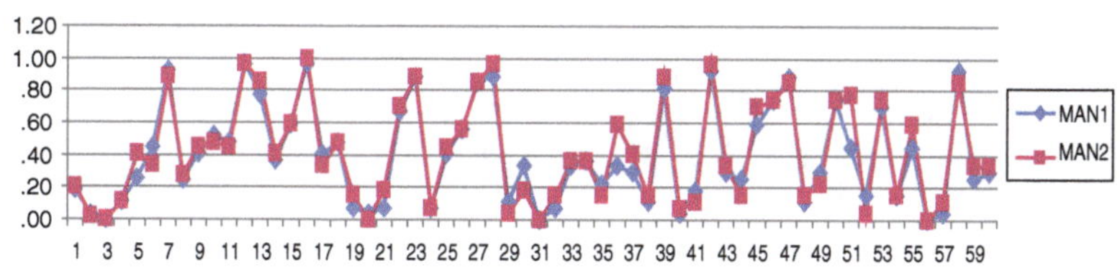

Fig. 13.2 How men were represented

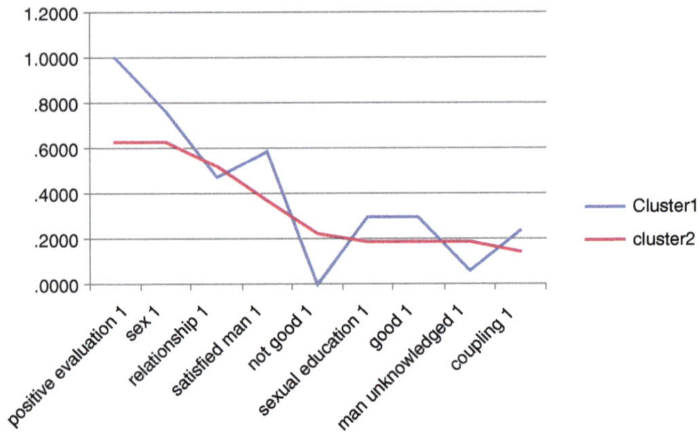

Fig. 13.3 Comments related to the first drawing (cluster analysis)

dimension, in respect to the A4 paper, was of medium size in "men 2," while for "men1" it was bigger (Fig. 13.3).

Two clusters emerged: one associated with a positive image, the other not depicting a positive image. Of the subjects, 63 % depicted the first drawing positively ($p < 0.001$), arising from the fact that in 76.5 % of the cases it was considered to favor the sexual act ($p < 0.05$); and that the man was satisfied (58.8 % of the cases; $p < 0.01$). The girls perceived the first drawing positively ($p < 0.001$), remarking that this was because of the specific sexual education (29.4 %, $p < 0.05$) they had received and they used the adjective "good" (29.4 %, $p < 0.05$). For the second group (who did not depict a positive image), the girls stated that the relationship of a couple is "not good" (60 % of the cases; $p < 0.001$) because there is no male knowledge of the practice (40 %, $p < 0.05$) (Fig 13.4).

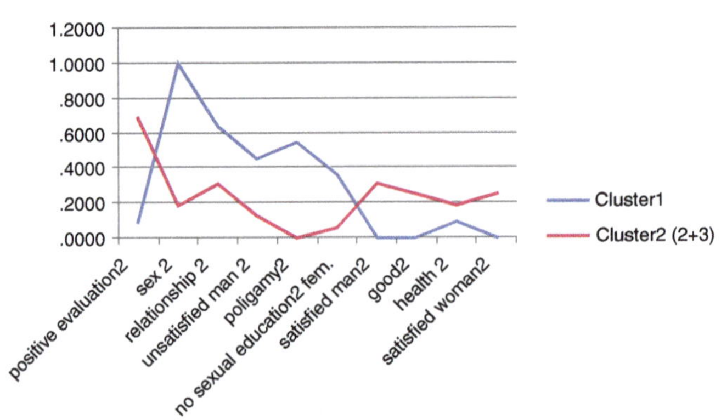

Fig. 13.4 Comments related to the second drawing (cluster analysis)

Two clusters emerged: 16 of the participants portrayed women who had not had GS performed in a negative light, and 11 participants portrayed them positively ($p < 0.01$). The women who had depicted negative images claimed this was because: a) it compromises sexuality (100 %, $p < 0.01$); b) the partner is dissatisfied (45.5 %, $p < 0.05$); c) he, therefore, is more prone to polygyny (54.5 %, $p < 0.001$); d) the women do not receive an appropriate sexual education (36.4 %, $P < 0.05$). Among those who portrayed "non manipulation" positively, there was also the conviction that the partner is satisfied anyway (31.3 %, $p < 0.05$).

13.7 Discussion and Conclusions

The analysis of a complex practice like GS has proved to be somewhat problematic for several reasons, which are mainly connected to the fact that the practice is disappearing so quickly (over the course of one generation) from the customs and traditions of the Venda. In fact, multiple contradictions emerged between the various age and gender subgroups, and also within the same age groups analyzed here, indicating that the phenomenon is very dynamic and that its discontinuation is highly controversial (as is the case whenever a custom is discontinued from one generation to the next). Anthropologists are well aware that the discontinuation of an important cultural trait is painful, both at collective and individual level. In fact, our findings furnish some clues, especially regarding what is expressed by the drawings. The representations of a non-manipulated woman, for example, suggests that she has sexual problems (as symbolized by depictions of the hair), an excessive control of her instinctual life (neck), sensations of guilt (hands), and low self-confidence (due to the position in which she is represented at the top of the drawings).

The representations of men (when they are portrayed with an elongated woman), on the other hand, tend to manifest self-confidence, expansion, and aggressiveness. These attributes can contrast with those found in images depicting a non-elongated woman, as their position at the top of the drawing indicates low self-confidence. It is interesting to note that some cultural aspects cannot be eliminated: sexuality is culture-driven, and any changes must also take the unconscious into account.

The finding that non-manipulated girls are more prone to sexual problems, low self-confidence, and a sense of guilt is symptomatic. The fact that missionaries usually stigmatize GS as a form of masturbation to be proscribed may play a role in these findings. The interviews show that, in the past, manipulated girls never felt any guilt about GS, as it was so widely accepted. Even if virginity was a "value," the strict rules transmitted during the *vhusha* were probably not in contrast with the physiology of a growing young woman. Today, with the abandonment of *u'kwevha* and the disappearance of the IS, no sexual education is furnished to the girls, so they can only find out the facts about sex from friends and the media, with all the possible distortions that are well known in the western countries, to which we can add a vague reminiscence of events long past that, as we have seen, are still working.

The fact that GS disappeared in one generation only permits some reflections. Contrarily to what happened to male circumcision (which is still considered to be a "value" among Venda males, and, therefore, is widely performed), GS is disappearing, which is mostly due to the pressures of the several churches that have settled in the area. They have replaced local sacred traditions with new "sacred" beliefs, which are interpreted to be more "modern" and somehow more practical by the Venda and, therefore, were quickly adopted.

If, in the past, the sexuality of women was considered to be "functional" to male sexuality (women had to be virgins when they married, but with elongated *labia* to assure more satisfaction to their man), they are now under pressure from other'messages'. Some of them, such as those conveyed by missionaries, could be seen as traditional (for example, the importance of virginity before marriage), but they are still assumed by women because they understand that some other messages carried by religious sects could free them from their condition of subjection to the male, and become more independent. In practice, this would mean having a job and, therefore, a higher social value. For other young women, with a weak or absent adherence to religious beliefs, the dismissal of *u'kwevha* created a "cultural hole" that will be filled by what we could define as being the Western style "acculturation," in practice the shoddy and the waste spread by media. This aspect clearly emerged in the interviews. For example, it was stated that the younger generations are more promiscuous, and virginity is no longer considered to be a "value" in the Venda region.

The price that the new generation must pay for such a rapid cultural change is potentially very high–from personal problems (related to the emotional sphere that could lead to psychological problems) to the risks associated with sexually transmitted diseases in a country where the HIV/AIDS rate of infection is incredibly high. If the data regarding male circumcision among the Venda and those regarding GS is compared, there is an apparent contradiction: the difference between the so-called boys' and girls' initiation schools (Malisha et al. 2008). First of all, to be initiated is necessary to belong to a structure of power, and usually women are not, as they were historically exchanged by males. The fact that these kinds of institutions are disappearing for females and not for their gender counterpart is a clue that they were not structures of power for women. Therefore, it is much better is to call them "introductory" schools for girls, as stated before. Then, GS is at present regarded as being an "old and derisible" practice.

At this point, it is necessary to mention that throughout South Africa, and in the Venda area in particular, women make up only a small part of the formal workplace. When women do work, they are paid less and have less financial stability than men. In order to keep a partner, women refuse to demand monogamy (and, among other demands, the use of condoms) (Hjort 2006). In practice, women tend to grant the wishes of their partners.

Male circumcision is maintained because it is a way for men to assert their masculinity; therefore, it must be inculcated to the new generations through an intervention symbolically and practically affecting the most important male part: the penis. With an "engraved spear" (as it is locally said), a male is believed to be not only more attractive to women but also more prolific.

For women, we can imagine a different scene due to the different and conflicting socio-cultural messages with which they are currently bombarded. From one side, they are inundated with media messages of female beauty and the consequent rewards on achieving this standard. Other messages put emphasis on the virtues of independence and autonomy for women, while traditional duties require their dependence that can be traced back in their curvaceous and large-breasted bodies. However, the deforming mirror of codified rules for physique are now changing even for African women, as the degree of dissatisfaction with the body is rising (Dionisio et al. 2010); for example, in the (formal) workplace, voluptuous women are perceived to be less competent and less intelligent than non-curvaceous women. Regarding the form of their external genitalia, if the *labia minora* stretching was highly considered two generations ago, it was lost under the influence of Christianity that required converts to abstain from a number of customs (e.g., polygynous marriage, the inheritance of wives, pre- and extra-marital sexual intercourse, sacrificial rituals, and so on). As Western missionaries are generally anti-sexual, genital manipulation was seen as being a form of masturbation, to be banned in a more active way than MC (that instead is considered to restrain onanism).

As a woman who manipulated her genitalia at a younger age was more sexually confident and disposed than a non-manipulated and self-possessed girl, it was not difficult to get rid of the practice of female IS, with the reciprocal satisfaction of local males (who in this way maintained their control over women in a world that was changing women's status) and missionaries (who considered the practice to be "tribal"). Women adhered for multiple reasons because missionaries conveyed several messages, freeing women from further obligations: for example, the daughters in a Christian family can become independent and obtain a greater say in the economic affairs, and even become eligible for inheritance. These aspects of modernity were very attractive. We can imagine that, for Venda women, the phantom of the so-called "male universal sexual desire" (Cresto-Dina 2010) changed from a traditional to a Western-driven one. This did not happen for males, who continue to imagine that a "spear" without the prepuce is the best tool to satisfy women who, on the other hand, require circumcision of their partners because this is the "hard core" of a consolidated tradition: another aspect of "male universal sexual desire" at work.

Acknowledgments We are very grateful for their invaluable help to Professor Pia Grassivaro Gallo (University of Padua), to the editors and to all the participants in the research project.

References

Benso L (1979) The independent Venda. Pretoria, Benso

Blacking J (1964) Black background. The childhood of a South African girl. Abelard-Schuman, New York

Cresto-Dina D (2010). Lo specchio deformante. La Repubblica, 8 July, p 33

Dionisio E, Biague F, Bagnol B, Zecchinato C, Scarcella F, Viviani F (2010) Body image in a Cohort of South African youngsters. In: Longhusrt G et al. (eds) Proceeding book of the 27th ICPAFR Symposium, KwaDlanzegwa, p 33
Fabbris L (1997) Statistica multivariata. Analisi esplorativa dei dati. Mc-Graw-Hill, Milan
Hammond-Tooke WD (1974) The Bantu-speaking people of Southern Africa. Routledge & Kegan P, London
Hjort L (2006) Sexism, youth and HIV in South Africa. http://www.alternatives.ca/eng/our-organization/our-publications/analysis-and-articles
Junod HA (1927) The life of a South African tribe. Macmillan, London
Krige EJ, Krige JD (1943) The realm of a rain-queen. A study of the pattern of lovedu society. Juta & Company limited, Capetown
Lestrade GP (1927) Some notes on the ethnic history of the Bavenda and their Rhodesia affinities. S Afr J Sci 24:487
Lévi-Strauss C (1970) Dal miele alle ceneri. Il Saggiatore, Milan
Machover K. (1949) Il disegno della figura umana. Florence, OS
Malisha L, Maharaj P, Rogan M (2008) Rites of passage to adulthood: traditional schools in the context of HIV/AIDS in the Limpopo Province, South Africa. Health Risk Soc 10(6):585–598
Miles MB, Huberman AM (1994) Qualitative data analysis: a sourcebook of new methods. Sage, Thousand Oaks
Stayt HA (1968) The Bavenda. F. Cass & Co, Capetown
Warmelo NGV (1932) Ethnological publications Vol. III. Contributions towards Venda history, religion and tribal ritual. The Government Printer, Pretoria
West M (1976) Abantu. An introduction to the black people of South Africa. Cape. C. Struik, Capetown
www.southafrica.info/about/geography/province.htm
www.southafrica.info/about/geography/limpopo.htm
www.nationmaster.com/encyclopedia/vhembe-district-municupality
www.britannica.com/EBCHECKED/topic/625046/venda
www.unpo.org/menbers/7912

Author Biography

Erika Dionisio is a graduating student, Department of Applied Psychology, University of Padua. She was involved in a field qualitative research on genital modifications in the Venda region in South Africa, and she collected data on body image from South African students. Padua, Italy.

Franco Viviani a physical anthropologist, is Professor of Anthropology at the Departments of Philosophy, Sociology, Pedagogy and Applied Psychology (FISPPA) and Human Movement Studies, University of Padova. He has published papers and articles both on male and female circumcision. Padua, Italy.

Chapter 14
Male Circumcision Among the Venda of Limpopo (South Africa)

Erika Dionisio and Franco Viviani

Abstract In order to collect raw data on male circumcision (MC) in the Limpopo region of South Africa, in Spring 2009 a semi-structured and open-ended interview was conducted on 27 male subjects of various ages, all of them circumcised and belonging to the Venda ethnic group. The main conclusions from the interviews are as follows:

(a) The practice is still carried out among the majority of the male population;
(b) Contrary to female expansive interventions on genitalia, which are now disappearing among the Venda population, MC is still widely carried out in the area considered;
(c) Nowadays the operation is often carried out in day-hospitals regimen as opposed to in the Bush (performed by traditional operators). If the operation is performed in the Bush, however, a health worker often supervises the rite;
(d) These small changes (location and operator) are due to hygienic reasons, mainly to the quite high prevalence of HIV in the region;
(e) However, the ritual is one of the most important moments in a boy's life: a rite of passage, making him a "man," and enabling him to have status in the community, have sexual relations, in the belief that MC will enhance his sexual capacities.

Keywords Male circumcision • South Africa • Venda • Limpopo • Initiation school • Ritual • Culture • HIV/AIDS

E. Dionisio · F. Viviani (✉)
Anthropology, University of Padua, Padua, Italy
e-mail: franco.viviani@unipd.it

E. Dionisio
e-mail: franco.viviani@unipd.it

F. Viviani
FISPPA and Department of Human Movement Studies, University of Padua, Padua, Italy

G. C. Denniston et al. (eds.), *Genital Cutting: Protecting Children from Medical, Cultural, and Religious Infringements*, DOI: 10.1007/978-94-007-6407-1_14,

14.1 Introduction

The Venda (also called BaVenda or Vhavenda), with a population estimated at about 1,000,000, are concentrated in locations from approximately longitude 29°40′–30°50′ E. and latitude 22°20′–23°10′ S., in the mountainous and rugged Zoutpansberg district in the Northern Transvaal (Stayt 1968). This is officially the Thulamela district of the Vhembe municipality of the Limpopo province in the Republic of South Africa. In conventional usage, the region is called Venda, the people are called Vhavenda (singular Muvenda) and their language is called Tshivenda, which has more affinity with the Niger-Congo linguistic cluster (other members of this cluster are the Shona in Zimbabwe and the Lozi in Zambia). It is a composite people who have gradually welded into a whole, incorporating different groups, but now speaking a common language with different dialects (Lestrade 1927), inserted into the Bantu linguistic family (Hammond-Tooke 1974). Immigrant groups came with their chiefs from the north at about the end of the seventeenth century. All the Venda history is family or clan history, but like their neighbors, they are the result of a combination of biotopic influences and hybridization, perhaps tempered by genetic drift.

During the most part of the last century, the whole of Venda consisted of mutual independent kingdoms, polarized around a few powerful dynasties. But when genealogies are traced back, they are extremely brief, with no exception, and all of them start with the founder who first came into the country. For subsistence, they were devoted mainly to agriculture; skilled in pottery, woodwork, basketry, weaving, and skin dressing; and excelled in metalwork. Due to both their linguistic differentiation from other groups and their marginal location, there exists a stereotype among the surrounding populations: Venda are identified as mystical, very secretive people, with an extraordinary focus on witchcraft (McNeill 2009). This popular belief was reinforced recently, when ritual murders increased in the area (Comaroff and Comaroff 2004).

Regarding the raising of children, peculiar differences from neighboring groups were not noted, apart from their method of bringing up children in the 12–15 age groups. Children built their own play-village (*mahundwani*), a miniature representation of their village, and they acted as if they were in a real village. Adult routine life was copied, for example, infants were borrowed from the real villages to act as babies; a chief was elected, and boys took wives. Adolescents returned home at night to sleep (West 1982): a very interesting way to prepare children for adulthood.

Regarding male circumcision (MC), in the overwhelming majority of cases, anthropologists agree that this is not a traditional Venda practice (Grant 1905; Wheelwright 1905; Junod 1927; Harries 1929; Hammond Tooke 1974). According to West (1982), it started at the beginning of the last century, probably by imitation, as it was dangerous for an uncircumcised man to travel through the neighboring Sotho territory: he was likely to be caught and detained by force and MC was performed on him. For Blacking and Huffman (1982), it was brought to Western Venda in the 1860s. According to Stayt (1968), the rite started to attract smaller tribes to a prominent clan and became widespread after 1904. It is reported that neighboring BaLemba groups declared that the Venda adopted MC for purely mercenary purposes, copying their ritual (Stayt 1968, page 126).

The word *murundu* (circumcision lodge) is used by BaLemba groups, and *per extenso*, is used to signify both MC and boys' "initiation school." For boys, the procedure of the ritual does not differ from that of other groups, as it is a custom commonly associated with the so-called "boys' initiation school" (IS), which exist in many parts of South Africa. A fundamental feature of the initiation school is that the boys should be separated from the community. Usually a hut or lodge is built in a difficult-to-reach place that is "taboo" for women. It must be noted that around fifty years ago, two types of IS existed for boys: the *murundu* (the circumcision lodge), and the *thondo,* the school through which all boys were obliged to pass in order to reach manhood. Little by little *murundu* drove the *thondo* out of existence (Stayt 1968), probably because MC is the central act separating a boy from his childhood and the two schools existing side by side were amalgamated in most parts of the Venda region. Originally, the *thondo* was the school for the upper classes (for sons of the royal family and aristocracy) but, before its disappearance, it was customary for all boys to attend this school.

During the period following MC, the initiates are taken to the seclusion lodge. A main feature of the initiation school is the administration of various hardships or ordeals (boys are forbidden to eat meat or drink water, they have uncomfortable sleeping conditions, and sometimes they are beaten). The other main characteristic is the formal teaching given by the men of the group. Singing and dancing are also important. At the end of the IS, the lodge, with all its contents, is burnt down. The circumcised boy now has a different status, even if he is not considered to be a proper adult.

Ancient reports describe *murundu,* which had no fixed time, occurring in Winter (probably to prevent haemorrhages) at intervals of about five years. The school lasted for three months. The structure was erected in the bush and close to a river. The site was consecrated by a medicine man, and enclosed by a thorn fence with two openings—one for the boys and one for the adults. Different huts were also built for the old men and the initiates.

When the decision to hold a *murundu* was made, the news spread around the area and the boys were taken to the site. In ancient time, the boys went there after reaching puberty; later on, the ages decreased (probably because the *thondo* was assimilated, where the boys were younger). The boys' heads were shaved before leaving home.

The operation was carried out by a medicine man and the operator's face was masked. The boy sat on a stone and the hand of the medicine-man's assistant covered his eyes, while the assembly accompanied the operation with a tumult of shouting, so as to overwhelm the cries that the initiate may utter. After the prepuce was removed, the wound was wrapped up for couple of days in leaves believed to have curative power. When all the acolytes had been operated on, their faces were painted with white stripes, they rested all the afternoon, then they were allowed to lead into the *murundu.* This was all was accompanied by song and dance. The initiates were sometimes submitted to ordeals to reinforce them.

Throughout the *murundu* boys were not supposed to drink water, and had to eat in complete silence. Then boys were requested to memorize some "sacred" formulas, with lessons followed by dancing. This period usually lasted two months. The following month was devoted to the teaching of tribal norms and values and the performance of ritual dances. However, as much of the information was given in unusual and dramatic circumstances and in an obscure and esoteric way, it was not granted that the boy was able to understand its meaning. Later ceremonies, with the assistance of a teacher, were often necessary to reinforce what had been taught. Then the boy returned home.

MC, according to Stayt (1968), was not a preparation for marriage, nor a declaration of puberty, but was "a powerful agent in forming a centralizing intertribal bond of mutual interest and friendship" (page 136). The boys' schools had the purpose of equipping and entitling the initiate to accept the roles that maturity would bring. Over time the rite has changed, due to the pressures of missionaries, who persuaded converts to avoid sacrificial rituals and other traditional practices and customs. Other changes have recently occurred in the ritual, since the ritual is now performed in health facilities due to the fear of HIV.

14.2 Materials and Methods

Twenty-seven male Venda, living in the Vhembe area, aged 23–80 years, were interviewed. They were interviewed with a 35-item, semi-structured, and open-ended interview, using the person-to-person format. Of these, 85.2 % were married and had an average of 7.5 offspring (minimum 3, maximum 12). The high number of children is due to the Venda polygynous system of marriage. The various items included questions regarding the modalities in which MC was performed (who, when, where, why); propositions aiming to understand variants and changes with respect to the traditional form reported in literature; personal evaluations regarding the practice; and other questions related to MC (i.e., the social importance of MC, its role in sex life, whether or not their male offspring should be circumcised, and so on).

14.3 Results

For 74.1 % of the respondents, the term *murundu* coincided with MC, while for 18.5 % it signified an IS. An alternative term is *hogo*. *Murunduni* or, alternatively *hogoni*, means to participate in the IS for males. All of them claimed that the practice was not only a Venda feature, as it was found in neighboring populations (i.e., the Sotho group was mentioned in 70.4 % of interviews). All of them affirmed that MC is a bloody and painful collective rite, performed on all male children at the average age of 9 or 10 (63.0 %), and that it is part of an IS. All the subjects agreed that the father was essential in teaching sexual education to his male offspring, and all the respondents were inclined to submit their children to the rite. In 59.3 % of the cases, the meaning of *murundu* had been explained to them by their fathers and/or grandfathers during childhood. The mother was excluded, as the participants assigned her the traditional role of raising children (77.8 %).

Of the participants, 61.5 % said they never talk about sexual affairs with their peers, and 96.3 % were convinced that MC gave more sexual pleasure to women during sexual intercourse, and that uncircumcised men could create problems for the couple (77.8 %), mostly because of female sexual dissatisfaction. In 51.9 % of the cases, uncircumcised men were believed to be more prone to (unspecified) sicknesses, and those who did not submit to the practice were labeled as being "weak" (25.9 %) or "stupid" (22.2 %); while a circumcised man was highly valued as he showed courage (44.4 %), and was a "true man" (44.4 %). In order to understand the role of taboos and the differences between the subjects who do talk about sexual affairs and/or MC and those who never talk about these topics, we asked the participants whether uncircumcised men are more prone to sickness or not: the results were non-significant ($X^2 = 2.7$; df = 1; N.S.).

As the majority of the subjects (77.8 %) assigned a traditional role to women, i.e., to raise children, the sample was subdivided into those over and those under 50 years of age in order to understand if differences existed between age groups. No differences emerged ($X^2 = 0.3$; df = 1; N.S.) regarding the role assigned to women in relation to age. Regarding the questions aimed at collecting information on how MC changed over time, 96.3 % of the subjects mentioned two dialectal expressions as an alternative to *murundu*: *mula* and *hogo*. However, not all subjects were accurate in their responses, so it is only possible to sketch a general frame of the practice as follows (at least for the Vhembe area). *Murundu* is still widespread, in this part of South Africa.

Today, many parents prefer to send their sons to a hospital, but the son is not considered to be a "true" man if a female nurse operates on him. Some of those interviewed mentioned the fact that missionaries have struggled hard against MC, but without success, as parents strongly request it.

The Vhemba variant requires the erection of a lodge, with poles, straw, and grass, in a place carefully chosen beforehand, usually in the winter, in mountainous forests and close to a river or stream. *Thava* means "mountain," *thavani* means "in the mountains," and the term, in a figurative way, means also "at the chief kraal" or to participate in the boys' IS. A fence surrounds the building, with entries being called *khareni*. Poles are put into the ground facing the lodge: the boys must be as respectful to these poles as if they were their ancestors. Sometimes a skin is hung on them, representing the bear of an old man.

The site is located in a hidden place (*hamadala*), and nobody must see what happens in it, especially women. The boys are taken there by the elders of the villages and are received by the *mudabe*, a young instructor assisting them during the ceremony. Girls prepare the food for the boys, which is placed close to the hut (called *dzikhareni*) and is taken by the *mudabe* later on. It is forbidden for the initiates to eat salted or flavored food, or to drink water, as it is believed that these are not "healthy" for the operation. Meat is ordinarily forbidden.

The operator, usually a medicine man, is called *maine* (or *who-maine*). The place where MC is performed can be called *hogoni* or *milani*. Boys are operated on, one by one, by the *maine* under the grip of helpers, usually in the morning. The other initiates cannot see what is going on. Their eyes are closed (*tsihotola*) by the hands of helpers. The boy sits on notched stones called *mano a tshikadzi* (cat's teeth), named in this way because, when the boy is operated on, he feels a strong pain "as if sharp teeth were biting him." The position taken by the boy is sometimes called *vhadabe*, the cutting is called *u'geda*, while the circumcised penis is called *u'vhada pfumo* (engraved spear), meaning that the penis is now prepared like the tip of a spear.

During the painful operation, a lot of blood is lost (*munege*) and the boys can sometimes collapse (in this case it is said that the boy has been struck by a ram–*diwa nga nngu*). Only two of the participants mentioned the fact that the boy can die. The penis is then covered with the leaves of the African black wood (*muuluri*), whose leaves are called *rathelo*. From then on, the operated part is called *mutshila wa nngu* (the sheep tail). The cut prepuce is laid in a horn. When all interventions have been performed, other substances (believed to have magical powers) are added (the mixture is called *lutala*) to the horn containing the prepuces and then burnt. This "medicine" is believed to protect from the "shadows."

For two weeks, early in the morning, the circumcised boy must stay close to a fire, with his back to it, and let that the fresh air coming from the east cure the wound. Then the boys go hunting with the *mudabe* and collect wood. If they see a woman, they must cry out, so as to frighten her so she moves away. During this period, special instructions containing traditional norms and laws (*milayo*) are recited and repeated. Songs and dances are performed (Netshitangani, 2005). At night the Venda warrior songs are learnt. The main teachings are about the Venda beliefs (*vhutuka or vhutuga*) regarding sex. This means not only talking about sex, but also how to have sexual intercourse with women and how to get them pregnant. Uncircumcised boys are called *mashuvhuru*; those circumcised without *milayo* are labelled as *manngoda*; while *mudabe* or *whabade* is the term designated for the "real men."

When the IS ends, the lodge is burnt down and the boys must return home without looking back, as they could get burnt, too. When they get home, they are smeared with lemon and are covered with adornments (*vhulungu ha mpakato*).

14.4 Discussion and Conclusions

The Venda culture is a clear example of an aggregate of meanings, which has been built up over time through the addition, selection, and elimination of various meanings; with social dynamics rapidly changing values and norms under the pressure of economic and political adaptation strategies. Among the Venda, MC is an interesting cultural trait, as it was established under the constraining forces of contiguous populations and quickly became a "tradition"; as the terms to name procedures and passages are linguistically very rich, so are the rituals and the accompanying ceremonies characterizing the whole *murundu*, and its widespread presence among male Venda. At present, the practice is still popular and all the subjects that we interviewed expressed the desire to maintain it. This is in contrast to what happened to the female counterpart, where interventions on genitalia quickly faded (more or less in one generation), due to several reasons probably connected to the changing female role in a rapidly changing society. This suggests that MC is pursued for reasons of masculinity and that this ritual could only be modified by reversing beliefs regarding masculinity. This is a very difficult task in South Africa, where 30 % of girls' first sexual experiences are forced, as women and girls are seen as being "less worthy" than males, and they simply have to be respectful and obey the sexual desires of their partners (Hjort 2006). This tendency clearly emerged in our sample, as there were no distinctions between older and younger subjects on the questions aiming to better understanding the male attitude towards the other gender.

Beliefs regarding masculinity are strongly associated with MC because it is the main way to socialize and strengthen these beliefs in pre-pubescent boys. Even if the boys do not fully understand the essence of this tradition (to be socially accepted as males), they undergo this very painful practice under the pressure of peers and adults. This is reinforced linguistically: an uncircumcised man is a *mashuvuru*, a "weak man" unable to "satisfy women in bed," but the term expresses other subtle nuances, suggesting indolence, childishness, and effeminacy. A circumcised man, on the other hand, is a *vhadabe*, a "true man," a strong and courageous individual who is able to perform well "in bed." Practically all our subjects were convinced that MC enhances sexual pleasure and that women prefer circumcised men, mainly so they can be sexually satisfied.

MC, therefore, is regarded as a procedure through which a boy acquires social status, enhances his opportunities for sexual relations (as he can be chosen by women), together with his sexual and reproductive capacities. In this context, it will be very difficult to start an anti-circumcision campaign. In some of the interviews, it emerged that the missionaries' efforts to ban MC were unsuccessful. There was a little change in attitude when government agencies introduced the use of individual and septic instruments to lessen the risk of contracting HIV and other sexually transmitted infections because now, mostly in town, boys are hospitalized.

The role of ethnicity and social stratification is important in South Africa, where the definition of a population like "the Venda" by one set of criteria, such as language, often does not coincide with other limits, such as chiefdoms, mode of subsistence, political boundaries, and migrations. In this marginal part of the country, changes are slow; this area was not involved in the big socio-economic changes that occurred in other parts of South Africa due to industrialization, foreboding migrations (Gluckman 1960; Maher 1994). The social stratification therefore shows slow variations; the same is true of the rituals with anthropopoietic function like *murundu*.

Furthermore, MC is widely practiced in all South Africa, and efforts have been made to reduce its risks, which are mainly due to the fact that boys are operated on by a "traditional" surgeon, and that the removal of the foreskin is done without anesthetic, and is performed in secluded IS that do not provide even minimal hygienic conditions (Peltzer et al. 2008a, b; Mayatula and Mavundla 1997). Almost all the Venda adjacent groups practice MC, and the prestige associated to the European way of life is not appealing for males. And, we cannot forget that MC is a widespread practice in America.

The medical consequences of MC are surely known but underestimated. For example Sidley (1996) found that in the Cape Province alone, during 1995, 34 deaths, 12 penis amputations, and 743 hospitalizations for septic wounds were recorded due to MC carried out in traditional ways. In the same Province, 26 eighteen-year-old boys were submitted to reconstructive surgery in 1996 after a botched MC (Hofvander 2004). Mogotlane et al. (2004), and Kanta (2004) described all the possible consequences of traditional MC. Some of them are botched MC, infections of the wounds, gangrene of the penis, severe hemorrhage, dehydration, respiratory infection, disability, and death. In this context, IS are very important in providing sexual information, but they often fail to provide relevant information for adopting healthy sexual behaviors in the age of HIV/AIDS, as demonstrated by Malisha et al. (2008). To our knowledge, no data on the consequences of clumsily-performed MC in the Venda area is available. It therefore is not difficult to imagine that in the IS the traditional surgeon is not provided with adequate training; that the living conditions of these schools (cold and dusty) are unhealthy for boys; that the pre-existing abnormalities or illnesses of the initiated are not considered; doubts persist about the sterility of the surgical instruments (often used and reused); and that the aftercare of the boys and all the critical cases after surgery are not adequately managed.

Traditional beliefs are still working in the area, for example, the cause of a sickness (HIV/AIDS included) and those of a death are never openly mentioned, and no death is "natural" (except for the very old and the very young). Most of the people believe that something or someone was directly responsible for a person's early passing (McNeill 2009). Furthermore, this could be due to witchcraft or to the contact with a thing, in particular condoms. The popular belief is as follows: if a condom is filled with warm water and left in sunlight, white "worms" will hatch inside, and that the contact with these worms will transmit the virus (Boer and Mashamba 2009). Until recently in some parts of the Venda area, AIDS (whose name is never mentioned because of the social stigma) was rumored to be spread by young women aiming to prevent it. These denials and obfuscations can be partially ascribed to the government's misguided approach to the AIDS pandemic of the recent past (mostly a denialist stance). Clearly, the silence of authorities permitted the rise of gossip and rumors, as happens when a world of fantasies, fears, and ideas are built around matters that cannot be spoken about openly.

Since the demise of apartheid in 1994, the political/economic changes that have occurred in the whole country have led to a "re-traditionalization of customs," as "many perceive the post-apartheid era as one of emergency" (McNeill 2009, page 5), a process that has ignited old rivalries and dominates the political landscape. Bearing this in mind, changes are difficult, and all the prevention policies based on an inadequate understanding of the wider context are attempts doomed to fail. Adequate and effective prevention campaigns for HIV/AIDS are very difficult; not to mention the efforts to ban MC. Perhaps, an involvement of the IS leaders is necessary, as they should be at the forefront of initiations that—at least—should be performed under sterile and controlled conditions. They could also provide information for a more complete and adequate sex education, especially about the sexually transmitted diseases.

References

Blacking J, Huffman TN (1982) The great enclosure and domba. Man 20(3):542–545

Boer H, Mashamba MT (2009) Gender power imbalance and differential psychosocial correlates of intended condom use among male and female adolescents from Venda, South Africa. Br J Health Psychol 12(1):51–63

Comaroff J, Comaroff JL (2004) Notes on afromodernity and the neo world order: an afterword. In: Weiss B (ed) Producing African futures: ritual and reproduction in a neoliberal age. Brill. Leiden, pp 329–348

Gluckman M (1960) Anthropological problems arising from the African industrial revolution. In: Southall A (ed) Social changes in modern Africa. Oxford University Press, London

Grant W (1905) Magato and his tribe. J Roy Anthropol Inst 4:267

Hammond-Tooke WD (1974) The Bantu-speaking peoples of southern Africa. London and Boston: Routledge and Kegan P. Publ

Harries CL (1929) The Laws and customs of the BaPedi and cognate tribes of the Transvaal. Johannesburg, Hortors Limited

Hjort L (2006) Sexism, youth and HIV in South Africa. http://www.alternatives.ca/eng/our-organization/our-publications/analysis-and-articles

Hofvander Y (2004) Violations against children in the name of religion and tradition. Is there a way out ? Syllabus of abstracts, VIII International symposium on circumcision and human rights. Padua, Sep 2–4, 2004

Junod HA (1927) The Life of a South African Tribe. MacMillan, London

Kanta XGM (2004) Traditional male circumcision and initiation into manhood: legal, health and environmental perspectives. Gonubie, Impilo ya Bantu Health Dev Projects, Eastern Cape

Lestrade GP (1927) Some notes on the ethnic history of the BaVenda and their Rhodesia affinities. S Afr J Sci 24:486–495

Maher V (1994) Questioni di etnicità. Rosenberg and Sellier, Turin, pp 15–32

Malisha L, Maharaj P, Rogan M (2008) Rites of passage to adulthood: traditional schools in the context of HIV/AIDS in the Limpopo Province, South Africa. Health, Risk Soc 10(6):585–598

Mayatula V, Mavundla TL (1997) A review on male circumcision procedures among the South African black. Curationis 20(3):16–20

McNeill FG (2009) "Condoms cause AIDS": poison, prevention and denial in Venda, South Africa. Afr Aff 1–18:0. doi:10.1093/afraf/adp020

Mogotlane SM, Ntlangulela JT, Ogunbanjo BG (2004) Mortality and morbidity among traditionally circumcised Xhosa boys in the Eastern Cape Province. Curationis 27(2):57–62

Netshitangani K (2005) Songs of the Venda Murundu Schools. In: Christine L (ed) The world of South African music. Cambridge Scholar Press, Newcastle upon Tyne, pp 245–249

Peltzer K, Nqeketo A, Petros G, Kanta XGM (2008a) Evaluation of safer male circumcision training programme for traditional surgeons and nurses in the Eastern Cape, South Africa. Afr J Tradit Complement Altern Med 5(4):346–354

Peltzer K, Nqeketo A, Petros G, Kanta XGM (2008b) Attitudes of preinitiates towards traditional male circumcision in the context of HIV in Eastern Cape, South Africa. Soc Behav Pers 36(8):1023–1034

Sidley P (1996) Botched circumcision led to arrest for murder. Br Med J 313:647–650

Stayt HA (1968) The Bavenda. F Cass and Co, Capetown

West M, Morris J (1982) Abantu. An introduction to the black people of South Africa. C Struik Publ, Cape Town, pp 89–198

Wheelwright CA (1905) Native circumcision lodges in the Zoutpansberg district. J Roy Anthropol Inst 4:252

Author Biography

Erika Dionisio A graduating student, Department of Applied Psychology, University of Padua. She was involved in a field qualitative research on genital modifications in the Venda region in South Africa, and she collected data on body image from South African students. Padua, Italy.

Franco Viviani A physical anthropologist, is Professor of Anthropology at the Department of Human Movement Studies and at the Department of Philosophy, Sociology, Pedagogy and Applied Psychology (FISPPA), University of Padova. He has published papers and articles both on male and female circumcision. He is the NOCIRC of Italy representative. Padua, Italy.

Chapter 15
Critique of African RCTs into Male Circumcision and HIV Sexual Transmission

Gregory J. Boyle

Abstract On the basis of three seriously flawed sub-Saharan African randomized clinical trials into female-to-male (FTM) sexual transmission of HIV, in 2007 WHO/UNAIDS recommended circumcision (MC) of millions of African men as an HIV preventive measure, despite the trials being compromised by irrational motivated reasoning, inadequate equipoise, selection bias, inadequate blinding, problematic randomization, trials stopped early with exaggerated treatment effects, and failure to investigate non-sexual transmission. Several questions remain unanswered. Why were the trials carried out in countries where more intact men were HIV+ than in those where more circumcised men were HIV+? Why were men sampled from specific ethnic subgroups? Why were so many men lost to follow-up? Why did men in the intervention group receive additional counselling on safe sex practices? The *absolute reduction* in HIV transmission associated with MC was only 1.3 % (without even adjusting for known sources of error bias). *Relative reduction* was reported as 60 %, but after correction for lead-time bias alone averaged 49 %. In a related Ugandan RCT into male-to-female (MTF) transmission, there was a 61 % *relative increase* (6 % *absolute increase*) in HIV infection among female partners of circumcised men, some of whom were not informed that their male partners were HIV+ (also some of the men were not informed by the researchers that they were HIV+). It appears that the number of circumcisions needed to infect a woman (Number Needed to Harm) was 16.7, with one woman becoming infected for every 17 circumcisions performed. As the trial was stopped early for "futility," the increase in HIV infections was not statistically significant, although clinically significant. In the Kenyan trial, MC was

This article was first published by Thomson Reuters in the Journal of Law and Medicine and should be cited as Boyle GJ, Hill G. Sub-Saharan African randomised clinical trials into male circumcision and HIV transmission: Methodological, ethical and legal concerns. (2011) 19 JLM 316. For all subscription inquiries please phone, from Australia: 1300 304 195, from Overseas: +61 2 8587 7980 or online at www.thomsonreuters.com.au/catalogue. The official PDF version of this article can also be purchased separately from Thomson Reuters.

G. J. Boyle (✉)
Faculty of Humanities and Social Sciences, Bond University, Queensland, Australia
e-mail: gregb@bond.edu.an

G. C. Denniston et al. (eds.), *Genital Cutting: Protecting Children from Medical, Cultural, and Religious Infringements*, DOI: 10.1007/978-94-007-6407-1_15,

associated with at least four new incident infections. Since MC diverts resources from known preventive measures and increases risk-taking behaviors, any long-term benefit in reducing HIV transmission remains dubious.

Keywords Randomized clinical trials • HIV/AIDS • Sexual transmission • Male to female transmission • Female to male transmission • Researcher bias • External validity

15.1 Background

Three randomized clinical trials (RCTs) tested the efficacy of male circumcision (MC) to reduce female-to-male (FTM) sexual transmission of HIV in South Africa, Kenya, and Uganda. (Auvert et al. 2005; Bailey et al. 2007; Gray et al. 2007) At the time when these trials were approved, it was deemed that they were needed to test the hypothesis that MC would lead to a decreased risk of HIV acquisition among men. The risk–benefit ratio was judged acceptable by all Institutional Review Boards (IRBs) involved, and men were allowed to (and many did) decline participation. It was reported that MC reduces FTM sexual transmission of HIV. Evidence from a parallel RCT into male-to-female (MTF) sexual transmission of HIV in Uganda suggested that MC *increases* MTF transmission of HIV. Alarmingly, this evidence appears to have been ignored by WHO/UNAIDS in recommending the promotion of MC (Wawer et al. 2009). In the MTF trial, women were unwittingly exposed to HIV infection since male sexual partners who submitted to MC were already HIV+. Several women subsequently became HIV+, raising concerns about informed consent. In real-life settings, HIV testing cannot be assured and will not always occur prior to the circumcision intervention. The present critique raises several methodological, ethical and legal concerns with these trials, suggesting that the decision by WHO/UNAIDS to recommend MC as an HIV-preventive measure was unwarranted.

While the “gold standard” for medical trials is the randomized, double-blind placebo-controlled trial (RCT), (Sussman and Hayward 2010; Padian et al. 2010) the African trials suffered design and sampling problems, including problematic randomization and selection bias, inadequate blinding, lack of placebo-control (MC could not be concealed), inadequate equipoise, experimenter bias, attrition (673 drop-outs in FTM trials), not investigating MC as a cause of HIV transmission, not investigating non-sexual HIV transmission, as well as lead-time bias, supportive bias (circumcised men provided additional counselling sessions), participant expectation bias, and time-out discrepancy (restraint from sexual activity only by circumcised men). Men were randomized either to immediate or delayed MC groups, obfuscating long-term effectiveness. The number of crossovers and participants lost to follow-up differed between groups in all three FTM trials, and in the South African and Ugandan FTM trials group sizes were somewhat discrepant.

Despite excessively large sample sizes (producing statistically significant effects that were trivial), the actual number of HIV+ circumcised vs. intact men was small, but almost identical across the FTM trials (20, 22, 22) versus (49, 47, 45), raising questions as to whether these were three separate trials or three arms of the same trial? The Ugandan MTF trial was stopped early after 25 (17 *in MC group*) *previously uninfected women became HIV+*. MC was associated with a 61 % *relative increase* (6 % *absolute increase*) in HIV transmission, (Wawer et al. 2009) leading Wawer et al. to caution that, *Condom use after male circumcision is essential for HIV prevention* (Wawer et al. 2009). What is the purpose of MC if condom use is still needed to prevent sexual transmission of HIV?

Although the Cochrane review asserted that no further studies into MC and HIV sexual transmission are needed, (Siegfried et al. 2009) the epidemiological evidence shows that MC does not reduce HIV sexual transmission in several sub-Saharan African countries, including Cameroon, Rwanda, Lesotho, Malawi, Tanzania, Ghana, and Swaziland, all of which have a higher prevalence of HIV infection among circumcised men (Young 2010; Gisselquist 2007). Clearly, much epidemiological evidence does not support the WHO/UNAIDS decision to recommend the genital cutting of millions of African men as a putative HIV preventive measure.

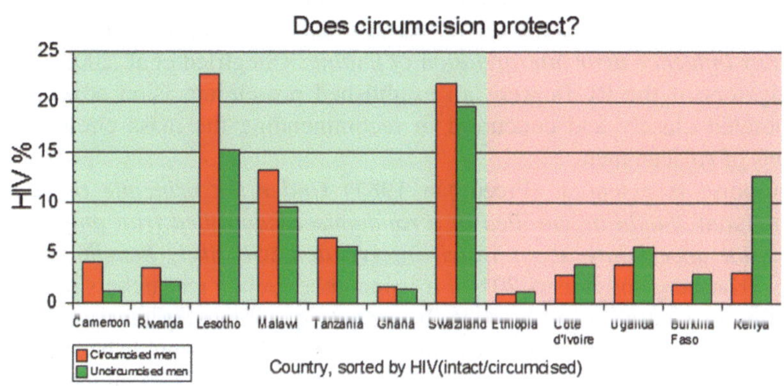

From www.circumcstitions.com (retrieved 4 July 2011; reproduced with permission from the author Hugh Young, email: hugh@buzz.net.nz).

15.2 Methodological Concerns

15.2.1 Factors Jeopardizing Internal Validity

Several factors may jeopardise internal validity of RCTs, including (1) researcher expectation bias, (2) participant expectation bias, (3) inadequate double blinding, (4) lead-time bias, (5) selection and sampling bias, (6) experimental mortality, and (7) premature termination. Treatment effects are exaggerated when there are problems with participant allocation (e.g., allocation concealment; allocation schedule), exclusion of certain participants from analyses, and early termination of trials. Inadequately concealed trials may exaggerate ORs by 41 % (plus additional 17 % if lack of double-blinding) (Schulz et al. 1995). These internal validity problems are discussed below in relation to each of the four trials.

1. Researcher expectation bias

The principal investigators had a history of co-authoring papers promoting MC (e.g., Gray and Wawer have co-authored more than 100 joint papers) indicating their close collaboration (Mehta et al. 2009). The names of no fewer than 14 co-authors appeared on the reports of both Ugandan trials, (Gray et al. 2007; Wawer et al. 2009) suggesting the two trials were not independent. Analysis of the references cited in common across the four trials also reveals substantial overlap (Auvert: 17 out of 34 = 50 %; Bailey: 19 out of 50 = 38 %; Gray: 17 out of 27 = 63 %; Wawer: 7 out of 18 = 39 %).

Claims by Auvert et al. (2005) as to *the long-term protective effect of MC* when the trials were terminated prematurely, and that, *If women are aware of the protective effect of MC, this awareness could…[encourage] males to become circumcised* suggest a lack of equipoise. A Cochrane Review warned, *researchers' personal biases and the dominant circumcision practices of their respective countries may influence their interpretation of findings* (Siegfried et al. 2003). The lead investigators of the RCTs were all established pro-circumcision advocates who collaborated closely and concurred in recommending the mass circumcision of millions of African men.

Equipoise is essential. (Freedman 1987) *Under the principle of equipoise, a participant should be enrolled in a randomised controlled trial only if there is substantial uncertainty about which intervention will likely benefit the participant…* (Karlberg and Speers 2010). It is incumbent upon researchers to start from a position of neutrality and balance. In order to quantitatively measure equipoise, an empirical analysis of references cited in each of the four published reports was undertaken based on content deemed pro-circumcision (MC recommended as beneficial), neutral (e.g., articles pertaining to statistical procedures), or anti-circumcision (MC not recommended), respectively. As Table 15.1 shows, each of the RCT reports cited observational studies suggesting a benefit of MC, but not even one of the observational studies showing either no effect of MC on HIV transmission (13 studies) or a higher incidence of HIV among circumcised men (4 studies) were cited (Young 2010). Omission of contradictory evidence prevented a balanced

Table 15.1 Analysis of cited references

	Auvert	Bailey	Gray	Wawer
Pro-MC	24 (70.6 %)	36 (72 %)	19 (70.4 %)	12 (67 %)
Anti-MC	2 (5.9 %)	1 (2 %)	0 (0 %)	0
Neutral	8 (23.5 %)	13 (26 %)	8 (29.6 %)	6 (33 %)
Total	34	50	27	18

consideration of the available empirical evidence, suggesting the trials lacked equipoise and were biased from the very outset.

Chi square analyses (with Yates' correction) of the number of cited references deemed to be pro-MC versus. anti-MC (Chi squares for Pro-MC versus Neutral vs. Anti-MC shown in parentheses) for each of the four trials provide evidence of pre-existing pro-circumcision bias.

Auvert $\chi^2 = 16.96(1df), p < 0.001$ $(\chi^2 = 20.66(2df), p < 0.001)$
Bailey $\chi^2 = 31.24(1df), p < 0.001$ $(\chi^2 = 35.60\,(2df), p < 0.001)$
Gray $\chi^2 = 17.06(1df), p < 0.001$ $(\chi^2 = 18.33(2df), p < 0.001)$
Wawer $\chi^2 = 10.08(1df), p < 0.001$ $(\chi^2 = 10.13(2df), p < 0.01)$

In the South African report, two anti-MC references were mis-cited either as neutral (Siegfried et al. 2005) or as pro-MC (Kim et al. 1999) so that 25/34 (74 %) of the references were cited in support of MC. In the Kenyan report, only one anti-MC reference was cited, but incorrectly as being neutral (Magoha 1999). In both Ugandan reports, no references opposing MC were cited. In none of the reports was even a single reference cited as opposing MC, in contrast to the more than 70 % of citations supporting MC. Not acknowledging the published evidence showing no prophylactic benefit of MC suggests selective reporting and *confirmation bias*. Admittedly, investigator bias in favor of the hypothesis probably was not the only factor that led to these trials given the growing desperation to stem the terrible HIV/AIDS epidemic in sub-Saharan Africa.

2. Participant expectation bias

Participants were informed that previous studies suggested a potential benefit of MC. Presumably the trial authors would argue that this was a requirement of disclosure, but why did they not also inform participants that other observational studies had shown no benefit of MC? Why was this contradictory evidence withheld from the prospective participants? Asking leading questions may have influenced the men's decisions to participate. Indeed, Auvert et al. remarked that *59 %... of uncircumcised men said that they would be circumcised if it reduced their chance of acquiring HIV and STDs*. Did the researchers help create a demand for MC by implying that it would help to protect men against HIV and STIs? (Dowsett and Couch 2007).

3. Inadequate double blinding

Since MC cannot be concealed, double blinding, which reduces observer bias and placebo effects, was not possible in the African trials (Schulz et al. 1995). As Wawer et al. conceded, *In view of the surgical nature of the intervention, neither participants nor study clinicians could be masked to assignment group* (Wawer et al. 2009). Also, some researchers had access to the data. In the South African trial, *BA analysed the data with RS, with inputs from JST* and *at each visit to the centre the nurse completed a questionnaire after the genital examination...* (Auvert et al. 2005). In the Kenyan trial, *...some participants divulged their circumcision status...* (Bailey et al. 2007). Knowing men's circumcision status may have influenced their questionnaire responses. Clearly, it is not possible to conduct such trials to the same standards as a double-blind placebo-controlled trial taking place in a laboratory setting.

4. Lead-time bias

Men in the intervention group had less time to become HIV infected since effectively they were out of the trials for up to two months while their circumcision wounds (portals for HIV infection) healed. This occurred early in the trials, thereby amplifying lead-time bias. HIV incidence rate ratios (RRs) adjusted for lead-time bias of two months have been calculated using SAS (Version 8.2; SAS Institute, Cary, North Carolina) (Van Howe 2010). Auvert's RR of 0.40 after adjustment was found to be 0.46 (95 % CI 0.23–0.77 %; $p = 0.003$), Bailey's RR of 0.47 after adjustment was found to be 0.52 (95 % CI 0.31–0.87 %; $p = 0.012$), while Gray's RR of 0.49 after adjustment was found to be 0.56 (95 % CI 0.34–0.93 %; $p = 0.026$). Thus, the relative protection against HIV (1-RR) across the three trials decreased to a mean of 49 %, showing that the claimed 60 % protective effect of MC is an overstatement. That the *absolute* reduction of 1.3 % was statistically but not clinically significant (relevant from a policy implementation perspective) has been overlooked in the RCT reports, where only the *relative* reduction in HIV transmission has been highlighted. The statistical significance was most likely an artifact due to the excessively large sample sizes in the two comparison groups (5,411 men circumcised; 5,497 controls) wherein the studies were overpowered thereby producing a statistical effect when the absolute effect was unimportant.

5. Selection and sampling bias

Pre-screening and participant self-selection may have produced non-equivalent comparison groups and undermined internal validity. Volunteers were not a population-based random sample since religious or ethnic groups already circumcised necessarily were excluded. Presumably, the trials were located in areas where MC was uncommon in order to recruit adequate sample sizes. Since many unemployed men were financially rewarded for participating, it is likely that samples were skewed towards men from lower SES backgrounds.

There were more at-risk men in the delayed circumcision (control) groups in the South African (+36) and Ugandan (+48) FTM trials, raising questions about the allocation of participants. In the South African trial, the two groups differed significantly on background variables including age ($\chi^2 = 4.58$ (1df), $p < 0.05$), religious affiliation ($\chi^2 = 9.36$ (2df), $p < 0.01$), and ethnic group ($\chi^2 = 12.84$ (2df), $p < 0.01$). There was also a significant between-group difference for ethnic group ($\chi^2 = 12.84$ (2df), $p < 0.01$) in the Kenyan trial, suggesting that, in both trials, participants from different tribal backgrounds were differentially admitted into the comparison groups. In the Ugandan FTM trial, participants allocated to the MC group received significantly more counselling ($\chi^2 = 6.02$ (1df), $p < 0.02$).

In both the South African and Ugandan FTM trials, a higher prevalence of STIs and genital disorders was reported within the control groups. Since HIV is more likely to co-occur with other STIs, (Fleming and Wasserheit 1999) it is likely that the control groups were at greater risk of acquiring new HIV infections, irrespective of any preventive effect of MC. Why were there significant between-group differences on these background variables? In the South African trial, only men who produced three positive Enzyme-Linked Immunosorbent Assay (ELISA) tests were classified as HIV+. The screening approach, which comprised one ELISA test and two confirmatory ELISA tests using different testing approaches, represents WHOs' current testing strategy for low- to middle-income countries. Since men with one or two positive ELISA tests were regarded as HIV−, how many false negatives (HIV+ men) were assigned to the respective groups? However, even if some HIV+ men were erroneously considered to be HIV−, it would only affect the study results if the majority of these men were randomized to the delayed circumcision arm.

6. Experimental mortality

Participant loss (missing data) was considerably greater than the number of new HIV infections (South Africa: 151 vs. 49 intact men, 100 vs. 20 circumcised men; Kenya: 92 vs. 47 intact men, 87 vs. 22 circumcised men; Uganda: 133 vs. 45 intact men, 140 vs. 22 circumcised men). While losses exceeded incident cases, it appears that losses were relatively comparable between study arms. However, it remains unclear whether there was a high proportion of new incident HIV+ infections among those lost to follow-up in the MC group. Men who submitted to MC but who subsequently became HIV+ may have become disillusioned and dropped out, differing from those who completed follow-up evaluations. Which participants were not followed up and their HIV status not reported? *The problem with both the lost-to-follow-up and non-sexual transmission numbers is that they are unknown, thereby creating uncertainty, and reducing confidence in the estimate of the treatment effect* (Van Howe RS, 12 March 2011, "personal communication").

7. Early termination

Truncated RCTs produce exaggerated effect sizes (Montori et al. 2005; Mills and Siegfried 2006; Bassler et al. 2010) and amplify lead-time bias (Pocock and White 1999). Even though Gray et al. acknowledged that *trials that are stopped early could overestimate efficacy when compared with subsequent studies,* (Gray et al. 2007) all three FTM trials were stopped early, thereby exaggerating effects. In addition, Auvert et al. conceded that *adjustment cannot fully account for the confounding effect associated with partial follow-up*. Claims based on trials stopped early for benefit should be viewed with caution. Subsequently, Bailey reported that the "protective effect" of MC in the Kenyan trial had been sustained over 4.5 years (Bailey et al. 2010). This assertion is difficult to evaluate since it was based on the analysis of incomplete *observational data*. As Van Howe (12 March 2012, "personal communication") pointed out, *No one knows the trajectory the data would take in the next 20 years because the studies were stopped prematurely (as soon as they reached statistical significance, although the effect size was inconsequential). The bottom line is that the three African RCTs had a very serious missing data problem, to the point where the results are basically worthless.*

8. Statistical significance versus clinical significance

The three FTM trials, while significant in the statistical sense, were not significant in any clinically important or meaningful real-life sense. The RCT investigators failed to investigate non-sexual sources of HIV infections, they built-in lead-time bias, and may have coerced the largely unemployed participants in the trials with inducements of monetary payments. *Inexplicably, WHO, UNAIDS, and various medical journal editors continue to advocate the circumcision solution even though they know the science is invalid* (Van Howe RS, 10 March 2011, "personal communication"). In the RCT reports, why was the relative reduction highlighted rather than the absolute reduction, thereby giving the misleading impression that MC could actually reduce HIV sexual transmission, wen the evidence actually indicated that MC resulted in a negligible risk reduction (ARR)? The trials found nothing of any clinical significance and after adjusting for sources of error bias, any statistically significant effect would have disappeared entirely.

While the results of the RCTs were "statistically" significant, the Absolute Risk Reduction (ARR) was so small as to be almost meaningless. The studies all had nearly identical methods and shared the same built-in forms of bias, all of which increased the estimated treatment effect. As Van Howe pointed out (10 March 2012, "personal communication"),

> *The first big problem was that half of the men did not get HIV from sexual contact, so that would reduce the absolute risk reduction from 1.3 to 0.65 %. The lead-time bias would reduce the ARR by another 17–0.54 %. Early stoppage of studies is associated with an over estimate of treatment effect by 30 %, so the ARR becomes 0.38 %. There is also the expectation bias in both the researchers and participants and the Hawthorn effect this produced. This could have reduced the treatment effect by another 10 % at least, so the ARR is now 0.34 %.*

Van Howe further commented (12 March 2011, "personal communication") that,

> *This does not even account for the missing data problem in which there were several men lost to follow-up for every man who became infected. The accepted approach to missing data is to calculate the extremes and note that the truth lies within that range. If one assumes that all the men in the control group lost to follow-up became HIV+ and none of the intervention group became infected, the RRs in the three studies would be: Auvert: 0.10, 95 % CI = 0.07–0.16; Gray: 0.07, 95 % CI = 0.04–0.11; Bailey: 0.14, 95 % CI = 0.09–0.2. If all the men in the intervention group lost to follow-up became HIV infected and none of the men lost to follow in the control group were to become infected relative risks would be: Auvert: 2.52, 95 % CI = 1.81–3.51; Gray: 5.60, 95 % CI = 4.33–7.71; Bailey: 3.13, 95 % CI = 2.25–4.35. For the Ugandan FTM trial (Gray et al.) the relative risk ranged from 0.07 to 5.60. This is a huge range, suggesting that the number lost to follow-up was excessive and what happened to these men (what we don't know) could easily increase the reported risk estimates. The bottom line is these studies have a very serious missing data problem, to the point where the results are basically worthless.*

The NNT for the unadjusted 1.3 % is 1/0.013 or 76.9, so that 77 men would gain no benefit whatsoever from circumcision. If we use the adjusted ARR estimate of 0.34, then the NNT is 294.1, so it is obvious that the vast majority of African men submitting to circumcision would receive absolutely no

HIV-preventive benefit whatsoever. Thus, for every HIV infection (theoretically) averted, 294 men would have a highly sensitive part of their penis destroyed and suffer the consequences of short-term and/or long-term complications, including reduced sexual sensitivity/function, as well as possible life-long psychological distress (PTSD).

The Ugandan MTF trial was stopped prematurely as soon as it became apparent that the absolute increase in risk was 6 %. The number of circumcisions needed to infect a female partner (Number Needed to Harm) suggests that for every 17 male circumcisions performed, another female partner became infected with HIV. Why has this clinically important finding apparently been overlooked by WHO/UNAIDS in their recommending mass circumcision programs? *Considering that there are more effective methods of prevention available that do not remove body parts and increase the risk to female partners, why is circumcision even part of the discussion? The money could be better spent on clean medical equipment and needles, condoms, and secondary prevention with ARTs* (Van Howe RS, 12 March 2011, "personal communication").

15.3 Factors Jeopardizing External Validity

The RCT reports provided inadequate information about external validity, including methodological flaws in experimental design and procedures, non-representative sampling (e.g., sampling from mostly poorly educated, impoverished African men), reporting of *relative* rather than the *absolute* efficacy of MC, and inadequately investigating confounding factors (e.g., non-sexual transmission of HIV via skin piercing procedures such as injections, transfusion, etc.). Also, the reports of the FTM trials failed to acknowledge adverse effects of the circumcision interventions (e.g., four new incident HIV infections related to MC in the Kenyan trial) (Gisselquist 2007; Rothwell 2005; Van Spall et al. 2007; Moher et al. 2010; Gisselquist 2009).

Many problems in generalizing results from the trials to the real-world context have been documented (Green et al. 2008, 2010; McAllister et al. 2008). Since the men enrolled in the trials were not representative of the respective populations at large (at least in the South African and Kenyan trials, where data was provided), it is difficult to generalize the findings. Certain ethnic sub-groups were disproportionately represented in the MC and control groups (South Africa: Sotho 49.0 and 47.3 %, Zulu 32.8 and 38.1 %; Kenya: Luo 98 and 99 %; Uganda: no ethnicity data provided). In South Africa, the major ethnic groups consist of Zulu (21 %), Xhosa (17 %) and Sotho (15 %)—so that the Xhosa were under-represented. In Kenya, the main ethnic groups are Kikuyu (22 %), Luhya (14 %), Luo (13 %), Kalenjin (12 %), and Kamba (11 %), so that the Luo were over-represented. Green et al. (2010) concluded that *Effectiveness in real-world settings rarely achieves the efficacy levels found in controlled trials, making predictions of subsequent cost-effectiveness and population-health benefits less reliable… Recommending mass circumcision by generalizing from the particular RCTs to the diverse populations of Africa highlights problems of external validity.*

Furthermore, there has been inaccurate and irresponsible reporting of the trials in the medical literature (e.g., by Peter Piot, former UNAIDS Head in the *Lancet* and by Helen Epstein in the *BMJ*) (Fox and Thomson 2010). Fox and Thomson stated that *Our concern is that such partial reporting of the trials will impact on the role that circumcision is perceived to play in HIV prevention...in perpetuating erroneous beliefs...that circumcision offers immunity to AIDS... If the contexts of the African trials can be so poorly represented in the medical literature, it is no surprise that accounts in the popular press are still more misleading* (Fox and Thomson 2010).

Men enrolled in the immediate MC groups received two years free medical treatment plus supportive counselling and safe-sex advice, difficult to provide in any large-scale "roll out" of MC in sub-Saharan Africa. WHO had specifically cautioned that the FTM Kenyan and Ugandan findings might not generalize to real world settings (Statement on Kenyan 2006). The RCTs were premised on the untested assumption that men who have sex with men (MSM) are extremely rare in Africa and that the HIV epidemic is primarily heterosexual in nature. Evidence suggests this is not the case, (Beyrer et al. 2009; Brody and Potteratt 2003; Roehr 2010; Wakabi 2007) weakening the findings of the RCTs since MC is not effective in preventing HIV transmission among MSM, as the USA epidemiological evidence clearly demonstrates (Millet et al. 2007, 2008). The assumption of heterosexuality is problematic with the African trials. Participants were deemed heterosexual because they *said* they were. In sub-Saharan Africa, capital punishment has been advocated for sodomy making it unlikely that men would willingly admit to homosexual activity. Not controlling for MSM confounded the RCT findings. The American doctors conducting these trials were offering perhaps the only medical attention many of these men were ever likely to receive making it unlikely that they would admit to homosexual activity if it meant being denied this medical attention. With their multiple flaws, these circumcision trials could not be described as the "gold standard" (Young 2010).

Alarmingly, the United States Centers for Disease Control and Prevention (CDC) recently has been considering a recommendation for *routine infant* MC as an HIV-preventive measure in the USA (where homosexual activity is the predominant mode of HIV transmission), ignoring the fact that the RCTs only investigated HIV transmission among heterosexual adults. *Recognition of the potential pitfalls in the transition from clinical trials to effective public health policy is particularly crucial given attempts...by the [CDC] to extrapolate from the three African trials to inform US domestic policy, notwithstanding how typical modes of HIV transmission in the USA are radically different from the model of sexual transmission assumed in the African trials* (Fox and Thomson 2010).

The WHO/UNAIDS recommendation also failed to heed the Cochrane Review, (Siegfried et al. 2009) which noted that further research is required to assess the feasibility, desirability, and cost-effectiveness of MC implementation within local contexts (i.e., external validity and effectiveness in real-life settings, rather than the contrived experimental settings under which the RCTs were carried out).

15.4 Ethical and Legal Concerns

15.4.1 Circumcision as a Cause of HIV Infection

One of the major problems with scaling up these trials is that quality control is not feasible, particularly in relation to MC itself being a possible cause of HIV transmission (Brewer et al. 2007; Zulu et al. 2006). *Possible paths for HIV transmission during circumcision include skin-piercing instruments reused without sterilization, and multidose vials of local anaesthetic contaminated with HIV from a previous patient… [which] might have infected participants with HIV in Kenya* (Gisselquist 2009). Auvert et al. acknowledged *the possible impact of surgery on HIV acquisition as a result of sexual activity during the healing phase following circumcision….* (Auvert et al. 2005) and subsequently, all the lead investigators cautioned that following MC, *…men should delay intercourse to limit the potential for increased HIV risk until complete wound healing* (Mehta et al. 2009). In the Ugandan MTF trial, Wawer et al. cautioned that, *Female acquisition of HIV…occurred in a higher proportion of couples who resumed sex early…strict adherence to sexual abstinence during wound healing and consistent condom use thereafter must be strongly promoted…* (Wawer et al. 2009).

Wawer et al. acknowledged that *…circumcision of HIV-infected men did not reduce transmission of HIV to female partners…* MC was associated with a relative 61 % increased transmission of HIV to female sexual partners. During the 6 month follow-up, 25 new-incident HIV infections occurred among female partners (17 in MC group). However, in an apparent example of irrational *motivated* reasoning, (Kunda 1990). Wawer et al. concluded that *Male circumcision programmes…confer an overall benefit to women* (Wawer et al. 2009). This dissonance suggests a preconceived bias in favour of MC. How can becoming infected with HIV be viewed as a "benefit to women"? Why weren't the women informed that their male partners were HIV+ so that they could take steps to protect themselves? Not informing women that they were at risk of HIV infection would seem unethical. It is regrettable that Wawer et al. the IRBs, and institutions involved did not investigate (which would have been legally required if the trial had been conducted in the United States) since previously uninfected women actually became HIV+ following their participation in the trial.

15.4.2 Non-Sexual Transmission of HIV

The trials did not report on non-sexual transmission of HIV from use of non-sterile surgical and other skin-piercing instruments such as re-use of contaminated scalpels, contaminated injection syringes, contaminated blood transfusions (or other blood exposures from contaminated multi-use vials, etc.) likely to occur in any real-life scaling up of MC (Gisselquist 2008; Gisselquist et al. 2004, 2002). *In the South African trial, 23 (of 69) incident infections occurred in men who reported no unprotected sex. …in Uganda, 16 (of 67) infections occurred in men who reported no sex partners (6 infections) or 100 % condom use (10 infections)*

(Gisselquist 2007). Clearly, *the authors did not control for other sources of HIV transmission such as blood transfusions or exposure through infected needles… circumcision may not be as effective at decreasing HIV transmission as the article suggests* (Vines 2006). Since some men acquired HIV having reported no unprotected sexual exposures, the RCT authors had a duty of care to investigate such non-sexual transmission. *These studies, with their ignored evidence (on sexual exposures) and missing evidence (on blood exposures and on HIV status of sexual partners), launched programs to circumcise millions of African men* (Gisselquist 2007).

15.5 Contradictory Evidence

What does the frequently cited "60 % *relative* reduction" in HIV infections actually mean? Across all three FTM trials, of the 5,411 men subjected to MC, 64 (1.18 %) became HIV+. Among the 5,497 controls, 137 (2.49 %) became HIV+, so the *absolute* decrease in HIV infection was trivial, being only 1.31 %, which was statistically but not clinically significant (see discussion above).

The claimed efficacy of MC in reducing HIV transmission has been contradicted by at least 17 observational studies (Green et al. 2008, 2010; Thomas et al. 2004; Mor et al. 2007). To take just one example, Mor et al. in an epidemiological study of 58,598 men found no relationship between MC and HIV transmission (Mor et al. 2007). In at least Cameroon, Ghana, Lesotho, Malawi, Rwanda, Swaziland, and Tanzania, HIV is more prevalent among circumcised men (Young 2010; Gisselquist 2007; Chao et al. 1994; Urassa et al. 1997). In Malawi, the HIV rate is 13.2 % among circumcised men (9.5 % among intact men), while in Cameroon the HIV rate is 5.1 % among circumcised men (1.5 % among intact men). If MC reduces HIV transmission, as the RCT authors would have us believe, then why is HIV prevalence much higher in the USA (where most men are circumcised) than in developed countries where most men are intact? (e.g., Europe, Scandinavia, United Kingdom) (Boyle and Hill 2011)

Viral load and genital ulcers are predictors of the risk of heterosexual transmission of HIV (Quinn et al. 2000). Langerhans cells in the foreskin produce Langerin, which blocks transmission of HIV (de Witte et al. 2007). Moreover, *Langerhans cells occur in the clitoris, the labia and in other parts of both male and female genitals, and no one is talking of removing these in the name of HIV prevention* (Dowsett and Couch 2007). Indeed, *A lowered risk of HIV infection among [5297] circumcised women* has been reported (Stallings and Karugendo 2005). Why weren't trials also undertaken into the alleged HIV-preventive efficacy of female circumcision (FC) to test how randomly allocating women to immediate vs. delayed FC groups could "benefit" women by showing that FC is an effective HIV preventive measure?

Auvert et al. speculated that *Male circumcision provides a degree of protection against acquiring HIV infection equivalent to…a vaccine of high efficacy…widespread MC could lead to a strong reduction of the spread of HIV* (Auvert et al. 2005). In Thailand, a vaccine provided about six times the protection against HIV as that claimed for MC (across all modalities of transmission, not just sexual), and for both males and females, not just for sexually active men (Rerks-Ngarm et al. 2009). Also, 1 % Tenofovir microbicide gel applied to the genital mucosa (using mucosal immunity) was found to result in a 37–45 % reduction in actual risk of HIV infection (Karim et al. 2010). Ironically, circumcised men may not benefit from Tenofovir treatment because their preputial mucosa has been excised. Since there was no test of the efficacy of MC vs a vaccine of high efficacy, the claims by Auvert et al. were entirely speculative. Thus,

> *...a 60 % reduction...among circumcised men...does not mean that those men are really "protected" against HIV...the choice is either using condoms consistently, with extremely low risk of becoming infected, or being circumcised, with relatively high risk of becoming infected... Concluding that "male circumcision should be regarded as an important public health intervention for preventing the spread of HIV" appears overstated...it is unlikely to have a major public health impact...* (Garenne 2006).

15.5.1 Lack of Fully Informed Consent

It appears that researchers controlled the information available to men so that provision of fully informed consent may have been compromised. In Uganda, the Kampala *Monitor* reported men as saying, *I have heard that if you get circumcised, you cannot catch HIV/AIDS. I don't have to use a condom...* (Ajwang 2007). A Brazilian Health Ministry official (Simao) stated, *the WHO and UN HIV/AIDS program...gives a message of "false protection" because men might think that being circumcised means that they can have sex without condoms without any risk, which "is untrue"* (VivirLatino and April 2007). Ugandan President Museveni denounced claims that MC could reduce HIV transmission, saying that it sends out a misleading and dangerous message, *...that if you are circumcised, you are less likely to catch AIDS even if you behave recklessly. Now what sort of message is that?* (Cooke 2006) Risk compensation following MC has been demonstrated in large-scale empirical studies (Laumann et al. 1997; Pinkerton 2001). Having being stopped early for benefit, the RCTs gave inflated estimates of efficacy, which unduly influenced the subsequent advocacy of mass circumcision programs in sub-Saharan Africa. Indeed, *risk compensation by HIV-infected circumcised men will substantially increase the risk of transmission to their sex partners...the failure of models to account for increased STI risk due to risk compensation likely inflates estimates of averted HIV infections* (Kalichman et al. 2007). Is it ethical to give men a false sense of security?

15.5.2 Participant Inducement

As most participants were unemployed, paying them and providing two years free medical care was clearly a substantial inducement. Inducing impoverished men to submit to amputation of a normal functional sexual body part in the absence of any pre-existing pathology is unethical. (Price 1997; Boyle et al. 2002; Todd 2001). *Financial inducements are equivalent to coercion… If benefits to the patient are so self evident, why are payments or gifts thought to be necessary*? (Raffle and Morgan 1998) The prepuce is a highly erogenous part of the penis (Sorrells et al. 2007; Taylor et al. 1996; Cold and Taylor 1999). All four RCTs failed to acknowledge the significant bodily injury caused by the irreversible amputation and the resultant possible long-term adverse psychosexual effects (Boyle et al. 2002; Johnson 2010). The African RCTs inflicted bodily harm in the absence of pathology, violating the first tenet of ethical medical conduct: *Primum Non Nocere* (First Do No Harm), which may be tantamount to criminal assault (Boyle et al. 2000).

Do IRBs have lower standards when considering experiments in Africa as compared with the USA? *Double standards exist within developed and developing countries, depending on illness conditions, social status of participants, national health priorities* (Wassenaar 2007). Does the USA medical establishment regard poor black African men as an expendable resource to be exploited? (Wakabi 2007) *Participants from developing countries may have little or no alternative means of treatment other than that offered through clinical trials… Poverty, limited or no education…may question the validity of the informed consent procedure in this group of patients* (Verástegui 2006).

Although all participants were alleged to have been HIV- prior to the FTM trials, Bailey et al. admitted, *We cannot exclude the possibility that any of these individuals were actually HIV+ at baseline, and that their [HIV] infection was not detected* (Bailey et al. 2007). Auvert et al. stated that it was *unethical to inform participants of their HIV status without their permission...[and]...unethical to deter from participating in the study potentially at-risk men who did not want to know their HIV status* (Auvert et al. 2005). But, how could any reputable IRB consider it ethical to withhold information about HIV status since some HIV+ men unknowingly infected their female sexual partners? (Wawer et al. 2009) In the USA, individuals are not permitted to participate in a trial without being willing to know their HIV test results. Even when men did hear their HIV results, the investigators did not warn their female sexual partners (Edwards et al. 1998).

Why was there such a brief "cooling off" period for men allocated to the MC group? The surgery was carried out almost immediately after randomization ensuring that participants had little time to change their minds. Bailey et al. stated that *886 (64 %) had their procedures on the day of randomisation…* Why were the circumcisions carried out with such undue haste? The lack of an adequate "cooling off" period would seem unethical. Fully informed consent required that men be made aware that MC might not have any prophylactic benefit. Did the RCT investigators make this explicit to the participants?

15.6 Discussion

Assertions by Auvert et al. that MC *prevented six out of ten potential infections* Auvert et al. 2005 mask a much smaller, non-significant *absolute* reduction in risk (1.3 %). MC is not a cost effective means of reducing HIV transmission,

(McAllister et al. 2008) and any long-term effectiveness in sub-Saharan Africa will not be known for many years (Garenne 2008). Is it *right to circumcise a whole population or a considerable part of it, when many will not benefit from the intervention, for example, because they do not engage in risky sexual behaviour* (Dekkers 2009). While the RCT investigators advocated mass circumcision of African men, *many of their assertions are reminiscent of statements made by fervent proponents of routine neonatal circumcision…exaggerating the alleged advantages, ignoring potential harms, and giving the impression that circumcision is no more than a simple intervention comparable to a vaccination* (Dekkers 2009). Mass circumcision programs inevitably result in complications not generally acknowledged (Muula et al. 2007). *There are always concerns about the safety of MC in sub-Saharan African health systems… The lack of basic instruments and inadequate supplies were identified as crucial limitations in facilitating provision of safe MC…* (Mattson et al. 2004).

Why was a "roll-out" of mass circumcision recommended by WHO/UNAIDS when it was known when the RCT findings were exaggerated due to early termination? Overstating the effectiveness of MC in preventing HIV transmission can only result in public health efforts being misdirected (Boyle 2003; Boyle 2004). For example, Auvert et al. made the claim that *Our study is also the first experimental study demonstrating that surgery can be used to prevent an infectious disease…this finding is an* a posteriori *proof of the use of MC to improve hygiene…* However, as the USA epidemiological experience illustrates, circumcised men will still acquire HIV, transmit HIV to their sexual partners, and die from AIDS. It is inevitable that mass circumcision programs will result in new HIV infections associated with the surgery itself (Brewer et al. 2007; Zulu et al. 2006). Provision of free medical care and sanitary settings would be well nigh impossible to implement in mass circumcision programs. What counselling and compensation will be provided for men who undergo MC but who subsequently become HIV+? The evidence suggests that mass circumcision programs may exacerbate the HIV epidemic among women (Wawer et al. 2009). Under these circumstances, it would be irresponsible and unethical to advocate mass circumcision programs in sub-Saharan Africa (Green et al. 2010). Since HIV transmission in sub-Saharan Africa is largely by non-sexual means, including blood exposures, use of non-sterile surgical instruments, and contaminated injection syringes, (Gisselquist 2007; Gisselquist et al. 2002) overstating the efficacy of MC can only result in public health efforts being misdirected. It is inevitable that mass circumcision programs will cause new HIV incident infections due to the unnecessary circumcision surgery itself.

The trials failed to acknowledge that safe sex practices, provision of free medical care, payment of participants, use of non-representative samples, and sanitary settings are not generally available in mass circumcision programs (Edwards et al. 1998). Men who become HIV+ after undergoing MC would likely become disillusioned and angry. What counselling and compensation will be provided for such men who submit to MC thinking that they will be protected from HIV infection? Mass circumcision programs in sub-Saharan Africa are likely to exacerbate the HIV/AIDS epidemic among women (Wawer et al. 2009). Wasting scarce resources on MC is unethical, when more effective preventive measures devoid of surgical risks are available. Antiretroviral drugs (ART) can reduce HIV transmission by 92 % (Bernstein et al. 2004). Another promising approach may be the use of FDA-approved drugs found to destroy the HIV virus via "lethal mutagenesis". *[A] combination of two clinically approved drugs, decitabine and gemcitabine, reduced HIV infectivity by 73 %...increased mutation frequency decreases infectivity through lethal mutagenesis* (Clouser et al. 2010). These drugs don't merely reduce viral levels (like ART), but actually eliminate the HIV virus from the body (Weinstein et al. 2010),[1] Now that these FDA-approved drugs can be added to the list with ART, use of condoms, abstinence, and more sanitary healthcare provision, the promotion of MC is even less ethical (Weller and Davis-Beaty 2002).

Several countries (e.g., Uganda, Brazil, Rwanda, Thailand) have reduced their HIV rates without recourse to MC.[2,3] However, according to Gray et al. 2007 *We estimate that about 67 circumcisions are needed to prevent one HIV infection.* Extrapolating from this NNT, if the target is to circumcise 38 million men in Africa, then MC would have no HIV-preventive effect for $66/67 \times 38{,}000{,}000 = 37{,}432{,}834$ men. Even accepting the exaggerated FTM effect sizes reported by the RCT investigators, for every 100 men circumcised, $66/67 = 98.5$ men would receive no HIV-preventive benefit. In countries where HIV prevalence is lower than in Uganda, the NNT would even be higher. Thus, it appears that almost 37.5 million men are to be circumcised for no HIV-preventive gain whatsoever. Furthermore, how can mass circumcision programs be justified if circumcised men still need to use a condom and practice safe sex to prevent HIV infection and other STDs?

15.7 Conclusions

The RCT lead authors all held pre-existing beliefs as to the "benefits" of MC and cited articles that supported their pro-MC opinions (Gifford 1995). One wonders whether contradictory evidence was also omitted in their IRB submissions? When undertaking research into MC, full disclosure of personal beliefs indicative of likely biases should include professional, religious, political, and cultural affiliations, as well as one's own circumcision status (Goldman 2004). Making unwarranted recommendations in relation to circumcision policy raises the vista of future legal litigation (Giannetti 2000). WHO/UNAIDS has uncritically accepted the African FTM reports as conclusive and have recommended MC as an HIV-preventive measure despite substantial contradictory evidence, including the Wawer et al. RCT itself which showed a 61 % relative increase (6 % absolute

---

[1] HIV virus neutralised with new antibodies http://news.ninemsn.com.au/article.aspx?id=7926291.

[2] The "ABCs" of HIV prevention 2002.

[3] HIV and AIDS can be stopped, World Vision Australia. http://www.worldvision.com.au/wvconnect/content.asp?topicID=19.

increase) in HIV transmission from circumcised men to their female sexual partners, some of whom were not informed that their male partners were HIV+. Even though 25 previously uninfected women became HIV+, incongruously, Wawer et al. still recommend mass circumcision of African men as a putative HIV prevention measure. Under any reasonable interpretation of ethical principles, the Wawer et al. trial was unethical in not telling some of the men that they were HIV+ and not warning some female sexual partners of HIV+ men that they were at risk of HIV infection.

All four RCTs failed to adhere to the first tenet of ethical medical conduct, *Primum Non Nocere* (*First Do No Harm*), since men were subjected to amputation of a normal functional body part (a significant sexual injury) (Bensley and Boyle 2001, 2003). None of these trials would have been granted IRB clearance in developed countries such as the USA, suggesting ethical double standards (Gisselquist 2009). Research that directly harms participants by inflicting a destructive amputation of a normal, healthy, functional body part with potential psychosexual adverse effects (Boyle et al. 2002) and/or by exposing participants and their sexual partners to a potentially life-threatening disease such as HIV is unethical. In light of the problems with clinical equipoise, methodology, MC as a cause of HIV infection, non-sexual transmission of HIV, unethical procedures, and lack of external validity, the African RCTs were of limited utility in evaluating the HIV-preventive effectiveness of MC (Benson and Hartz 2000; Concato et al. 2000; Sanson-Fisher et al. 2007; Van Spall et al. 2007; Vandenbroucke 2008; Dekkers et al. 2010). Accordingly, *the understandable haste to find a solution to the HIV pandemic means that the promise offered by preliminary and specific research studies may be overstated. This may mean that ethical concerns are marginalised. Such haste may also obscure the need to be attentive to local cultural sensitivities, which vary from one African region to another, in formulating policy concerning circumcision* (Fox and Thomson 2010).

Mass circumcision programs in sub-Saharan Africa may translate into worse plight for women and, because of risk compensation, also a greater risk to circumcised men. WHO/UNAIDS has uncritically and irresponsibly accepted the methodologically flawed reports of FTM trials as conclusive and has recommended MC despite contradictory evidence, including the Ugandan RCT which showed increased MTF transmission of HIV (Wawer et al. 2009). In light of the many methodological, ethical, and legal flaws in the trials, the WHO/UNAIDS recommendation to roll out mass circumcision programs in sub-Saharan African countries was not justified.

MC is a dangerous distraction and waste of scarce resources that should be used for known preventive measures (e.g., condoms have an 80 % effectiveness) (Weller and Davis-Beaty 2002). As Professor Johan Karlberg, MD, PhD, Director of the Clinical Trials Research Centre at the University of Hong Kong stated, *In my view the main problem with such trials is that it will be difficult to understand/study the sexual behavior of the participants; any group difference in the occurrence of HIV can thus be due to this confounding factor. If such a trial confirms that circumcision has a significant but still small effect in the HIV rate the message will be that 'we do not need to protect ourselves.' But safe sex should instead be promoted whatever the trial outcome is. For those reasons I do believe that such trials are neither scientifically nor ethically sound* (Karlberg 2010). A further serious oversight is that the low public health gains and possible short-term and long-term harms arising from implementing mass circumcision programs in sub-Saharan Africa have not been addressed by the trial investigators (Lie and Miller 2011). Also, the serious missing data problem, combined with all the other known sources of error bias discussed above, basically means that these trials are worthless in terms of informing the debate on male circumcision and any putative FTM reduction in HIV sexual transmission (Van Howe and Storms 2011). Alarmingly, the Ugandan MTF trials started to show an increase in HIV infections among the female sexual partners of HIV+ men, which appears to have been ignored by WHO/UNAIDS in recommending that millions of African men should undergo invasive, damaging circumcision. As Altman posited, *What then, should we think about researchers who... misinterpret their results, report their results selectively, cite the literature selectively, and draw unjustified conclusions? We should be appalled* (Altman 1994).

Acknowledgments The author wishes to acknowledge the assistance of George Hill, Vice-President for Bioethics and Medical Science, Doctors Opposing Circumcision, Seattle, Washington 98107, USA.

Appendix

The following studies either show no relationship with circumcision status or a higher risk in circumcised men.
No relationship between HIV infection and circumcision status (13 studies)

1. Hira SK, Kamanga J < Mcuacua R, et al. Genital ulcers and male circumcision as risk factors for acquiring HIV-1 in Zambia. *J Infect Dis* 1990; 161:584–5.
2. Pépin J, Quigley M, Todd J, et al. Association between HIV-2 Infection and genital ulcer diseases among male sexually transmitted disease patients in The Gambia. *AIDS* 1992; 6:489–93.
3. Bollinger RC, Brookmeyer RS, Mehendale SM, et al. Risk factors and clinical presentation of acute primary HIV infection in India. *JAMA* 1997; 278:2085–9.
4. Chiasson M, Stoneburner RL, Hildebrandt DS, et al. Heterosexual transmission of HIV-1 associated with use of smokable freebase cocaine (crack). *AIDS* 1991; 5:1121.
5. Carael M, Van De Perre, PH, Lepage PH, et al. Human immunodeficiency virus transmission among heterosexual couples in Africa. *AIDS* 1988; 2:201–5.
6. Moss GB, Clemerson D, D'Costa L, et al. Association of cervical ectopy with heterosexual transmission of human immunodeficency virus: results of a study of couples in Nairobi, Kenya. *J Infect Dis* 1991; 164:588–91.
7. Allen S, Lindan C, Serufilira A, et al. Human immunodeficiency virus infection in urban Rwanda: demographic and behavioral correlate in a representative sample of childbearing women. *JAMA* 1991; 266:1657–63

8. Seidlin M, Vogler M, Lee E, et al. Heterosexual transmission of HIV in a cohort of couples in New York City. *AIDS* 1993; 7:1247–54.
9. Konde-Lule JK. Bergley SF, Downing R. Knowledge attitudes and practices concerning AIDS in Ugandans. *AIDS* 1989; 3:513–18.
10. Van de Perre P, Clumeck N, Steens M, et al. Seroepidemiological study on sexully transmitted diseases and hepatitis B in African promiscuous heterosexuals in relation to HTLV-III infection. *Eur J Epidemiol* 1987; 3:14–8.
11. Quigley M, Munguti K, Grosskurth H, et al. Sexual behavior patterns and other risk factors for HIV infection in rural Tanzania: a case control study. *AIDS* 1997; 11:237–48.
12. Hudson CP, Hennis AJM, Kataaha P, et al. Risk factors for the spead of AIDS in rural Africa, hepatitis B and syphilis in southwestern Uganda. *AIDS* 1988; 2:255–60.
13. Laumann EO, Masi CM, Zuckerman EW. Circumcision in the United States: prevalence, prophylactic effects, and sexual practice. *JAMA* 1997; 277:1052–7

A higher risk of HIV infection in circumcised men (4 studies)

1. Barongo LR, Borgdorff W, Mosha FF, et al. The epidemiology of HIV-1 infection in rural areas, roadside settlements and rural villages in Mwanza Region, Tanzania. *AIDS* 1992; 6:1521–8.
2. Grosskurth H, Mosha F, Todd J, et al. A community trial of the impact of improved sexually transmitted disease treatment on the HIV epidemic in rural Tanzania: 2. Baseline survey results. *AIDS* 1995; 9:927–34.
3. Chao A, Bulterys M, Musanganire F, et al. Risk factors associated with prevalent HIV-1 infection among pregnant women in Rwanda. National University of Rwanda-Johns Hopkins University AIDS Research Team. *Int J Epidemiol* 1994; 23:371–380.
4. Urassa M, Todd J, Boerra JT, et al. Male circumcision and susceptibility to HIV infection among men in Tanzania. *AIDS* 1997; 11:73–80 [study 1].

The orange part of each of the three right-hand bars (below the dotted lines) represents the much-hyped "60 % protection" conferred by circumcision. If just those men, whose HIV status is unknown, proved in fact to be HIV+ (red), circumcision would certainly have no protective effect whatever, but it would not take all of them to reduce the effect below statistical significance.

All three trials had significant numbers "lost from study", their HIV status unknown (yellow + orange bars in the graphs below)—100 circumcised men (6.5 %) in South Africa, 87 (10 %) in Kenya, and 140 (3.5 %) in Uganda. (The figures are presented confusingly in the published reports because the men did not all enter the trials together, but each trial was stopped at a stroke).

Those figures are high enough in themselves to cast doubt on the validity of the results, but circumcised men who found they had HIV would be disillusioned with the trials and less likely to return. It would take only 25, 25, and 23 such men respectively to completely nullify the trials, and fewer to render the results non-significant.

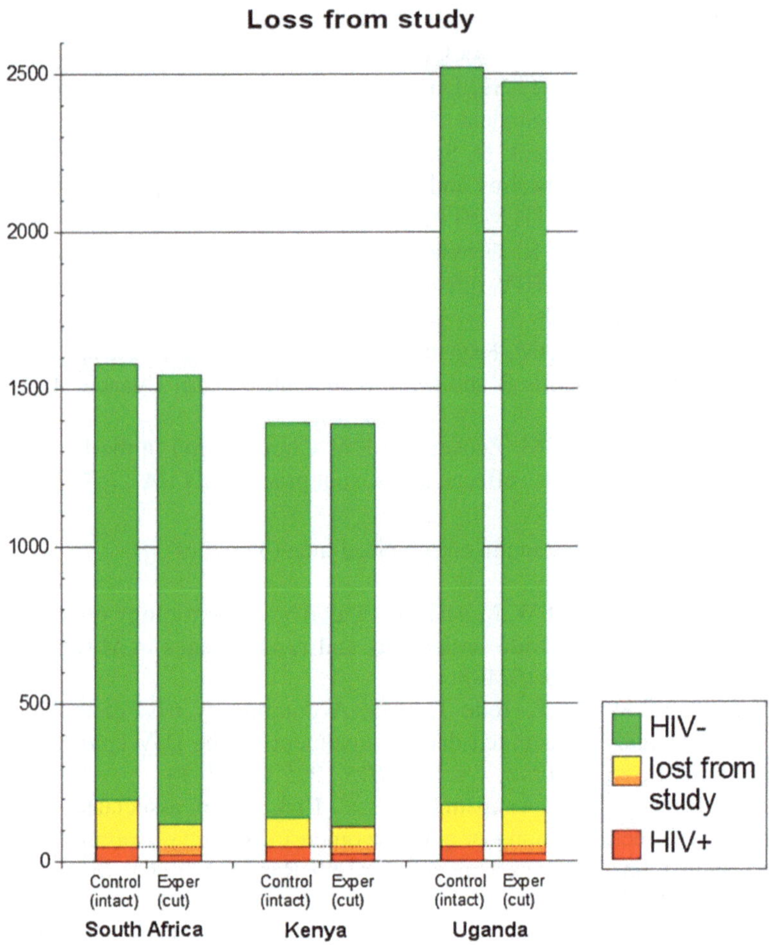

From www.circumcstitions.com (retrieved 4 July 2011; reproduced with permission from the author Hugh Young, email: hugh@buzz.net.nz).

References

Ajwang J (2007) Uganda: HIV—circumcision isn't enough, Monitor (Kampala), 10 April. http://allafrica.com/stories/200704091186.html

Altman D (1994) The scandal of poor medical research. BMJ 308:383–384

Auvert B, Taljaard D, Lagarde E et al (2005) Randomized, controlled intervention trial of male circumcision for reduction of HIV infection risk: the ANRS 1265 trial. PLoS Med 2(11):e2

Bailey RC, Moses S, Parker CB et al (2007) Male circumcision for HIV prevention in young men in Kisumu, Kenya: a randomised controlled trial. Lancet 369(9562):643–656

Bailey RC et al. (2010) The protective effect of adult male circumcision against HIV acquisition is sustained for at least 54 months: results from the Kisumu, Kenya trial. IAC, Abstract FRLBC101

Bassler D, Briel M, Montori VM et al (2010) Stopping randomized trials early for benefit and estimation of treatment effects: systematic review and meta-regression analysis. JAMA 303(12):1180–1187

Bensley GA, Boyle GJ (2001) Physical, sexual, and psychological impact of male infant circumcision: an exploratory study. In: Denniston GC et al. (eds) Understanding circumcision: a multi-disciplinary approach to a multi-dimensional problem Kluwer/Plenum, NY

Bensley GA, Boyle GJ (2003) Effects of male circumcision on female arousal and orgasm. New Zealand Med J 116:595–596

Benson K, Hartz AJ (2000) A comparison of observational studies and randomized, controlled trials. N Engl J Med 342(25):1878–1886

Bernstein HB, Kinter AL, Jackson R et al (2004) Neonatal natural killer cells produce chemokines and suppress HIV replication in vitro. AIDS Res Hum Retroviruses 20(11):1189–1195

Beyrer C, Trapence G, Motimedi F et al (2009) Bisexual concurrency, bisexual partnerships, and HIV among Southern African men who have sex with men (MSM). Sex Transm Infect 86(4):323–327

Boyle GJ (2003) Issues associated with the introduction of circumcision into a non-circumcising society. Sex Transm Infect 79:427–428

Boyle GJ (2004) Male circumcision and risk of HIV-1 infection. Lancet 363:1997

Boyle GJ, Hill G (2011) "The case for boosting infant male circumcision in the face of rising heterosexual transmission of HIV"...and now the case against. Med J Aust 194(2):99

Boyle GJ, Svoboda JS, Price CP et al (2000) Circumcision of healthy boys: criminal assault? J Law Med 7:301–310

Boyle GJ, Goldman R, Svoboda JS et al (2002) Male circumcision: pain, trauma and psychosexual sequelae. J Health Psychol 7:329–343

Brazil says no to circumcision (2007) VivirLatino, 3 April 2007. (Retrieved Dec. 26, 2010). URL. http://www.circumcisionandhiv.com/2007/04/brazil_rejects_.html

Brewer D, Potterat JJ, Robert JM et al (2007) Male and female circumcision associated with prevalent HIV infection in virgins and adolescents in Kenya, Lesotho, and Tanzania. Ann Epidemiol 17:217–226

Brody S, Potteratt JJ (2003) Assessing the role of anal intercourse in the epidemiology of AIDS in Africa. Int J STD AIDS 14:431–436

Chao A, Bulterys M, Musanganire F et al (1994) Risk factors associated with prevalent HIV-1 infection among pregnant women in Rwanda. National university of Rwanda-Johns Hopkins university AIDS research team. Int J Epidemiol 23(2):371–380

Clouser CL, Patterson SE, Mansky LM (2010) Exploiting drug repositioning for discovery of a novel HIV combination therapy. J Virol 84(18):9301–9309

Cocks T (2006) Ugandan president rejects circumcision study, Independent Online, 22 Dec, 2006. URL. http://www.iol.co.za/index.php?set_id=1&click_id=3016&art_id=qw1166790421634B225 (Retrieved Dec. 26, 2010)

Cold CJ, Taylor JR (1999) The prepuce. BJU Int 83(Suppl. 1):34–44

Concato J, Shah N, Horwitz RI (2000) Randomized, controlled trials, observational studies, and the hierarchy of research designs. N Engl J Med 342(25):1887–1892

Dowsett GW, Couch M (2007) Male circumcision and HIV prevention: is there really enough of the right kind of evidence? Reprod Health Matters 15(29):33–44

de Witte L, Nabatov A, Pion M et al (2007) Langerin is a natural barrier to HIV-1 transmission by Langerhans cells. Nat Med 13:361–371

Dekkers W (2009) Routine (non-religious) neonatal circumcision and bodily integrity: a transatlantic dialogue. Kennedy Inst Ethics J 19(2):125–146

Dekkers M, von Elm E, Algra A et al (2010) How to assess the external validity of therapeutic trials: a conceptual approach. Int J Epidemiol 39:89–94

Edwards SJL, Lilford RJ, Hewison J (1998) The ethics of randomised controlled trials from the perspectives of patients, the public, and healthcare professionals. Br Med J 317(7167):1209–1212

Fleming DT, Wasserheit JN (1999) From epidemiological synergy to public health policy and practice: the contribution of other sexually transmitted diseases to sexual transmission of HIV infection. Sex Transm Infect 75(1):3–17

Freedman B (1987) Equipoise and the ethics of clinical research. N Eng J Med 317(3):141–145
Fox M, Thomson M (2010) HIV/AIDS and circumcision: lost in translation. J Med Ethics 36:798–801
Garenne M (2006) Male circumcision and HIV control in Africa. PLoS Med 3(1):31
Garenne M (2008) Long-term population effect of male circumcision in generalised HIV epidemics in sub-Saharan Africa. Afr J AIDS Res 7(1):1–8
Giannetti M (2000) Circumcision and the American academy of pediatrics: should scientific misconduct result in trade association liability? Iowa Law Rev 85:1507–1568
Gifford F (1995) Community-equipoise and the ethics of randomized clinical trials. Bioethics 9(2):127–148
Gisselquist D (2007) Points to consider: responses to HIV/AIDS in Africa, Asia, and the Caribbean. Adonis & Abbey, London
Gisselquist D (2008) Denialism undermines AIDS prevention in sub-Saharan Africa. Int J STD AIDS 19:649–654
Gisselquist D (2009a) HIV infections as unanticipated problems during medical research in Africa. Accountability Res 16:199–217
Gisselquist D (2009b) Double standards in research ethics, health-care safety, and scientific rigour allowed Africa's HIV/AIDS epidemic disasters. Int J STD AIDS 20(12):839–845
Gisselquist D, Rothenberg R, Potterat J et al (2002) HIV infections in sub-Saharan Africa not explained by sexual or vertical transmission. Int J STD AIDS 13:657–666
Gisselquist D, Potterat JJ, Brody S (2004) Running on empty: sexual co-factors are insufficient to fuel Africa's turbocharged HIV epidemic. Int J STD AIDS 15:442–452
Goldman R (2004) Circumcision policy: a psychosocial perspective. Paediatr Child Health 9(9):630–633
Gray RH, Kigozi G, Serwadda D et al (2007) Male circumcision for HIV prevention in men in Rakai Uganda: a randomised trial. Lancet 369(9562):657–666
Green LW, McAllister RG, Peterson KW et al (2008) Male circumcision is not the HIV 'vaccine' we have been waiting for! Fut HIV Ther 2(3):293–299
Green LW, Travis JW, McAllister RG et al (2010) Male circumcision and HIV prevention: insufficient evidence and neglected external validity. Am J Prev Med 39(5):479–482
Johnson M (2010) Male genital mutilation: beyond the tolerable? Ethnicities 10(2):181–207
Karlberg JPE (2010) Personal communication (email). University of Hong Kong.
Karlberg JPE, Speers MA (2010) Reviewing clinical trials: a guide for the ethics committee. Karlberg JPE, Hong Kong
Kalichman S, Eaton L, Pinkerton S (2007) Circumcision for HIV prevention: failure to fully account for behavioral risk compensation. PloS Med 4(3):e138
Karim QA, Karim SA, Frohlich JA et al (2010) Effectiveness and safety of Tenofovir gel, an antiretroviral microbicide, for the prevention of HIV infection in women. Science 329(5996):1168–1174
Kim DS, Lee JY and Pang MG (1999) Male circumcision: A South Korean perspective. Brit J Urol Int 83:28
Kunda Z (1990) The case for motivated reasoning. Psych Bull 108(3):480–498
Laumann EO, Masi CM, Zuckerman EW (1997) Circumcision in the United States: prevalence, prophylactic effects, and sexual practice. JAMA 277:1052–1057
Lie RK, Miller FG (2011) What counts as reliable evidence for public health policy: the case of circumcision for preventing HIV infection. BMC Med Res Methodol 11:34
Magoha GA (1999) Circumcision in various Nigerian and Kenyan hospitals. East Afr Med J 76: 583
Mattson CL, Muga R, Poulussen R, Onyango T, Bailey RC (2004) Feasibility of medical male circumcision in Nyanza province. Kenya. East Afr Med J 81:320–335
McAllister RG, Travis JW, Bollinger D et al (2008) The cost to circumcise Africa. Int J Men's Health 7(3):307–316
Mehta SD, Gray RH, Auvert B et al (2009) Does sex in the early period after circumcision increase HIV-seroconversion risk? Pooled analysis of adult male circumcision clinical trials. AIDS 23(12):1557–1564
Mills E, Siegfried N (2006) Cautious optimism for new HIV/AIDS prevention strategies. Lancet 368:1236

Millet GA, Ding H, Lauby J et al (2007) Circumcision status and HIV infection among black and Latino men who have sex with men in three US cities. J Acquir Immune Defic Syndr 46(5):643–650

Millet GA, Flores SA, Marks G et al (2008) Circumcision status and risk of HIV and sexually transmitted infections among men who have sex with men: a meta-analysis. JAMA 300(14):1674–1684

Moher D, Hopewell S, Schulz KF et al (2010) CONSORT 2010 explanation and elaboration: updated guidelines for reporting parallel group randomised trials. Br Med J 340:c869

Mor Z, Kent CK, Kohn RP et al (2007) Declining rates in male circumcision amidst increasing evidence of its public health benefit. PLoS ONE 2(9):e861

Montori VM, Devereaux PJ, Adhikari NK et al (2005) Randomized trials stopped early for benefit: a systematic review. JAMA 294:2203–2209

Muula AS, Prozesky HW, Mataya RH et al (2007) Prevalence of complications of male circumcision in Anglophone Africa: a systematic review. BMC Urol 7:4

Padian NS, McCoy SI, Balkus JE et al (2010) Weighing the gold in the gold standard: challenges in HIV prevention research. AIDS 24(5):621–635

Pinkerton SD (2001) Sexual risk compensation and HIV/STD transmission: empirical evidence and theoretical considerations. Risk Anal 21:727–736

Pocock S, White I (1999) Trials stopped early: too good to be true? Lancet 353:943–944

Price C (1997) Male circumcision: an ethical and legal affront. Bull Med Ethics 128:13–19

Quinn TC, Wawer MJ, Sewankambo N et al (2000) Viral load and heterosexual transmission of human immunodeficiency virus type 1. Rakai project study group. N Engl J Med 342(13):921–929

Raffle AE, Morgan K (1998) Financial inducements are equivalent to coercion. BMJ 316(7128):394

Rerks-Ngarm S, Pitisuttithum P, Nitayaphan S et al (2009) Vaccination with ALVAC and AIDSVAX to prevent HIV-1 infection in Thailand. N Engl J Med 361(23):2209–2220

Roehr B (2010) How homophobia is fuelling Africa's HIV epidemic. BMJ 340:c2245

Rothwell PM (2005) External validity of randomised controlled trials: "to whom do the results of this trial apply?". Lancet 365:82–93

Sanson-Fisher RW, Bonevski B, Green LW et al (2007) Limitations of the randomized controlled trial in evaluating population-based health interventions. Am J Prev Med 33(2):155–161

Schulz KF, Chalmers I, Hayes RJ et al (1995) Empirical evidence of bias. Dimensions of methodological quality associated with estimates of treatment effects in controlled trials. JAMA 273:408–412

Siegfried N, Muller M, Volmink J et al. (2003) Male circumcision for prevention of heterosexual acquisition of HIV in men (Cochrane Review). In: The Cochrane Library, Issue 3, Update Software, Oxford

Siegfried N, Muller M, Deeks et al (2005) HIV and male circumcision-A systematic review with assessment of the quality of studies. Lancet Infect Dis 5:165

Siegfried N, Muller M, Deeks JJ et al. (2009) Male circumcision for prevention of heterosexual acquisition of HIV in men. Cochrane Database Syst Rev 2 (CD003362). URL: http://onlinelibrary.wiley.com/o/cochrane/clsysrev/articles/CD003362/frame.html

Sorrells ML, Reiss JL, Snyder MD et al (2007) Fine-touch pressure thresholds in the adult penis. BJU Int 99:864–869

Stallings RY, Karugendo E (2005) Female circumcision and HIV infection in Tanzania: for better or for worse? 3rd IAS conference HIV pathogen and treatment, Rio de Janeiro, Brazil, 24–27 July

Statement on Kenyan and Ugandan trial findings regarding male circumcision and HIV (2006) WHO, Geneva, Switzerland, December 13. http://www.who.int/mediacentre/news/statements/2006/s18/en/index.html (Retrieved Oct. 15, 2010)

Sussman JB, Hayward RA (2010) An IV for the RCT: using instrumental variables to adjust for treatment contamination in randomised controlled trials. BMJ 340:c2073

Taylor JR, Lockwood AP, Taylor AJ (1996) The prepuce: specialized mucosa of the penis and its loss to circumcision. Br J Urol 77:291–295

The "ABCs" of HIV prevention: report of a USAID technical meeting on behavior change approaches to primary prevention of HIV/AIDS (2002) 17 Sept

Thomas AG, Bakhireva LN, Brodine SK et al. (2004) Prevalence of male circumcision and its association with HIV and sexually transmitted infections in a U.S. navy population. Abstract no. TuPeC4861. Presented at the XV international AIDS conference, Bangkok, Thailand, 11–16 July 2004

Todd C (2001) Research participation and financial inducements. Amer J Bioethics 1(2):60–61

Urassa M, Todd J, Boerra JT et al (1997) Male circumcision and susceptibility to HIV infection among men in Tanzania. AIDS 11:73–80

Vandenbroucke JP (2008) Observational research, randomised trials, and two views of medical science. PLoS Med 5(3):e67

Van Howe RS (2010) Analysis of the circumcision/HIV randomised clinical trials. Unpublished manuscript

Van Howe RS, Storms MR (2011) How the circumcision solution in Africa will increase HIV infections. J Pub Health Africa 2:e4. doi:10.4081/jphia.2011.e4

Van Spall HG, Toren A, Kiss A et al (2007) Eligibility criteria of randomized controlled trials published in high-impact general medical journals: a systematic sampling review. JAMA 297(11):1233–1240

Vines J (2006) Major potential confounder not addressed. PLoS Med 3(1):e63

Verástegui EL (2006) Consenting of the vulnerable: the informed consent procedure in advanced cancer patients in Mexico. BMC Med Ethics 7:13

Wakabi W (2007) Homophobia is fuelling the AIDS epidemic in Africa. CMAJ 177(9):1017

Wassenaar D (2007) Double standards in research ethics. Case-studies: informed consent and vaccine to treat rotavirus. EU forum on ethics, research and globalisation. Brussels

Wawer MJ, Makumbi F, Kigozi G et al (2009) Circumcision in HIV-infected men and its effect on HIV transmission to female partners in Rakai, Uganda: a randomised controlled trial. Lancet 374:229–237

Weinstein RS, Weinstein MM, Alibek K et al (2010) Significantly reduced CCR5-tropic HIV-1 replication in vitro in cells from subjects previously immunized with vaccinia virus. BMC Immunol 11:23

Weller SC, Davis-Beaty K (2002) Condom effectiveness in reducing heterosexual HIV transmission. Cochrane Database Syst Rev Issue 1 Art. No. CD003255

Young H (2010) False assumptions. BMC Public Health 10:209. URL: http://www.circumstitions.com/HIV.html (Retrieved Dec. 23, 2010)

Zulu K, Bulawo ND, Zulu W (2006) Circumcision razor a preventative tool or a strategic vector in the transmission of HIV? A case of Zambia. Poster presented at XVI international AIDS conference, Toronto, Canada, 13–18 August 2006

Author Biography

Gregory J. Boyle, PhD (Delaware), PhD (Melbourne), DSc (Queensland) is a Fellow, Australian Psychological Society and, Fellow, Association for Psychological Science. Gold Coast, Queensland, Australia.

Chapter 16
Randomized Controlled Trials for HIV/AIDS Prevention Among Men in Africa: Untraced Infections, Unasked Questions, and Unreported Data

David Gisselquist

Abstract Outside sub-Saharan Africa HIV infects 0.3 % of adults, primarily men who have sex with men (MSM) and injection drug users (IDU). In Africa, 5 % of adults are infected with HIV, with MSM and IDUs accounting for only small minorities of infections. HIV prevalence is higher in Southern Africa, in women, and in adults aged 30–40 years. For more than 25 years, researchers have not identified what is different about HIV risks and transmission in Africa that allows such terrible epidemics. Much of the research into HIV risks in Africa has been conducted through randomized controlled trials (RCTs) of interventions for HIV prevention. This review of RCTs among men (and a parallel review including RCTs among women) examines how a massive research effort has not yet explained Africa's HIV epidemics. A search identified 21 RCTs that followed more than 43,000 men in Africa and observed more than 900 incident infections. For 9 interventions, HIV incidence was significantly lower among men who received the intervention than among other men; four of these interventions provided antiviral drugs for pre-exposure prophylaxis, and three circumcised men. Despite some encouraging results, information from these 21 RCTs is insufficient to guide HIV prevention in Africa. With few exceptions, RCTs did not identify sexual partners who infected men, or report incidence in men with and without unprotected sex, injections, or other skin-piercing events. Studies thus cannot say why interventions succeeded or failed, or why men in Africa have such high risk for HIV. Moreover, the projected impact of apparently successful interventions is limited not only by incomplete information about what happened during the trials but also by conflicting evidence and/or practical difficulties. No study team has made their data available for others to analyze, and only one details what data was collected. Some procedures were ethically dubious; for example, 5 studies followed men who did not know their wives were infected. Governments of countries that host research should insist on defensible ethics and on better science to explain their HIV epidemics.

D. Gisselquist (✉)
Independent researcher and consultant, Hershey, PA, USA
e-mail: david_gisselquist@yahoo.com

G. C. Denniston et al. (eds.), *Genital Cutting: Protecting Children from Medical, Cultural, and Religious Infringements*, DOI: 10.1007/978-94-007-6407-1_16,

Keywords Randomized controlled trials (RCTs) • HIV/AIDS • Prevention • Interventions • Ethics • Immunodeficiency • Injection drugs

16.1 Introduction

Africa's Unexplained HIV Epidemics: The virus that caused the global HIV/AIDS epidemic very likely crossed from a chimpanzee to a human in southeastern Cameroon around 1900; this information comes from sequencing HIV and simian immunodeficiency viruses (SIV) from non-human primates (Gisselquist 2008). The first person infected was probably a cut hunter or butcher. SIV likely passed to humans many times during the millennia that humans lived near chimpanzees, but then never spread; apparently sexual transmission alone was not enough to spread HIV into an epidemic.

In the early 20th century, several rare HIV infections in humans did not die out, but rather spread with the aid of unsafe injections for sleeping sickness and other diseases (Pépin et al. 2010) to thousands of people in French and Belgian colonies in Central Africa. Even so, with high mortality and morbidity from other causes, the epidemic was invisible in Africa. AIDS was first identified as a new disease in the United States (US) in 1981 among men who have sex with men (MSM) and injection drug users (IDUs). Within a year, doctors recognized that Africans were also dying of AIDS.

HIV epidemics in sub-Saharan Africa are not only older, but also different. Only 0.3 % of adults are HIV-positive outside Africa, compared to 5 % in Africa (UNAIDS 2010). In most countries outside Africa, HIV infects more men than women, and MSM and IDUs account for most infections. For example, the US Centers for Disease Control and Prevention (CDC) estimates that 87 % of HIV-positive men in the US in 2008 were MSM or IDUs (Centers for Disease Control and Prevention 2009). In contrast, HIV in Africa attacks the general population; MSM and IDUs account for only small minorities of infections.

The worst HIV epidemics are found in nine countries in Southern Africa, where 11–26 % of adults are HIV-positive (Botswana, Lesotho, Malawi, Mozambique, Namibia, South Africa, Swaziland, Zambia, and Zimbabwe). Although HIV in Africa infects more women than men, the difference narrows in those over 30 years old. In recent national surveys, HIV prevalence among men aged 35–39 years exceeds 40 % in Swaziland, 30 % in Botswana, Lesotho, and Zimbabwe, and 20 % in Zambia (see Table 16.1).

Foreign experts commonly blame Africa's AIDS disasters on sex. If that is so, then HIV would have to transmit much more extensively and efficiently through penile-vaginal sex in Africa than elsewhere. After more than 25 years, experts are still debating how that can be so. Suggested explanations include promiscuity, lack of circumcision, other common infections that facilitate HIV transmission, and unspecified "unique biological factors" (Pettifor et al. 2010, p. 242).

Importantly, sexual behavior in Africa appears to be more conservative than in the US or Europe. For example, a 2006 review reported a "comparatively high

Table 16.1 HIV infections in men in Southern Africa

Country, year	% of men that are HIV-positive	
	15–49 years	35–39 years
Botswana, 2004	20.0	33.3
Lesotho, 2009	18.0	35.4
Malawi, 2004	10.2	18.4
Mozambique, 2009	9.2	14.2
South Africa, 2008	Not available	18.5
Swaziland, 2006–2007	19.7	44.9
Zambia, 2007	12.3	22.4
Zimbabwe, 2005–2006	14.5	32.1

Source Demographic and Health Surveys and AIDS Indicator Surveys (Measure DHS. Demographic and health Surveys. Available at:http://www.measuredhs.com/start.cfm. Accessed 29 August 2011); national surveys for Botswana (National AIDS Coordinating Agency 2005) and South Africa (Shisana et al. 2009). No survey is available for Namibia

prevalence of multiple partnerships in developed countries, compared with… African countries" (Wellings et al. 2006, p. 1723). Recent national surveys among youth aged 18–24 years in the US and South Africa found that young men and women in the US were more likely to have had vaginal sex, had a lower age of coital debut, used condoms less, and had more lifetime sex partners than young men and women in South Africa (Pettifor et al. 2010).

The Research Puzzle: The puzzle posed by Africa's HIV epidemics—how HIV could infect so many people who are neither MSM nor IDUs—remains unsolved. This leads to a second puzzle: How is it that researchers have failed for more than 25 years to find out what is happening in Africa?

HIV transmission requires events—sexual contact or blood contact through skin-piercing procedures or wounds—that most people can remember. Thus, anyone who meets and talks with adults with new infections should be able to elicit short lists of events that might have led to their infections. From such information, researchers could establish the source of many infections by tracing and testing sexual partners and possible blood contacts. But that has not happened.

16.2 Review of RCTS for HIV Prevention Among Men in Africa

Much of the research effort has been channeled into randomized controlled trials (RCTs) of interventions to prevent HIV. These RCTs recruit HIV-negative participants, then randomly assign them to one of two study "arms"—an intervention arm where participants receive the intervention, and a control arm where they do not. The RCTs then follow and retest participants to see if those in the interventions arm had lower HIV incidence. To explain why interventions succeeded or failed, RCTs should also identify the risks that account for HIV incidence.

Although many other studies have followed men and women in Africa to look at risks for HIV, RCTs characteristically test and follow participants more closely than other studies, and are thereby a potential source of good information on risks. This present review of RCTs for HIV prevention among men in Africa—and a companion review of RCTs for HIV prevention among men and women (Gisselquist 2011)—seeks to explain how a massive research effort could have failed to find what is different about HIV transmission in Africa that allows and sustains such horrible HIV epidemics.

This review continues a long-running critique of HIV research for not doing what is needed to explain Africa's epidemics. In 1991, Packard and Epstein criticized the "narrowing of research" into risks for HIV in Africa (Packard and Epstein 1991, p. 781). Nineteen years later, Potterat noted frequent "unexpected and disappointing results" in "the long lineage of RCTs in sub-Saharan Africa," and called for more detailed information about both sexual and blood risks (Potterat 2010, p. 23).

Literature Search: This review considers all trials for HIV prevention among young and adult men in Africa that assess impact by HIV incidence, and that have reported at least partial results through August 2011. The search for RCTs began with a list from a previous review (Padian et al. 2010), followed by a review of my own records, referrals from colleagues, and a 26 August 2011 search of trial registries, as follows: Australian New Zealand Clinical Trials Registry (advanced search condition and intervention: acquired immune deficiency syndrome, prevention; 2 records returned, no additional trials); University Hospital Medical Information Network Clinical Trials Registry (search region: Africa; 5 records, no additional trials); ISRCTN (search term: Africa; 135 records, no additional trials); WHO's International Clinical Trials Registry Platform (search terms: HIV and Africa; 330 records, no additional trials); and ClinicalTrials.gov (search terms: HIV and Africa; 304 studies returned, no additional trials).

Because this review focuses on risks for HIV incidence, I exclude one trial that measured success by HIV prevalence (Cowan et al. 2010) and include two that assessed success by composite measures of incidence of conventional sexually transmitted infection (STI) with or without HIV, but that also measured HIV incidence (The NIMH Collaborative HIV/STD Prevention Trial Group 2010; Dow 2011).

Scale and Focus of RCTs for HIV Prevention Among Men in Africa: This search identified 21 RCTs of interventions to prevent HIV among men in Africa (Table 16.2). Some trials recruited women as well as men, and several recruited adults in other countries; in such cases, this review extracts data for men in Africa only, as reported or estimated from reported data (see the Appendix). Trials span nearly a quarter century, with the first initiated in 1987 and the latest data from 2011.

These 21 trials followed a total of more than 44,000 men for more than 89,000 person-years (PYs) and observed more than 900 incident (new) infections (Table 16.3). Seventeen RCTs recruited men from the general population (e.g., from rural communities, work places, schools), accounting for 90 % of follow-up time and 85 % of incident infections. Three RCTs that recruited only discordant couples accounted for 9.6 % of follow-up time and 15 % of infections. One RCT recruited 88 MSM in South Africa; no study focused on men at high risk because of injection drug use (IDU).

Two of 21 RCTs (Kamali et al. 2003; Baeten and Celum 2011) tested two interventions each, for a total of 23 interventions. The types of interventions studied most intensively are: information, education, and communication (IEC) with 10 interventions, 53 % of follow-up time, and 39 % of incident infections; and STI treatment with 5 interventions. After excluding double-counting (two interventions combined IEC with STI treatment), 12 RCTs with a net total of 13 IEC and/or STI interventions accounted for 72 % of follow-up time and 64 % of incident infections.

Four RCTs testing circumcision accounted for 21 % of follow-up time and 26 % of infections. All other RCTs together accounted for 7–8 % of both follow-up time and incident infections.

16.3 Review Findings: Prospective Impact of Interventions on HIV in Africa

One important result from RCTs for HIV prevention is the relative risk (RR) for HIV incidence in the intervention vs. the control arm. For example, if 10 of 100 men in the intervention arm acquire HIV in a year vs. 15 of 100 men in the control arm, the RR for HIV incidence among men receiving the intervention is 0.67 (=10 per 100 PYs/15 per 100 PYs). But even if an intervention has a low RR, success cannot be credited to the intervention without knowing how men in both arms acquired HIV, to see whether and how the intervention was the factor that made the difference. Furthermore, the usefulness of interventions with low RRs depends as well on other factors—such as expense, and whether its extension to the public would have other negative impacts.

For these 23 interventions, study teams report 18 relative risks (RR) for HIV incidence in the intervention vs. the control arm (Table 16.4). Two additional RRs can be calculated from reported data (see notes to Table 16.2 and explanations in the Appendix). The three missing RRs are from a trial of IEC among school-aged youth in Tanzania that observed too few infections to produce a useful statistic (only 5 in more than 13,000 PYs) (Ross et al. 2007); and two trials that monitored but did not report HIV incidence (The NIMH Collaborative HIV/STD Prevention Trial Group 2010; Dow 2011; McClellan et al. 2010). Eight RRs combine results for men and women in Africa, while two are from cohorts including adults from Brazil, Ecuador, India, Peru, the US, and/or Thailand (see notes to Table 16.2).

Eleven interventions had no apparent impact, with RRs not significantly less than 1. Nine had RRs significantly less than 1, which suggests they might be useful for HIV prevention. However, the potential impacts of the various interventions

Table16.2 Randomized controlled trials for HIV prevention among men in Africa

Participants, intervention, and reference	Location and study years	RR	Number followed	PYs of follow-up	Incidence: Cases	Incidence: Rate per 100 PYs	Follow-up interval with HIV test
General population men							
STI treatment (Grosskurth et al. 1995; Todd et al. 2006a)	TZ, 1991-94	<u>0.58</u>[a]	4,104[b]	8,208[b]	71	0.87[b]	2 years
STI treatment (Wawer et al. 1999)	UG, 1994-98	0.89	4,351	5,737	82	1.4	10 months
STI treatment, IEC (Kamali et al. 2003)	UG, 1994-2000	1.00	6,198[b]	18,682[b]	138[b]	0.74[b]	2 years
STI treatment, IEC (Gregson et al. 2009; Lopman et al. 2008)	ZI, 1998-2003	1.27[a]	1,672	4,916	98	1.99	3 years
Community IEC (Kamali et al. 2003)[c]	UG, 1994-2000	0.97[a]					
School-based IEC (Ross et al. 2007)	TZ, 1998-2002	NR	4,100	13,643[b]	5	0.04[b]	1.5 years
Credit, community IEC (Pronyk et al. 2006)	SA, 2001-05	1.06[a]	566[b]	1,755[b]	33[b]	1.9[b]	3 years
Workplace VCT, IEC[24] (Corbett et al. 2007)	ZI, 2002-04	1.49[a]	2,653[b]	4,493[b]	57[b]	1.27[b]	2 years
Opinion leader IEC (The NIMH Collaborative HIV/STD Prevention Trial Group 2010; McClellan et al. 2010)	ZI, 2002-07	NR	NR	NR	NR	4.89	1 year
Stepping Stones IEC (Jewkes et al. 2008; Michielsen et al. 2010)	SA, 2003-06	0.99	1,121	2,079[b]	28	1.38[b]	1 year
Cash for no new HIV, IEC[f]	MW, 2008-09	1	478[b]	956[b]	NR	NR	2 year

(continued)

Table 16.2 continued

Participants, intervention, and reference	Location and study years	RR	Number followed	PYs of follow-up	Incidence		Follow-up interval with HIV test
					Cases	Rate per 100 PYs	
Cash for no new STI, IEC (Dow 2011; de Walque et al. 2010)	TZ, 2009-10	NR	1,169[b]	1,052[b]	NR	NR	1 year
Circumcision (Auvert et al. 2005)	SA, 2002-05	0.40	3,128	4,693	69	1.43	3, 9 months
Circumcision (Bailey et al. 2007)	KY, 2002,06	0.47	2,784	4,416[b]	69	1.5[b]	3, 6 months
Circumcision (Gray et al. 2007)	UG, 2003-06	0.49	4,817	6,744	67	0.99	6, 12 months
Circumcision (Gray et al. 2007, 2009)	UG, 2004-07	0.58[b]	NR	2,927[b]	38[b]	1.3[b]	6, 12 months
PrEP with TDF/FTC (Thigpen et al. 2011)	BT, 2007-11	0.20	656	NR	12	NR	1 month
Vaccine (Gray et al. 2011)	SA, 2007-09	1.25[a]	441	829[b]	20	2.4[b]	3-6 months
Men in discordant couples							
STI treatment (Grosskurth et al. 1995; Hugonnet et al. 2002)[d]	TZ, 1991-94	NR	21	40	2	5.0	2 years
STI treatment (Wawer et al. 1999; Quinn et al. 2000)[d]	UG, 1994-98	1.26[a]	187	345	40	11.6	10 months
Acyclovir for HSV2 (Celum et al. 2010; Campbell et al. 2011;	BT, KY, RW, SA, TZ	0.92[ae]	2,218	3,009	88	2.9[b]	3 months
Lingappa et al. 2010)	UG, ZA, 2004-08						
PrEP with TDF (Baeten and Celum 2011)	KY, UG, 2008-11	0.45	2,943[b]	4,622[b]	36	0.8[b]	1 month
PrEP with TDF/FTC (Baeten and Celum 2011)[c]	KY, UG, 2008-11	0.17					1 month

(continued)

Table 16.2 continued

Participants, intervention, and reference	Location and study years	RR	Number followed	PYs of follow-up	Incidence: Cases	Incidence: Rate per 100 PYs	Follow-up interval with HIV test
ART as prevention (Cohen et al. 2011)	BT, BR, IN, KY, MW, TH, US, ZI, 2005-11	<u>0.11</u>[a]	556[b]	988[b]	18[b]	1.8[b]	1-3 months
High risk men							
PrEP with TDF/FTC (Grant et al. 2010)	BR, EC. PE, SA, TH, US, 2007-11	<u>0.56</u>[a]	88	NR	NR	NR	1-8 months

Note Underlined RRs are significantly less than 1.

Abbreviations ART antiretroviral therapy, *FTC*: emtricitabine, *IEC* Information, education, communication, *NR* not reported, *PrEP* oral pre-exposure prophylaxis, *PY* person-years, *RR* relative risk for HIV incidence in the intervention versus the control arm, *STI* sexually transmitted infection, *TDF* tenofovir disoproxil fumarate, *VCT* voluntary counseling and testing, *BR* Brazil, *BT* Botswana, *EC* Ecuador, *GH* Ghana, *IN* India, *KY* Kenya, *MW* Malawi, *PE* Peru, *RW* Rwanda, *SA* South Africa, *TH* Thailand, *US* United States, *TZ* Tanzania, *UG* Uganda, *ZA* Zambia, *ZI* Zimbabwe

[a]These RRs are from cohorts including women in Africa and/or adults in non-African countries

[b]These data are estimated from reported data as explained in the Appendix.

[c]The RRs in these rows are from RCTs with 2 interventions; data on all participants are reported in previous rows for the other intervention in each RCT

[d]The data in these rows are for men in discordant couples from RCTs reported elsewhere in this table that followed large cohorts of adults

[e]This RR for transmission within discordant couples excludes HIV acquired from other sources

[f]Kohler and Thornton, 2010, Conditional cash transfers and HIV/AIDS prevention: unconditionally promising? Available at: http://www-personal.umich.edu/~rebeccal/RebeccaLThornton/Home_files/KohlerThornton.CCTHIV.pdf. Accessed 26 August 2011, "unpublished"

Table 16.3 Scale and focus of RCTs for HIV prevention in among men in Africa

Men's risk profile, type of intervention	RCTs	Number of men	PYs of follow-up		Incident cases	
			Number	Percent	Number	Percent
All RCTs	21	>44,043	>89,749	100	>929	100
RCTs by men's risk profile						
General population	17	>38,238	>81,130	90	>787	85
Men in discordant couples	3	>5,717	>8,619	9.6	>142	15
Men in discordant couples[a]	5	>5,925	>9,004	10	>184	20
High risk men	1	88	NR	NR	NR	NR
Interventions						
IEC	10	>17,957	>47,576	53	>359	39
STI treatment	5	18,543	40,552	45	477	51
Circumcision	4	>10,729	18,780	21	243	26
PrEP	4	>3,687	>4,622	5.1	>36	3.9
Vaccine	1	441	829	0.9	20	2.2
ART as prevention	1	556	988	1.1	12	1.3

Abbreviations see notes to Table 16.2
Note Two RCTs combined STI treatment with IEC (see Table 16.2), and are listed in both the STI and IEC rows. Also, two RCTS had two intervention arms each (see Table 16.2). Thus, the number of interventions listed in this table exceeds the number of RCTs
[a]This row includes men in discordant couples in two RCTs (Grosskurth et al. 1995; Wawer et al. 1999; Hugonnet et al. 2002; Quinn et al. 2000) that followed large cohorts of adults (see Table 16.2)

Table 16.4 Summary of relative risks (RRs) for HIV incidence in intervention versus control arms

Type of intervention	Number of interventions	RRs for intervention versus control arm			Number of interventions without reported RRs
		Number of RRs significantly <1	Number of RRs not significantly <1	Median (range)	
All interventions	23	9	11	0.38 (0.11–1.49)	3
IEC[a]	10[a]	–	7[a]	1.00 (0.97–1.49)	3
STI treatment[a]	5[a]	1	4[a]	0.92 (0.58–1.27)	–
Circumcision	4	3	1	0.48 (0.40–0.58)	–
PrEP	4	4	–	0.36 (0.17–0.56)	–
Vaccine	1	–	1	1.25	–
ART	1	1	–	0.11	–

Abbreviations see notes to Table 16.2
[a]Two interventions combining STI treatment with IEC are listed in both rows (see Table 16.2)

depend on more than RRs. Following paragraphs briefly consider the implications of observed RRs for HIV prevention according to type of intervention. The failure of the vaccine (RR = 1.25) shows that Africans will have to rely on other interventions to stop HIV for the foreseeable future.

IEC: Among all types of interventions, IEC has received the most attention in these RCTs. This is appropriate, because risks for HIV infection unprotected sex and blood-to-blood contact—are easily recognized and often avoidable. Without a vaccine, HIV prevention relies heavily on people knowing and avoiding risks. Thus, the failure of IEC interventions—such as educational events for communities in Uganda and South Africa, and counseling workers to avoid HIV in Zimbabwe—is a serious problem.

Lack of impact from IEC is often blamed on the supposed failure of those who receive IEC messages to curtail sexual risks. Alternately, IEC may fail due to incomplete messages that do not mention important risks, such as injections, scarification, blood tests, and other skin-piercing events (Brewer 2011; Gisselquist and Correa 2011). As detailed in later sections in this review, RCTs have not reported enough information about sources of infections to determine why IEC interventions failed.

STI Treatment: The first RCT of STI treatment to reduce HIV transmission—in Mwanza, Tanzania, 1991–1994—reported that HIV incidence was 42 % less over 2 years in communities served by clinics that offered improved STI treatment. The RR = 0.58 in this trial was significantly less than 1 ($p = 0.007$) (Grosskurth et al. 1995). However, 8 subsequent RCTs of STI treatment reported non-significant RRs ranging from 0.7 to 1.53 (4 trials among men and women reported in Table 16.2, and four other trials among women only (Celum et al. 2008; Ghys et al. 2001; Kaul et al. 2004; Watson-Jones et al. 2008). The puzzle posed by these 9 RCTs is why the Mwanza trial appears to have been a success. One common explanation is that HIV in Mwanza was concentrated in promiscuous adults infected with both conventional STI and HIV, so that STI treatment had a big impact on HIV transmission. However, the facts do not agree: In Mwanza's baseline survey, the 10 % of men reporting the most partners in the previous 12 months had only 11 % of prevalent HIV infections among men; and the 10 % of women reporting the most partners had only 18 % of infections (Quigley et al. 1997). Another hypothesis is that the RCT's distribution of syringes, oral antibiotics, and benzathine penicillin to clinics in the intervention communities reduced HIV transmission through fewer and safer injections in the intervention arm (Grosskurth et al. 1995; Grosskurth et al. 2000; Gisselquist and Potterat 2003).

Taking all RCTs of STI treatment together, there appears to be no reason to expect that STI treatment would have any noticeable impact on Africa's epidemic. However, the reason for this failure cannot be determined without knowing the source of observed infections—did the infections come from sex with or without an STI, from injections to treat STI, or from other causes? As explained below, these studies do not say.

Circumcision: In late 2005, a trial of circumcision to protect men from HIV in South Africa reported lower HIV incidence among circumcised vs. intact men, with a significant RR of 0.40 (95 % confidence interval [CI] 0.24–0.68) (Auvert et al. 2005). In early 2007, two similar trials in Kenya and Uganda, reported similar results, with significant RRs of 0.47 (95 % CI 0.28–0.78) and 0.49 ($p = 0.006$), respectively (Bailey et al. 2007; Gray et al. 2007). Results from a fourth trial in Uganda, 2004–2007, show a not significant RR = 0.58 (95 % CI 0.30–1.12); the study team has not reported this RR, but has reported enough data to calculate it (see notes to Table 16.2 in the Appendix) (Gray et al. 2007; Gray et al. 2009).

Based on results from the South African trial (the trial with the lowest RR), circumcision advocates estimate that circumcising all African men by 2015 would reduce new HIV infections in Africa by 13 % over the next 20 years (Williams et al. 2006). However, other evidence suggests circumcision would have less impact on personal risk and on Africa's epidemics. For example, five other RCTs in this review report HIV incidence in circumcised vs. intact men in Africa (excluding the trial among MSM, for which the major risk is receptive anal sex); in four trials, HIV incidence in circumcised men ranges from 0.63 to 1.57 times incidence in intact men (none of the differences are significant); the fifth reports no significant difference but does not provide data (Table 16.5). Also, national surveys in more than a dozen African countries are almost equally likely to find higher HIV prevalence in circumcised than in intact men (Gisselquist 2008; Mishra et al. 2009; Garenne 2008).

Based on results from RCTs of circumcision reported in 2005–2007, WHO and UNAIDS in 2007 endorsed circumcision for HIV prevention, (WHO and UNAIDS 2007) and some donors have extended support to African governments to circumcise males, including infants (WHO 2010). However, the expected impact of mass circumcision on Africa's HIV epidemics remains controversial (Fox and Thomson 2010). One factor that feeds this controversy is missing information about what happened in the circumcision trials. Study teams that managed the trials not only failed to ask about or investigate all potential risks, but have also not reported all relevant collected information (see below).

Table 16.5 HIV incidence in circumcised vs. intact men in other RCTs in Africa

Study	Number of men	% circumcised	Incidence per 100 PYs Circumcised	Incidence per 100 PYs Intact	RR for HIV in circumcised vs. intact men (95 % confidence interval)
Improved STI treatment, TZ, 1991–1994 (Todd et al. 2006a)	440	26	NR	NR	1.57 (0.70–3.51)
Improved STI treatment, IEC, Zimbabwe, 1998-2003(Lopman et al. 2008)	1,672	6.3	1.91	1.99	0.96(0.42-2.20)
Mass STI treatment, UG, 1994–1998 (Wawer et al. 1999)	4,351	16	1.07	1.50	0.72 (0.37–1.39)
Acyclovir for discordant couples, BT, KY, RW, SA, TZ, UG, ZA, 2004–2008 (Celum et al. 2010)	2,218	45	1.17	1.85	0.63 (0.35–1.15)
Vaccine, SA, 2007–2009 (Gray et al. 2011)	441	29 → 54[a]	NA	NA	Not significant

NR not reported, *RR* relative risk; for Tanzania, 1991–1994, the table shows the reported adjusted odds ratios; for the other two studies, the table shows crude rate ratios calculated from reported data using an online program (VassarStats: website for statistical computation. Available at:http://faculty.vassar.edu/lowry/VassarStats.html. Accessed 26 June 2011)

[a]129 men were circumcised at baseline, and an additional 109 before the end of the trial

PrEP: Beginning in 2004, a series of RCTs have tested the potential for daily ingestion of antiviral drugs, or pre-exposure prophylaxis (PrEP), to prevent HIV infection. Trials have used tenofovir disproxil fumarate (TDF) with or without emtricitabine (FTC). In 2010, a trial of PrEP with TDF/FTC among MSM in South Africa and five non-African countries reported that men in the intervention arm were 44 % less likely to acquire HIV compared to men in the control arm, giving a significant RR = 0.56 (p = 0.005) (Grant et al. 2010). In early 2011, a trial of TDF/FTC among women in Kenya and Uganda reported no impact on HIV incidence, as well as an unexplained higher rate of pregnancy in the intervention arm (FHI 2011). Subsequently, two more trials reported RRs for TDF and TDF/FTC in men ranging from 0.17 to 0.45, all significantly less than 1, and similar results among women (Thigpen et al. 2011; Baeten and Celum 2011).

Considering previous experience with antivirals to protect health care workers exposed to HIV through needle stick accidents and to prevent mother-to-child transmission, there is little doubt that PrEP can prevent HIV. However, PrEP has drawbacks, including not only cost but also potentially serious side effects in some percentage of users. Furthermore, studies have not determined the reasons for low RRs—did PrEP interrupt sexual or blood-borne transmission? Without knowing where HIV infections are coming from, it is impossible to determine who is at highest risk, and therefore could get the most benefit from PrEP.

Antiretroviral Therapy as Prevention: In early 2011, an RCT among HIV discordant couples reported that treating the HIV-positive partner with antiviral drugs reduced HIV transmission to susceptible partners by 96 %, giving a significant RR = 0.04 for acquisition of HIV from an HIV-positive partner; this RR increases to 0.11 if one includes HIV acquired from other sources (Cohen et al. 2011). This result was not surprising, considering that other studies in Africa and elsewhere have reported low rates of sexual transmission from people taking antiviral drugs as well as from people with low viral loads (Attia et al. 2009). The report has stimulated debate about the potential role of treatment as prevention in Africa. Limits to the extension of this intervention include cost, people not knowing they are infected, and potential harm to HIV-positive adults from beginning antiviral treatment before it is required for their own health (Sonnabend 2011).

16.4 Review Findings: RCTs Provide Little Information on HIV Risks in Africa

All interventions proposed to reduce HIV transmission through sexual contact, although several such as PrEP could also block blood-borne transmission. To evaluate an intervention's success in stopping sexual transmission, an RCT must determine not only HIV incidence in the intervention and control arms, but also the proportions of infections coming from sex. The record of these 21 RCTs in collecting and reporting information to determine the source of observed incident infections is considered for three basic inquiries: (a) tracing and testing sexual partners of men who seroconvert; and (b) determining HIV incidence in men with and without sexual exposures and (c) with and without skin-piercing procedures.

Not tracing the source of incident HIV infections: Of the 926 incident infections recognized in these RCTs, more than 60 % were observed in men followed at intervals no longer than a year. In most trials, large majorities of men reported not more than one sex partner during a follow-up interval. Yet, no trial determined the HIV status of any sexual partner for any man with incident infection aside from women the study team was already following for the same study or for a related study.

Ten of 21 studies tested the primary partners for some or all men in the study (Table 16.6). However, 5 of these 10 studies have not reported the partner's HIV status for any men with new infections. These five studies include two circumcision trials in Uganda (Gray et al. 2007, 2009) that tested and followed more than 3,700 partners of approximately 6,500 men (including circa 5,500 HIV-negative men in the two circumcision trials) (Wawer et al. 2011; ClinicalTrials.gov 2007). Neither circumcision trial has reported the partner's HIV status for any of the combined 105 men with incident infections.

The other 5 RCTs reported that 178 men with incident HIV had primary partners with pre-existing infections. However, only 3 of these RCTs sequenced HIV to see if men acquired their infections from partners with similar HIV or from some other source. The RCT of acyclovir in discordant couples observed incident infections in 88 men; sequencing found that HIV from 58 men was similar to their partner's HIV (Campbell et al. 2011; Lingappa et al. 2010). The trial of antiretroviral therapy (ART) as prevention in discordant couples reported that 28 of 39 infections among men and women in 8 countries were genetically linked, (Cohen et al. 2011) but has not reported separate data for Africa; from reported data, I estimate that 11 infections in African men were genetically linked to their partner's HIV (see Appendix). An RCT of STI mass treatment that followed a large cohort of rural adults in Uganda identified HIV-positive primary partners for 50 women and 40 men with new infections; sequencing of HIV from 46 formerly discordant couples found that 42 couples had similar HIV (Quinn et al. 2000; Wawer et al. 2005); although the study did not specify the sex of partners with new and linked infections, I estimate that half or 21 were men. Thus, these three trials collectively established that 90 men (9.7 % of 926 men with new infections in 21 trials) had likely acquired their infections from sexual partners with similar HIV.

Not asking about or reporting sexual risks: To assess an intervention's success against sexual transmission, an RCT must determine the proportion of HIV infections acquired through sex. One line of inquiry to investigate this proportion is to compare incidence in men who report no possible sexual exposures to HIV (no sex partners or 100 % condom use) vs. men who report 1 or more partners or less than 100 % condom use. Whether self-reports can be trusted is another matter; in any case, self-reports should be solicited and reported along with results from any other efforts to determine men's sexual risks.

Table 16.6 Studies that determined the HIV-status of primary partners for at least some men

Study	Men with incident HIV infections: Total	With known HIV-positive partner	With linkage determined by genetic sequencing
Studies recruiting only discordant couples			
Acyclovir for HSV2, BT, KY, RW, SA, TZ, UG, ZA, 2004–2008 (Campbell et al. 2011; Lingappa et al. 2010)	88	88	58
ART as prevention, BT, BR, IN, KY, MW, TH, US, ZI, 2005–11 (Cohen et al. 2011)	18	18	11? (see text)
PrEP with TDF or TDF/FTC, KY, UG, 2008–11 (Baeten and Celum 2011)	36	36	No testing reported
Other studies including discordant couples			
Improved STI treatment, TZ, 1991–1994 (Todd et al. 2006a; Hugonnet et al. 2002)	71	2	Not tested
Mass STI treatment, UG, 1994–1998 (Wawer et al. 1999, 2005; Quinn et al. 2000)	82	40	21? (see text)
STI treatment with or without IEC, UG, 1994–2000 (Kamali et al. 2003)	138	NR	No testing reported
Circumcision, UG, 2003–2006 (ClinicalTrials.gov 2007; Gray etal. 2007; Wawer et al. 2011)	67	NR	No testing reported
Circumcision, UG, 2004–2007 (Gray et al. 2007, 2009; Wawer et al. 2011; ClinicalTrials.gov 2007)	38	NR	No testing reported
Cash for no new HIV, MW, 2006–2008[a]	NR	NR	No testing reported
Cash for no new STI, TZ, 2009–2010 (Dow 2011; de Walque et al. 2010)	NR	NR	No testing reported
Total for 10 studies	538	184	90

Abbreviations: see Notes to Table 16.2

[a]Kohler and Thornton, 2010, Conditional cash transfers and HIV/AIDS prevention: unconditionally promising? Available at: http://www-personal.umich.edu/~rebeccal/RebeccaLThornton/Home_files/KohlerThornton.CCTHIV.pdf. Accessed 26 August 2011, "unpublished"

Only 2 RCTs—both are trials of circumcision to protect men—report incident infections in men with and without reported unprotected sex during the relevant observation interval (the time from the last negative HIV test to the first positive test). In the South African trial, (Auvert et al. 2005) men who reported no unprotected sex acquired HIV at the rate of 1.11 per 100 PYs vs. 1.86 per 100 PYs for men who reported any unprotected sex (Table 16.7). The RR = 1.66 for HIV incidence in men with vs. without unprotected sex is significantly greater than 1, but just barely so. Using standard epidemiological analyses (see Note to Table 16.7), reporting any unprotected sex "explains" only 27 % of HIV incidence, leaving 73 % not explained by sex.

Similarly, in the circumcision trial in Uganda, 2003–2006, only 29 % of incident infections were statistically linked to reported unprotected sex (Gray et al. 2007). Moreover, in this trial, the RR of 1.63 for HIV incidence associated with reporting any vs. no unprotected sex is not significantly greater than 1.

The Kenyan circumcision trial collected information on sexual contacts and condom use, but has not reported sexual events in men with and without incident HIV infection—except for 7 men infected in the first 1–3 months (Bailey et al. 2007). Five of these 7 men reported no sexual partners from the beginning of the trial to their first HIV-positive test. Similarly, the second circumcision trial in Uganda, 2004–2008, has not reported sexual contacts and condom use for men with and without incident infections (Gray et al. 2009).

Not reporting basic information about sexual behavior means either failure to ask or failure to report collected information. Questionnaires are in the public domain for only one of 21 RCTs, the RCT of ART as prevention in discordant couples (Cohen et al. 2011);[1] the questions identified men with no sexual partner during follow-up, but not men with 100 % condom use. For another RCT, a

Table 16.7 Proportion of incident HIV associated with reported unprotected sex

Intervention, countries, years, reference	RR for any versus no unprotected sex (95 % confidence interval)	Cases with any versus no unprotected sex	Percentage of infections associated with any versus no unprotected sex (%)
Circumcision, South Africa, 2002–2005 (Auvert et al. 2005)	1.66 (1.00–2.75)	46 of 69	27
Circumcision, Uganda, 2003–2006 (Gray et al. 2007)	1.63 (0.93–2.86)	51 of 67	29

Note The percentage of HIV infections associated with any versus no unprotected sex (i.e., the population attributable fraction or PAF) is calculated from the relative risk (*RR*) and proportion of cases exposed (*CE*) with the standard formula: PAF = CE × [RR−1] / RR

[1] Statistical Center for HIV/AIDS Research and Prevention (SCHARP).052 Seattle: SCHARP, Fred Hutchinson Cancer Research Center, no date. Available at:https://atlas.scharp.org/cpas/Project/HPTN/052/begin.view. Accessed 28 August 2011.

journal article details the questions asked; the questions did not identify men with 100 % condom use or with any vs. no partners (Pronyk et al. 2006). For the other 19 RCTs in this review, there is no public record of what was asked. However, reading between the lines of articles that study teams have published, it's clear that many if not most RCTs asked men if they had any vs. no sex partners or practiced 100 % condom use during follow-up intervals, although study teams have not reported this information.

Not asking about or reporting blood-borne risks: Another inquiry into the proportions of men with incident HIV from sexual and non-sexual risks is to ask men at each follow-up visit about skin-piercing procedures (potential blood exposures) since their last visit. Even if study teams have no interest in blood exposures as risks for HIV, RCTs collect information on participants' instances of ill health (adverse events) and medical care to see if interventions cause health problems; studies also record procedures administered in study clinics as a part of the study protocol. See, for example, the protocol[2] and forms for collecting and reporting data[3] for the RCT of ART as prevention in discordant couples. Thus, RCTs routinely, if not systematically, collect information on injections, infusions, operations, and other skin-piercing medical procedures during follow-up.

Despite all this collected information, only 4 of 21 RCTs reported information about any skin-piercing or medical procedures in men with and without incident HIV infection (Table 16.8). Two studies reported medical injections. In Tanzania, 1991–1994, 27 of 50 men with incident HIV had received injections in a hospital, clinic, or elsewhere. Considering all injections together, men reporting any vs. no injections were 1.74 (95 % CI 0.97–3.13) times more likely to become HIV-positive, and 27 % of HIV incidence was statistically associated with injections (Todd et al. 2006a; Gisselquist 2006). In the only other study that reported injections versus HIV incidence, in Zimbabwe, 1998–2003, men who reported any injection during 3 years of follow-up were less likely to become HIV-positive than men who reported no injections (Lopman et al. 2005).

The South African circumcision trial reported HIV incidence in men with and without a composite measure of health-care exposures (having been transfused, injected, or hospitalized). Men with any of these risks were 1.7 times more likely to acquire HIV than other men (Auvert et al. 2006). The same study reported a 5.7 times greater risk for HIV incidence in men who visited a clinic for a genital condition compared to other men (Auvert et al. 2005); without tracing and testing sexual partners, this statistic may point to sexual risks, clinic risks, or genital symptoms due to primary HIV infection from any source. Finally, the Kenyan circumcision trial reported HIV incidence in 4 men 1 month after circumcisions

[2] Division of AIDS (DAIDS) HPTN 052: a randomized trial to evaluate the effectiveness of antiretroviral therapyplus HIV primary care vs. HIV primary care alone to prevent the sexual transmission of HIV-1 In serodiscordant couple, study documents. DAIDS Document ID: 10068. DAIDS, Washington, DC. Available at:http://www.hptn.org/research_studies/HPTN052StudyDocuments.asp#Protocol. Accessed 27 June 2011.

[3] See footnote 1.

Table 16.8 Incident HIV infections in men associated with skin-piercing procedures

Intervention, countries, years, reference	Skin-piercing procedure	RR (95 % confidence interval)	Cases exposed	PAF (%)
Improved STI treatment, Tanzania, 1991–1994 (Todd et al. 2006a, b; Gisselquist 2006)	Injection in hospital/clinic	1.94 (0.84–4.49)	22 of 50	21
	Injection elsewhere	2.47 (0.71–8.64)	5 of 50	6
Improved STI treatment and IEC, Zimbabwe, 1998–2003 (Lopman et al. 2005)	Injection	0.33 (0.07–1.46)	2 of 19	<0
Circumcision, South Africa, 2002–2005 (Auvert et al. 2005; Auvert et al. 2006)	Composite risk: blood transfusion, hospitalization, and/or injection	1.7 ($p = 0.092$)	15 of 69	9.5
	"Attending a clinic for a health problem related to the genitals"	5.73 (3.33–9.84)	21 of 69	25
Circumcision, Kenya, 2002–2006 (Bailey et al. 2007)	Circumcision		4 (see text)	

PAF and *RR* see notes to Table 16.7

provided by the study; 3 of the men reported no sexual events before testing HIV-positive (Bailey et al. 2007).

Despite their own reported evidence, none of the study teams concluded that injections, circumcisions, or other skin-piercing procedures accounted for substantial proportions of HIV infections.

16.5 Review Findings: RCTs Raise Ethical Issues

Some of the RCTs considered in this review demonstrate a double standard between what can be done in countries that fund these studies, and what study teams do in Africa. The ethical issues involved in these differential practices are controversial. The following comments present a brief introduction to selected issues only.

Not Telling Men they are HIV-Positive: In 1988, the US Office for Protection from Research Risks established the policy that "Individuals may not be given the option 'not to know' the result" of their HIV test (Public Health Service 1998). At least 11 RCTs in this review enrolled and followed men without telling some or all their HIV status at baseline or later (Table 16.9). If men asked, some studies would tell, while others sent them to testing services. For example, "Where participants (in a 1998–2003 RCT) indicate that they would like to be advised as to their own

Table 16.9 Examples of ethical issues in RCTs for HIV prevention among women

Intervention, location, study years, reference	Not telling men they are HIV-positive	Not warning men their partners are HIV-positive
IEC and/or STI treatment interventions		
Improved STI treatment, Tanzania, 1991-94 (Grosskurth et al. 1995; Hugonnet et al. 2002)	√	√
Mass STI treatment, Uganda, 1994–1998 (Wawer et al. 1999, 2005; Quinn et al. 2000)	√	√
Improved STI treatment and/or IEC, Uganda, 1994–2000 (Kamali et al. 2003)	√	√
School-based IEC for youth, Tanzania, 1998–2002 (Ross et al. 2007)	√	
Improved STI treatment with IEC, Zimbabwe, 1998–2003 (Gregson et al. 2009)	√	
IEC with credit, South Africa, 2001–2005 (Pronyk et al. 2006)	√	
IEC with workplace VCT, Zimbabwe, 2002–2004 (Corbett et al. 2007)	√	
IEC, opinion leader, Zimbabwe, 2002–2007 (The NIMH Collaborative HIV/STD Prevention Trial Group 2010; McClellan et al. 2010)	√	
IEC, Stepping Stones, South Africa, 2003–2006 (Jewkes et al. 2008; Michielsen et al. 2010)	√	
Circumcision		
South Africa, 2002–2005 (Auvert et al. 2005)	√	
Uganda, 2003–2006 (Gray et al. 2007; Wawer et al. 2011; ClinicalTrials.gov 2007)		√
Uganda, 2004–2007 (Gray et al. 2009; Wawer et al. 2011; ClinicalTrials.gov 2007)	√	√

HIV-1 serostatus, appointments will be arranged for them to visit a local clinic where a free counseling and testing service will be made available" (Gregson et al. 2009, p. 6 of Protocol S1). Over time, more RCTs adopted the practice of not enrolling participants who did not agree to hear their test results. For example, "willing to receive HIV results" was one of the inclusion criteria for participants in the circumcision trial in Uganda, 2003–2006, which was funded by the US government (ClinicalTrials.gov 2007). However, the same study team recruited men who did not want to hear their HIV results into a parallel trial funded by the Bill and Melinda Gates Foundation (ClinicalTrials.gov 2007; Wawer et al. 2007).

Not Warning Men Their Partners are HIV-Positive: US law requires states receiving federal funds for specific health programs "to require that a good faith effort be made to notify a spouse of a known HIV-infected patient that such spouse might have been exposed to the human immunodeficiency virus…" (DHHS 1996). At least 5 RCTs identified and followed discordant couples, including men who did not know their partners were infected, and women who did not know they were HIV-positive and thereby a danger to their husbands (Table 16.9). In 2000, the editor of the New England Journal of Medicine criticized one of these RCTs for not warning spouses at risk, noting that "such a study could not have been performed in the United States" (Angell 2000, p. 967). The study team explained, "this was a community-based trial that enrolled all consenting adults, the identification of couples...was done only retrospectively" (Quinn et al. 2000, p. 922). Several years later, a related study in the same community recruited, tested, and followed wives of HIV-negative men in two RCTs of circumcision to protect men; some of the women did not know they were infected (Gray et al. 2007, 2009; Wawer et al. 2011, 2007). The study team encouraged (Kairania et al. 2010) but did not insist that men and women in these trials receive their test results and share it with their partner.

Not Warning Partners When Men Seroconvert: Many RCTs in this review did not tell men with incident infections that they were infected, while others told men and offered or referred them to counseling. Based on practices common in Africa, counselors would not insist that men warn their partners, and would not warn partners if men did not. Thus, most RCTs in this review made no to modest efforts to ensure that partners of men with new HIV infections were aware of their risk.

Not Reporting and Investigating Unanticipated Problems: To protect research participants, US institutions managing research anywhere in the world that is funded from the US are ethically (and legally) obligated to investigate "unanticipated problems" among research participants that appear to be linked to their participation in research (Gisselquist 2009). The Kenyan circumcision trial, funded by the US and Canadian governments, recognized HIV infections in 4 men 1 month after circumcisions provided by the project. There is no evidence the study team reported or investigated these infections as unanticipated problems, as US regulations require.

16.6 Conclusions

This review leads to four conclusions and four linked recommendations.

Conclusion 1: Due to faulty design and implementation, these 21 RCTs do not explain why men (and women) in some African countries who are not MSM or IDUs are more than 100 times more likely to be HIV-positive than similar adults in Western Europe or the US. Notably, circumcision does not explain the difference, because it is already more common in Africa than Europe. Had study teams traced and tested sexual partners, and asked about and reported information on sexual and blood exposures, they could have explained not only why interventions failed or succeeded, but also what is different about HIV risks in Africa (Potterat 2010). These RCTs thus do not provide the information required to warn people about important risks, so they can protect themselves. Failure to trace and ask wasted not only money and time, but also the good faith and misfortune of participant men who acquired HIV infections.

Conclusion 2: Study teams have undermined the scientific process by not putting their data into the public domain (Pisani et al. 2010; Brewer et al. 2010). No study team has done so. With two exceptions, there is not even a public report of what was collected, so outsiders do not know what information was collected but not reported. Without the standard scientific discipline of disclosing data to allow others to critically examine proffered analyses, study teams may withhold data that does not fit favored hypotheses. For example, the study team that managed the RCT of STI treatment in Tanzania, 1991–1994, took more than 10 years to report data showing more than 20 % of incident HIV associated with injections (Todd et al. 2006a; Gisselquist 2006).

Withholding relevant data is particularly disturbing for the four RCTs of circumcision to protect men. The South African trial reported selected information on medical procedures as risks for HIV; the other three have reported no information on medical procedures. Circumcision trials in Kenya and in Uganda, 2004–2007, have not reported sexual behavior vs. HIV incidence (except for 7 men infected in the first 1–3 months in Kenya). Similarly, circumcision trials in Uganda, 2003–2006 and 2004–2007, have information on the HIV status of men's partners, but have not reported it. Incomplete reports from these RCTs energized programs intending to circumcise millions of African men.

Conclusion 3: Scientific failures are linked to ethical failures. Researchers who did not tell men when they acquired HIV infection, and did not then trace, test, and warn spouses and other sexual partners were not challenged to explain HIV incidence in men with no sexual exposures to HIV.

Conclusion 4: Scientific and ethical failures are systemic. Organizations funding the 21 RCTs in this review have accepted and supported such behavior for decades.

16.7 Recommendations

Recommendation 1: Governments of countries that host research should insist that researchers conform to the ethical standards of the funding country, along with any additional standards imposed by the host government. This means, inter alia, that studies should enroll only people who agree to hear their HIV test results—at baseline and during follow-up—and to share an HIV-positive result with their partner.

Recommendation 2: Governments of countries that host research should insist that all new studies of risks for HIV incidence are scientifically sound. Specifically, governments should insist that research teams: (a) publicly post questionnaires before the study begins; (b) include comprehensive questions about sexual and skin-piercing events; and (c) whenever an incident infection is observed, trace and test sexual partners and possible blood contacts. Such research could be expected to produce good information about all important risks within not more than 1–2 years. And to ensure that study teams do a good job, governments should also insist that they (d) post data for public access within a year after data collection is complete.

Recommendation 3: African governments should stop supporting infant circumcision to prevent HIV. Most of today's infants will not be sexually active for 15 years. With competent research and investigations (see recommendation 2), Africans will learn about all risks, which will allow them to avoid risks and stop new infections. Vaccines and other advances may also be expected over 15 years. It's a statement of despair to suppose that Africa will be facing the same HIV epidemic after another 1–2 decades.

Recommendation 4: African governments should withhold or suspend support for adult circumcision pending better information. At a minimum, governments should demand that: (a) the study teams for the four circumcision trials publicly report all protocols, questionnaires, and data; and (b) the Kenyan government investigates the possibility that unsterile procedures during circumcision infected 4 men in the Kenyan circumcision trial by tracing and testing others who attended the relevant clinics on the days the 4 men were circumcised. But that's not enough. Governments should also ask for adequate research to explain what is different in Africa that allows HIV to infect so many people. Only when men are aware of all risks for HIV—blood–borne as well as sexual—can they make informed choices about whether to be circumcised. Without knowing all of the important risks for HIV in Africa, circumcising millions of men is almost literally a stab in the dark.

Competing Interests: The author declares that he has no competing interests.

Acknowledgments I would like to thank Marilyn Milos, Hugh Young, and Devon Brewer for helpful advice after reading earlier drafts.

Appendix: Derivation of Estimated Data in Table 16.2

Studies with estimated data (data marked with superscript "b") in Table 16.2 are listed in this Appendix in the same order and with the same identifiers as in Table 16.2.

General population men

STI treatment, TZ, 1991–1994 (Grosskurth et al. 1995; Todd et al. 2006): Number of HIV-negative men is estimated as 48 % of HIV-negative adults from the proportion of men among all adults followed. Total PYs is estimated by multiplying men followed by 2 years (Grosskurth et al. 1995, p. 532). The incidence rate is estimated from reported infections in men (Todd et al. 2006, p. 460) and estimated PYs.

STI treatment, IEC, UG, 1994–2000 (Kamali et al. 2003): Number of men and men's PYs and incident cases are estimated as 45.5 % of totals for adults from the proportion of men in the recruited cohort. The incidence rate for men is estimated as the rate for all adults, calculated from reported PYs and incident cases (Kamali et al. 2003, pp. 648–649).

STI treatment, IEC, ZI, 1998–2003 (Gregson et al. 2009; Lopman et al. 2008): Numbers of men followed, PYs of follow-up, and incident infections are from Lopman et al. (2008).

IEC, TZ, 1998–2002 (Ross et al. 2007): PYs of follow-up in men in each arm are estimated from reported cases and incidence rates for men in each arm. The incidence rate for all men is estimated from estimated follow-up time and reported cases in men (Ross et al. 2007, p. 1950).

IEC, SA, 2001–2005 (Pronyk et al. 2006): Number of men followed is estimated as 44 % of adults followed from men's proportion of the recruited cohort. PYs is estimated from the reported 3.1 years average follow-up. Men's incident infections and incidence rate are estimated from the reported 142 infections among all adults, assuming that men's rate of incidence is 0.38 times women's rate, which is the ratio of reported baseline prevalence in men vs. women.

IEC, ZI, 2002–2004 (Corbett et al. 2007): Number of men and PYs followed are calculated as 88.4 and 90.5 % of totals for adults in the control and intervention arms, respectively, from the proportions of men in the recruited cohort. Incident infections and incidence rate for men are estimated from totals for men and women and the report that men's incidence rate was 1.73 women's rate (Corbett et al. 2007, pp. 486–487).

IEC, SA, 2003–2006 (Jewkes et al. 2008; Michielsen et al. 2010): PYs of follow-up and incidence rate for men in both arms combined are estimated from men's reported cases and incidence rates in each arm (Jewkes et al. 2008, p. 7) The RR for men is from Michielsen (Michielsen et al. 2010, p. 1200).

IEC, MW, 2006–2008 (Kohler and Thornton, 2010, Conditional cash transfers and HIV/AIDS prevention: unconditionally promising? Available at: http://www-personal.umich.edu/~rebeccal/RebeccaLThornton/Home_files/KohlerThornton.CCTHIV.pdf. Accessed 26 August 2011, "unpublished"): The RR is estimated from the reported coefficient of 0.001 for the intervention's impact on HIV status (table 5 in the reference). Number of men followed is estimated from the reported 1,312 men and women recruited, of which 45 % were men, 9 % were HIV-positive and 89 % were followed. PYs followed is estimated from the reported 2 years of follow-up multiplied by the estimated number of HIV-negative men.

IEC, TZ, 2009–2010 (Dow 2011; de Walque et al. 2010): Number of HIV-negative men followed is estimated from the reported 1,198 men followed, less 2.45 % HIV-positive men. PYs is estimated for the 1 year follow-up during which the intervention (cash for not testing positive for an STI) was delivered, assuming that 90 % are followed. These estimates ignore a second year of follow-up without the intervention.

Circumcision, KY, 2002–2006 (Bailey et al. 2007): PYs of follow-up is estimated from reported numbers tested at follow-up intervals (Bailey et al. 2007, p. 651). The incidence rate is estimated from reported cases and estimated PYs of follow-up.

Circumcision, UG, 2004–2007 (Gray et al. 2007, 2009): PYs of follow-up and infections are estimated by subtracting results previously reported for the UG,

2003–2006 circumcision trial (22 infections in 3,352.4 PYs in the intervention arm; 45 infections in 3,391.8 PYs in the control arm) (Gray et al. 2007) from totals for both Ugandan circumcision trials (36 infections in 4,825.5 PYs in the intervention arm; 69 infections in 4,864.0 PYs in the control arm) (Gray et al. 2009). The incidence rate and RR are calculated from infections and PYs. These estimates include approximately 2,000 PYs of follow-up time during 2006–2007 among men in the 2003–2006 trial that is additional to what the study team reported in 2007 (Gray et al. 2007).

Vaccine, SA, 2007–2009 (Gray et al. 2011): Total follow-up time for men and women combined is estimated as the sum of follow-up times in the intervention and control arms, which are estimated from 34 and 28 reported infections in the intervention and control arms, respectively, and incidence rates of 4.54 and 3.70 per 100 PYs in the intervention and control arms, respectively. Follow-up time for men is estimated as 55 % of total follow-up time from the reported percentage of men among participants. The incidence rate in men is estimated from the reported 20 infections in men and estimated follow-up time.

Men in discordant couples

STI treatment, BT, KY, RW, SA, TZ, UG, ZA, 2004–2008 (Celum et al. 2010; Campbell et al. 2011; Lingappa et al. 2010): Numbers of men followed and PYs of follow-up are from Celum and colleagues (Celum et al. 2010, p. 436). Number of incident infection is from Campbell and colleagues (Campbell et al. 2011). The incident rate is calculated from reported follow-up time and number of infections. The 58 linked infections in men are calculated as 53.7 % of 108 linked infections in men and women (Campbell et al. 2011, p. 9; Lingappa et al. 2010 p. 1).

PrEP, KY, UG, 2008–2011 (Baeten and Celum 2011): Number of men is calculated from men's reported 62 % of total 4,747 participants. Men's PYs of follow-up is estimated as 63 % of the reported 7,337 total PYs, allowing some women's follow-up time lost to pregnancy. Men's incidence rate is estimated from reported incident cases and estimated follow-up time.

ART as prevention, BT, BR, IN, KY, MW, TH, US, ZI, 2005–2011 (Cohen et al. 2011): Number of HIV-negative African participants is from Cohen and colleagues (Cohen et al. 2011, p. 498). Number of PYs of follow-up for African participants is estimated from follow-up time for all participants of 3,152.6 PYs [p. 500], assuming the percentage of follow-up time for Africans is similar to their reported 54 % of participants. Number of incident infections in Africans is estimated from Africans' reported 82 % (23/28) of linked infections and their reported greater rate of total vs. linked incidence, 2.3 vs. 1.6 per 100 PYs (supplementary material). Number of at-risk African men and men's PYs are estimated from estimated African totals and women's reported 58 % of infected partners in African couples. Number of total infections in African men is estimated from the estimated 33 total infections in Africans and African men's reported 0.88 lower HIV incidence versus African women. Number of linked infections in African men is estimated from the estimated 23 linked infections in Africans and African men's reported 0.69 lower incidence of linked infections vs. African women. The incidence rate is estimated from estimated infections and follow-up time.

References

Angell M (2000) Investigators' responsibilities for human subjects in developing countries. N Eng J Med 342:967–968

Attia A, Egger M, Muller M, Zwahlen M, Low N (2009) Sexual transmission of HIV according to viral load and antiretroviral therapy: systematic review and meta-analysis. AIDS 1397–1404

Auvert B, Taljaard D, Lagarde E, Sobngwi-Tambekou J, Sitta R, Puren A (2005) Randomized, controlled intervention trial of male circumcision for reduction of HIV infection risk: the ANRS 1265 trial. PLoS Med 2(11): e298

Auvert B, Sobngwi-Tambekou J, Taljaard D, Lagasrde E, Puren A (2006) Authors' reply. PLoS Med 3:e67

Baeten J, Celum C (2011) The partners PrEP study team. Antiretroviral pre-exposure prophylaxis for HIV-1 prevention among heterosexual African men and women: the partners PrEP Study (power point). In: 6th IAS conference on HIV pathogenesis, treatment and prevention, Rome, 17–20 July 2011

Bailey RC, Moses S, Parker CB. Agot L, Maclean I, Krieger JN, Williams CFM et al (2007) Male circumcision for HIV prevention in young men in Kisumu, Kenya: a randomised controlled trial. Lancet 369:643–656

Brewer DD (2011) Knowledge of blood-borne transmission risk is inversely associated with HIV infection in sub-Saharan Africa. J Infect Dev Ctries 5:182–198

Brewer DD, Potterat JJ, Muth SQ (2010) Withholding access to research data (letter). Lancet 375:1872

Campbell MS, Mullins JI, Hughes JP et al (2011) Viral linkage in HIV-1 seroconverters and their partners in an HIV-1 prevention clinical trial. PLoS ONE 6(3):316986. doi:10.1371/journal.pone.0016986

Celum C, Wald A, Hughes J et al (2008) Effect of acyclovir on HIV-1 acquisition in herpes simplex virus 2 seropositive women and men who have sex with men: a randomized double-blind, placebo-controlled trial. Lancet 371:2109–2119

Celum C, Wald A, Lingappa JR et al (2010) Acyclovir and transmission of HIV-1 from persons infected with HIV-1 and HSV-2. N Engl J Med 362:427–439

Centers for Disease Control and Prevention (2009) HIV surveillance report, 2009. CDC, Atlanta, 2011. Available at:http://www.cdc.gov/hiv/surveillance/resources/reports/2009report/pdf/table1.5a.pdf. Accessed 29 August 2011

ClinicalTrials.gov (2007) Trial of male circumcision: HIV, sexually transmitted disease (STD) and behavioral effects in men, women and the community. ClinicalTrials.gov identifier NCT00124878, last updated on 9 August 2007. Available at:http://clinicaltrials.gov/show/NCT00124878. Accessed 25 June 2011

ClinicalTrials.gov (2007) Male circumcision for HIV prevention in Rakai, Uganda. Last updated 23 August 2007. Available at:http://clinicaltrials.gov/ct2/show/NCT00425984. Accessed 28 June 2011

Cohen MS, Chen YQ, McCauley M et al (2011) Prevention of HIV-1 infection with early antiretroviral therapy. New Eng J Med 365:493–505

Corbett EL, Makamure B, Cheung YB et al (2007) HIV incidence during a cluster-randomized trial of two strategies providing voluntary counselling and testing at the workplace, Zimbabwe. AIDS 21:483–489

Cowan FM, Pascoe SJS, Langhaug LF et al (2010) The Regai Dzive Shiri project: results of a randomized trial of an HIV prevention intervention for youth. AIDS 24:2541–2552

de Walque D, Dow WH, Nathan R (2010) Evaluating conditional cash transfers to prevent HIV and other STIs in Tanzania (power point). In: 4th annual research conference on population, reproductive health, and economic development, Cape Town, 14–17 January 2010. Available at:http://poppov.org/Portals/1/documents/events/4thAnnConf/dewalque.pdf. Accessed 26 August 2011

Department of Health and Human Services (DHHS) (1996) A compilation of the Ryan White CARE Act of 1960, as amended by the Ryan White Care Act amendments of 1996 (Pub. L. No. 104-146). DHHS, Washington DC. Available at:http://www.caear.org/downloads/RW_1996_amendments.pdf. Accessed 3 January 2011

Dow W (2011) Presentation: evaluating conditional cash transfers to prevent HIV and other sexually transmitted infections (STIs) in Tanzania: 1 year post-intervention follow-up (abstract). In: 8th World Congress on Health Economics, Toronto, 10–13 July 2011

FHI (2011) FHI Statement on the Fem-PrEP HIV Prevention Study, 18 April 2011. Available at:http://www.fhi.org/en/Research/Projects/FEM-PrEP.htm. Accessed 19 April 2011

Fox M, Thomson M (2010) HIV/AIDS and circumcision: lost in translation. J Med Ethics 36:798–801

Garenne M (2008) Long-term population effect of male circumcision in generalized HIV epidemics in sub-Saharan Africa. Afr J AIDS Res 7:1–8

Ghys P, Diallo MO, Ettiegne-Traore V et al (2001) Effect of interventions to control sexually transmitted disease on the incidence of HIV infection in female sex workers. AIDS 15:1421–1431

Gisselquist D (2006) New information on the risks of HIV transmission in Mwanza, Tanzania (letter). J Infect Dis 194:536–537

Gisselquist D (2008) Points to consider: responses to HIV/AIDS in Africa, Asia, and the Caribbean. London: Adonis and Abbey. Available at:http://sites.google.com/site/davidgisselquist/pointstoconsider. Accessed 29 June 2011

Gisselquist D (2009) HIV infections as unanticipated problems during medical research in Africa. Accountability Res 16:199–217

Gisselquist D, Hutin Y. ed. (2003) Pilot testing the WHO tools to assess and evaluate injection practices. Geneva: WHO

Gisselquist D (2011) Randomized Controlled Trials for HIV/AIDS Prevention Among Men and Women in Africa: Untraced Infections, Unasked Questions, and Unreported Data. Available at Social Science Research Network: http://papers.ssrn.com/sol3/papers.cfm?abstract_id=1940999. Accessed 21 February 2013

Gisselquist D, Potterat JJ (2003) Confound it: latent lessons from the Mwanza trial of STD treatment to reduce HIV transmission. Int J STD AIDS 14:179–184

Gisselquist D, Correa M (2011) Don't Get Stuck with HIV: how to protect yourself during health care and cosmetic procedures. Available at: http://dontgetstuck.wordpress.com/. Accessed 30 August 2011

Grant RM, Lama JR, Anderson PL, McMahan V, Liu AY, Vargas L, Goicochea P et al (2010) Preexposure chemoprophylaxis for HIV prevention in men who have sex with men. NEJM 363:2587–2599

Gray RH, Kigozi G, Serwadda D, Makumbi F, Watya S, Nalugoda F, Kiwanuka N et al (2007) Male circumcision for HIV prevention in men in Rakai, Uganda: a randomized trial. Lancet 369:657–666

Gray RH, Serwadda D, Tobian AAR et al (2009) Effects of genital ulcer disease and herpes simplex virus type 2 on the efficacy of male circumcision for HIV prevention: analyses from the Rakai trials. PLoS Med 6(11):e1000187

Gray G, Allen M, Churchyard G et al (2011) Safety and efficacy of the HVTN 503/Phambili Study of a clade-B-based HIV-1 vaccine in South Africa: a double-blind, randomized, placebo-controlled test-of-concept phase 2b study. Lancet Infect Dis 11:507–515

Gregson S, Adamson S, Papaya S et al (2009) Impact and process evaluation of integrated community and clinic-based HIV-1 control: a cluster-randomised trial in Eastern Zimbabwe. PLoS Med 4: e102. Available at: http://www.plosmedicine.org/article/info%3Adoi%2F10.1371%2Fjournal.pmed.0040102. Accessed 13 December 2010

Grosskurth H, Mosha F, Todd J et al (1995) Impact of improved treatment of sexually transmitted diseases on HIV infection in rural Tanzania: randomized controlled trial. Lancet 346:530–536

Grosskurth H, Mwijarubi E, Todd J, Rwakatare M, Orroth K, Mayaud P. Cleophas B, Buve A, Mkanje R, Ndeki L, Gavyole A, Hayes R, Mabey D (2000) Operational performance of an STD control programme in Mwanza Region, Tanzania. Sex Trans Infect 76:426–436

Hugonnet S, Mosha F, Todd J, Mugeye K, Klokke A, Ndeki L, Ross D, Grosskurth H, Hayes R. (2002) Incidence of HIV infertion in stable sexual partnerships: a retrospective cohort study of 1802 couples in Mwanza Region, Tanzania. J Acquir Immune Defic Syndr 30:73–80

Jewkes R, Nduna M, Levin J et al (2008) Impact of Stepping Stones on incidence of HIV and HSV-2 and sexual behavior in rural South Africa: cluster randomized controlled trial. BMJ 337:a506

Kairania R, Gray RH, Kiwanuka N et al (2010) Disclosure of HIV results among discordant couples in Rakai, Uganda: a facilitated couple counselling approach. AIDS Care 22:1041–1051

Kamali A, Quigley M, Nakiyingi J et al (2003) Syndromic management of sexually transmitted infections and behavior change interventions on transmission of HIV-1 in rural Uganda: a community randomised controlled trial. Lancet 341:645–652

Kaul R, Kimani J, Nagelkerke NJ et al (2004) Monthly antibiotic chemoprophylaxis and incidence of sexually transmitted infections and HIV-1 infection in Kenyan sex workers: a randomized controlled trial. JAMA 291:2555–2562

Lingappa JR, Hughes JP, Wang RS et al (2010) Estimating the impact of plasma HIV-1 RNA reductions on heterosexual HIV-1 transmission risk. PLoS One 5:e12598, 1–7

Lopman BA, Garnett GP, Mason PR, Gregson S (2005) Individual level injection history: a lack of association with HIV incidence in rural Zimbabwe. PLoS Med 2:e37

Lopman B, Nyamukapa C, Mushati P, et al. (2008). HIV incidence in 3 years of follow-up of a Zimbabwe cohort – 1998-2000 to 2001-03: contributions of proximate and underlying determinants to transmission. Int J Epidemiol 37: 88-105

McClellan K, Patel R, Woelk G et al (2010) HSV and HIV prevalence and incidence among young men and women in Zimbabwe in the NIMH CPOL study. In: 18th conference on retroviruses and opportunistic infections, Boston, 27 February–2 March 2010. Available at:http://www.retroconference.org/2011/Abstracts/41282.htm. Accessed 6 April 2011

Michielsen K, Chersich MF, Luchters S et al (2010) Effectiveness of HIV prevention for youth in sub-Saharan Africa: systematic review and meta-analysis of randomized and nonrandomized trials. AIDS 24:1193–1202

Mishra V, Medley A, Hong R, Gu Yuan, Robey B (2009) Levels and spread of HIV seroprevalence and associated factors: evidence from national household surveys. DHS comparative reports no. 22. Macro International, Calverton

National AIDS Coordinating Agency (2005) Botswana AIDS impact survey II: statistical report. Central Statistical Office, Gaborone. Available at:http://www.cso.gov.bw/images/stories/HouseHold/stats_report.pdf. Accessed 29 August 2011

Packard RM, Epstein P (1991) Epidemiologists, social scientists, and the structure of medical research on AIDS in Africa. Soc Sci Med 33:771–794

Padian NS, McCoy SI, Balkus JE, Wasserheit JN (2010) Weighing the gold in the gold standard: challenges in HIV prevention research. AIDS 24:621–635

Pépin J, Labbé AC, Mamadou-Yaya F et al (2010) Iatrogenic transmission of human T cell lymphotropic virus type 1 and hepatitis C virus through parenteral treatment and chemoprophylaxis of sleeping sickness in colonial equatorial Africa. Clin Infect Dis 51:777–784

Pettifor AE, Levandowski BA, Macphail C et al (2010) A tale of two countries: rethinking sexual risk for HIV among young people in South Africa and the United States. J Adolesc Health 49:237–243

Pisani E, Whitworth W, Zaba B, Abou-Zahr C (2010) Time for fair trade in research data. Lancet 375:703–704

Potterat JJ (2010) Randomized, controlled trials for HIV/AIDS prevention in Africa: learning from unexpected results. Future Virol 5:21–24

Pronyk PM, Hargreaves JR, Kim JC et al (2006) Effect of a structural intervention for the prevention of intimate-partner violence and HIV in rural South Africa: a cluster randomized trial. Lancet 368:1973–1990

Public Health Service (PHS) (1998) Policy on informing those tested about HIV serostatus. PHS, Washington, DC. Available at:http://www.hhs.gov/ohrp/humansubjects/guidance/hsdc88jun.htm. Accessed 9 September 2007
Quigley M, Manguti K, Grosskurth H et al (1997) Sexual behaviour patterns and other risk factors for HIV infection in rural Tanzania: a case-control study. AIDS 11:237–248
Quinn TC, Wawer MJ, Sewankambo N, Serwadda D, Li C, Wabwire-Mangen F, Meehan MO, Lutalo T, Gray RH (2000) Rakai project study group: viral load and heterosexual transmission of human immunodeficiency virus type 1. N Eng J Med 342:921–929
Ross DA, Changalucha J, Obasi AIN et al (2007) Biological and behavioural impact of an adolescent sexual health intervention in Tanzania: a community-randomized trial. AIDS 21:1943–1955
Shisana O, Rehle T, Simbayi LC et al (2009) South African national HIV prevalence, incidence, behaviour and communication survey 2008: A turning tide among teenagers? HSRC Press, Cape Town. Available at:http://www.mrc.ac.za/pressreleases/2009/sanat.pdf. Accessed 29 August 2011
Sonnabend J (2011) Treatment as prevention: protecting patient autonomy (blog posting 7 June 2011). Available at: http://blogs.poz.com/joseph/archives/2011/06/treatment_as_prevent_1.html #comments. Accessed 23 June 2011
The NIMH Collaborative HIV/STD Prevention Trial Group (2010) Results of the NIMH collaborative HIV/sexually transmitted disease prevention trial of a community popular opinion leader intervention. J Acquir Immune Defic Syndr 54:204–214
Thigpen MC, Kebaabetswe PM, Smith DK et al (2011) Daily oral antiretroviral use for the prevention of HIV infection in heterosexually active young adults in Botswana: results from the TDF2 study (power point). In: 6th IAS conference on pathogenesis, treatment and prevention, Rome, 17–20 July 2011. Available at:http://pag.ias2011.org/PAGMaterial/IAS2011/PPT /596_640/tdf2%20study_ias2011%20-%20final.pptx. Accessed 25 August 2011
Todd J, Grosskurth H, Changalucha J et al (2006a) Risk factors influencing HIV infection incidence in a rural African population: a nested case-control study. J Infect Dis 193:458–466
Todd J, Grosskurth H, Hayes R (2006b) New information on the risks of HIV transmission in Mwanza, Tanzania: reply to Gisselquist (letter). J Infect Dis 194:537–538
UNAIDS (2010) UNAIDS Report on the Global Epidemic 2010. UNAIDS, Geneva. Available at: http://www.unaids.org/globalreport/Global_report.htm. Accessed 4 July 2011
Watson-Jones D, Weiss HA, Rusizoka M et al (2008) Effect of herpes simplex suppression on incidence of HIV among women in Tanzania. N Engl J Med 358:1560–1571
Wawer MJ, Sewankambo NK, Serwadda D et al (1999) Control of sexually transmitted diseases for AIDS prevention in Uganda: a randomized community trial. Lancet 353:525–535
Wawer MJ, Gray RH, Sewankambo NK et al (2005) Rates of HIV-1 transmission per coital act, by stage of HIV-1 infection, in Rakai, Uganda. J Infect Dis 191:1403–9
Wawer MJ, Serwadda D, Gray RH et al (2007) Randomized trial of male circumcision: STD, HIV and behavioral effects in men, women and the community. Protocol. Protocol stage 2, version 3b, 27 March 2007. Available at:http://www.plosmedicine.org/article/info%3Adoi%2F10.1371%2Fjournal.pmed.1000187#s6. Accessed 28 June 2011
Wawer MJ, Tobian AAR, Kigozi G et al (2011) Effect of circumcision of HIV-negative men on transmission of human papillomavirus to HIV-negative women: a randomized trial in Rakai, Uganda. Lancet 377:209–218
Wellings K, Collumbien M, Slaymaker E et al (2006) Sexual behavior in context: a global perspective. Lancet 368:1706–1728
WHO (2010) Scaling up male circumcision programmes in the Eastern and Southern Africa region. WHO, Geneva. Available at:http://www.who.int/hiv/pub/malecircumcision/country_progress_meeting_report_jun10.pdf. Accessed 25 June 2011
WHO, UNAIDS (2007) WHO and UNAIDS announce recommendations from expert consultation on male circumcision for HIV prevention. WHO press release 28 March 2007. Available at:http://www.who.int/hiv/mediacentre/news68/en/index.html. Accessed 25 June 2011
Williams BG, Lloyd-Smith JO, Gouws E et al (2006) The potential impact of male circumcision on HIV in sub-Saharan Africa. PLoS Med 3:e262

Author Biography

David Gisselquist PhD, received his degree in Economics from Yale University, with experience in anthropology and rural development. He has published more than 20 articles in medical journals on HIV in Africa and India. His history of unsafe health care and HIV, Points to Consider: Responses to HIV/AIDS in Africa, Asia, and the Caribbean, is available from Adonis and Abbey, London, and also for free download on-line at: http://sites.google.com/site/davidgisselquist/pointstoconsider. He has traveled and worked in Africa and Asia, and has assisted field research on HIV in India and Kenya. He co-edited a collection of country studies on injection practices Pilot-Testing the WHO Tools to Assess and Evaluate Injection Practices (Gisselquist and Hutin 2003), and has spoken at WHO and at international AIDS conferences. He is an independent researcher and consultant. Hershey, Pennsylvania, USA.

Chapter 17
Dangerous Myths and Tragic Misconceptions: Fighting HIV and AIDS Cases in Africa with Male Circumcision Strategies

Charles L. Geshekter

Abstract This chapter challenges the claim that African AIDS can be controlled through sexual behavior modification, male circumcision, or drugs. The symptoms that define AIDS cases in Africa (diarrhea, fever, weight loss and dry cough) make its profile decisively different from that in the West. To understand African illness over the past 30 years, the chapter examines the deteriorating political economies instead of scrutinizing peoples' sexual behavior. Field research in Somalia, Kenya, and South Africa and evidence from social sciences and public health are used to defuse African AIDS alarmism. A major portion of the billions of dollars spent "fighting AIDS" should be diverted to poverty relief, job creation, the provision of sanitation and clean drinking water, and aid for drought-stricken farmers, not squandered on male circumcision interventions. The chapter explains why the cure for African AIDS lies in an alternative explanation for what makes Africans sick in the first place.

Keywords HIV/AIDS in Africa • Behavior modification • Male circumcision • Poverty relief • Sanitation • Antibody tests

17.1 Introduction

Scientists and historians are seekers after the truth. As such, their deliberations need to be open to scrutiny and re-evaluation. An editorial in the *New Scientist* in January 2010 reminded scientists that their job was 'to test theories to destruction, which inevitably makes science adversarial at times. Dispute is good; consensus stultifies.' It concluded: 'If occasionally the emperors of the lab have no clothes,

C. L. Geshekter (✉)
Professor Emeritus, California State University, Chico, CA, USA
e-mail: charlesgeshekter@rethinkingaids.com

G. C. Denniston et al. (eds.), *Genital Cutting: Protecting Children from Medical, Cultural, and Religious Infringements*, DOI: 10.1007/978-94-007-6407-1_17,

someone has to say so... Scientists should welcome the outside world into check them out. Their science is useless if no one trusts it.'[1]

The *New Scientist* editorial was directed at climate scientists in the wake of recent controversies surrounding the data about global warming, and urged them to embrace debate rather than retreat from it. But this point could apply equally to the scientific debate about HIV/AIDS in Africa. This chapter provides a summary of my book-in-progress, *The Plague That Wasn't,* which is a critical history of the definition, diagnosis, and explanation for what is widely perceived as the 'AIDS epidemic' currently ravaging the African continent. It provides a context within which to critique recent studies that allege the protective benefits of male circumcision against HIV infection.

Historians recognize that complex issues sometimes solidify into myths that are tenaciously defended against new interpretations. Historical study combines the use of reason, evidence, and imagination to see things as they were and understand why they were that way. In medical history, scholars propose the variables they think caused changes in the health of a population and pinpoint the biological, ecological, and cultural factors that defined a disease over time. In the book, *The Plague That Wasn't,* I employ these methods to raise some important questions about the scientific and social assumptions underlying the discussion of, and policy response to, African AIDS.

My account shows how a set of research habits and medical beliefs were developed in the early 1980s to explain patterns of illness suddenly seen in a very small cohort of highly sexually active, heavy drug-ingesting urban gay men in the West. The explanation that came to be widely used was the 'single pathogen theory of AIDS.' From the start, there were key anomalies in the single pathogen theory, but it was widely accepted across western society. The Reagan Administration in 1984 endorsed the single pathogen theory to quell criticism that it was insensitive to gay men, and the gay community largely embraced the theory because it made AIDS 'everybody's disease,' in opposition to its initial characterization as a 'gay plague.'[2]

The acceptance of the single virus theory downplayed questions about the immuno-suppressive nature of the exchange of old pathogens in highly promiscuous urban gay enclaves, and the elevated levels of ingested toxins in the form of legal and illegal drugs, which featured highly in the party lifestyle of the gay sexual revolution of the 1970s and early 1980s.

---

1 Let the Sunlight In On Climate Change, *New Scientist* (January 30, 2010).

2 For an exposé of the fraud, waste, and abuse in the CDC's misleading campaign in the United States, see Amanda Bennett and Anita Sharpe, "AIDS Fight is Skewed by Federal Campaign Exaggerating Risks," *Wall Street Journal* (May 1, 1996) and David R. Boldt, "Aiding AIDS: The Story of a Media Virus," *Forbes Media Critic* (Fall 1996). The CDC believed that exaggerating the risks to the American people was the only way to enlist widespread support for funds to combat AIDS. Thus, the theme of its public service ad campaign launched in 1987 was, "If I can get AIDS, anyone can." In Australia, the so-called "Grim Reaper Campaign" was designed specifically to instill a new awareness and fear into people, See WHO Publications (2010).

In seeking the origins of AIDS or HIV in Africa, however, researchers readily assumed causal links among migratory labor patterns to urban areas, African sexual activities, and a variety of animal species. Following a novel definition established at the Bangui Conference of October 1985, sponsored jointly by the US Centers for Disease Control and Prevention (CDC) and the World Health Organization (WHO), western AIDS researchers clustered together the widespread clinical symptoms of ill health in impoverished parts of Africa, renamed them 'AIDS,' and proclaimed they were caused by risky heterosexual behavior. This conventional view of AIDS in Africa relied on a behavior modification paradigm that was wedded to an obsession about sexuality; it downplayed the political economy of poverty and disease.

A variety of social factors were soon mixed together. Some researchers claimed that truck drivers and prostitutes triggered the rapid spread of the African AIDS epidemic via migrations and urbanization. Others cited genital lesions, male demands for 'dry sex,' soldiers raping women, and unbridled male sexual desire as the causes. Some western feminist scholars seemed to embrace AIDS activism to promote an agenda that viewed men as the problem behind AIDS, and so changing men, while empowering women to negotiate safe sex, became the solution.[3]

Critical of the infectious viral theory of AIDS, my book explores how the causal equation of HIV = AIDS was born, sustained, and rendered impervious to alternative explanations. In explaining the biology of HIV, *The Plague That Wasn't* provides a synopsis of studies that show HIV tests are nowhere near as accurate as the manufacturers claim and indicates why many scientists remain uncertain as to what the tests really address.[4] The HIV/AIDS orthodoxy permits only one acceptable ideology among those who study this subject. Their refusal to consider alternative views and their open contempt for skepticism is anathema to the scientific method. This book shows that after all the billions of dollars spent on AIDS research, crucial aspects of HIV/AIDS science remain conflicted and misleading. The narrative raises fundamental questions about how AIDS science works in reality, the impropriety of permitting narrowly trained technical experts to set public health policies, and the extent to which journalists failed to scrutinize wrongdoing in their AIDS investigations.

17.2 AIDS in Africa

When it comes to questionable claims about HIV/AIDS, Africa is a fertile field where ludicrous notions abound about interspecies jumps, whether condom-less sex promotes the acquisition of HIV, and assertions that male circumcision protects against HIV transmission from heterosexual women. *The Plague That Wasn't*

---

[3] A valuable but largely ignored exception is Women's Health Interaction (1999).

[4] For a thorough review of HIV-antibody tests that demonstrates their initial approval for blood screening was never meant to serve as the basis to diagnose infection, see Bauer (2010).

reviews the past 30 years of African history, particularly as it relates to AIDS. It demonstrates how a combination of unreliable antibody tests, a clinical symptoms definition applicable to Africa but not to Europe or the United States, computerized models of dire projections set 20 years in the future yet repeatedly proven to be wrong, an obsession with African sexuality patterns, and a behavior modification agenda have done little to improve the health of Africans, let alone explain what was truly making them ill.

An examination of AIDS in Africa raises a number of scientific, medical, and historical questions. What do the initials 'HIV' and 'AIDS' actually mean? Why do they describe one set of symptoms in Africa and another in the West? What does a physician actually 'see' when he or she treats a patient who is then diagnosed with AIDS? In addressing these questions, my book attempts to explain what African AIDS is, the mechanisms that cause it, and how it may be avoided. I also provide an account of the actual recorded causes of morbidity and mortality in Uganda, Zimbabwe, and South Africa over the past 30 years. South Africa is home to the only major head of state, Thabo Mbeki, who seriously questioned the AIDS orthodoxy. A chapter on South Africa analyzes Mbeki's legitimate concerns about HIV/AIDS and debunks what readers will see were groundless accusations about the consequences of his dissidence.

This book's view of 'AIDS' in modern Africa differs sharply from the prevailing HIV/AIDS paradigm. I do not underestimate the anger it may generate. I am not an AIDS activist, physician, nurse, or health practitioner; and by expressing an opinion based on empirical data not congruent with the majority ideology regarding HIV/AIDS, *The Plague That Wasn't* may draw considerable fire. But as an historian, I must address the questions raised above with honesty and detachment. An historically and empirically based alternative paradigm challenges the doomsday predictions as an attempt to manipulate people's emotions through a relentless fear-mongering. The history of African AIDS is, in fact, less complicated and more understandable than are the behavioral, virological, and ideological constructs on which it is based.

This chapter emphasizes the need for accurate data and critical thinking about African AIDS. Billions of dollars have flowed freely to 'fight AIDS' through various initiatives from public and private sources, with little noticeable success. A generation of AIDS researchers has produced numerous investigations trying to demonstrate that AIDS can be transmitted heterosexually. But how closely are the studies read? And after careful review, what do they show? The first cases of AIDS were found in the West, but Africa is cited as the source of the infectious agent that causes AIDS. Confronting a belief system riddled with errors and distortions, I grew outraged watching a continent become saturated with scare stories, bogus statistics, absurd notions about sexuality, inflammatory posters, and assorted sexual imperatives.

With AIDS, there is a kind of reasoning backwards when attempting to explain HIV rates in Africa. If a cohort of people is said to be HIV-positive, then the infectious causes of that HIV—how it was acquired from another person—must be determined. The method of transmission is assumed to be through sexual behavior with someone else. Theories constructed to explain this acquisition dodge the fallibilities of the HIV test itself and ignore how differently its results may be interpreted from one lab or country or manufacturer to another. Instead, an AIDS virus is assumed to exist and be transmissible. Whenever its rates were determined at a certain frequency in an African population cohort, sexual activities were assumed to be the cause, without any empirical data to confirm that claim.

A task of the historian is to use reason, logic, and evidence to combat errors that distort reality or create unfounded fears. This study of African AIDS is rooted in a reconstruction of the political economy of poverty whose attendant public health effects and clinical symptoms grew alarmingly in the early 1980s. Within a few years, long-standing ailments that were the product of African poverty were being blamed on a sexually transmitted virus. With missionary-like zeal, condom manufacturers and AIDS fund-raisers attributed those symptoms to a (non-existent) 'African sexual culture.' In the late 1990s, Rev. Eugene Rivers of Boston launched a crusade to change African sexual practices, an effort reminiscent of Victorian voyeurs who equated black people with sexual promiscuity.

There were several crucial moments in this history of African AIDS. To understand those events, one must describe and analyze them in relation to one another in ways that were not immediately apparent or visible when they co-occurred in the 1980s. These myriad happenings became part of a modern social imagination, the construction of a myth, as AIDS was a key part of general perceptions about Africa and through which the continent has been 'studied' for the past three decades.[5]

One key moment was the political and cultural context in California and the United States, where the initial cases of Kaposi's sarcoma, pneumocystis *carinii* pneumonia, and ravaged immune systems among a tiny cohort of highly promiscuous, young, drug-using gay men were assumed to be caused the by sexual transmission of an infectious agent. The CDC/WHO conference in October 1985 produced an AIDS definition that has remained unchanged (even broadened slightly) as the basis for counting AIDS cases in Africa.

Around this time, events in 1984–1985 mobilized millions of people in Western countries to raise funds to alleviate starvation in Ethiopia, culminating with the Live Aid concert in 1985, an unprecedented fusion of rock music and philanthropy. Jonathan Benthall has analyzed several charitable, philanthropic, and humanitarian relief groups that he considers parts of a para-religious movement committed to a number of non-negotiable principles, developed and safeguarded by an inner core of loyalists whose style Benthall terms 'the skillful use of the technology of enchantment' (Benthall 2010). Using popular culture and the entertainment industry to tap western compassion was a model for raising funds to 'fight AIDS' in Africa, thereby further reinforcing the specious HIV/AIDS 'pandemic' on that continent.

[5] An examination of how this process occurs in the contemporary world is Taylor (2004).

A further key development was the end of the Cold War in 1989–1991 and the demise of the white supremacist regime in South Africa, which quickly brought about an inordinate focus on AIDS in that nation. Led by western AIDS researchers, international funding agencies, and local anti-apartheid activists, the country where a protracted, well-organized struggle against racism had finally ended was quickly transformed into the center of the 'fight against AIDS.'

17.3 Is There an Epidemic of African AIDS?

Is there an AIDS epidemic in Africa? I answer this question with care, precision, and historical examples. If we use the term 'AIDS' to refer in Africa to a patient who presents a series of clinical symptoms—weight loss, chronic diarrhea, prolonged fever, plus persistent cough or a history of herpes zoster—these symptoms have indeed increased in Africa since the 1980s. However, I have manifested some of these symptoms myself while conducting periods of field research in rural areas of Somalia. I did not engage in any sexual activities while in Africa, and when I returned home to California, the symptoms disappeared.

Drawing on empirical data from medical and public health sources, my book argues that those clinical signs of AIDS have far less to do with sexual behavior than with tuberculosis, malaria, protein anemia, improper waste disposal, unsanitary drinking water, malnutrition, and a variety of waterborne infections, all of which were widespread in Africa before 1985. The registration of African AIDS cases overlaps with malnutrition, diarrheal diseases, tuberculosis, and upper respiratory infections. That fact produced huge leaps in the claims of morbidity and mortality attributable to AIDS. In examining the AIDS statistics, I make use of orthodox and conventional research, together with an abundance of interdisciplinary writings of scientists, researchers, and journalists skeptical of the HIV-causes-AIDS orthodoxy. The statistical inconsistencies over AIDS cases in Africa are so staggering that most conventional claims should never be accepted at face value, or, for that matter, never be accepted at all, given the specious character of the HIV/AIDS paradigm.

For example, a recent study from Ghana bluntly admitted, 'In truth, the number of cumulative AIDS cases in the country is unknown and unknowable and the vast majority of those infected do not know that they are' (Oppong et al. 2006). When a small number of Kenyan prostitutes were found to be resistant to HIV despite frequent acts of unprotected sex with HIV-infected men, Dr. Anthony Fauci, director of the National Institute of Allergy and Infectious Diseases, offered this mind-boggling explanation:

> It could be that to maintain protection, people need nearly continual exposure to HIV so that antigens in the virus can constantly boost the immune system. Or perhaps sperm or semen somehow stimulates a relatively short-lived immunologic reaction in the women that protects them (Altman 2000).

Edward Hooper inventively traced the origins of AIDS cases to oral polio vaccines that were accidentally contaminated in the Congo, allegedly with tissues from a primate version of HIV (Hooper 1999). Other AIDS researchers explain HIV prevalence in Africa as the result of unbridled male predatory sexual prowess and women's lack of power to negotiate 'safe sex'.[6]

The most far-fetched speculation about the origins of African AIDS came from biologist Helen Epstein. In reviewing Hooper's book, Epstein imagined that the historical linkages might have proceeded as follows:

> *Perhaps* a hunter or butcher carrying a benign monkey virus gave blood at a blood bank or had an injection. *Perhaps* someone was transfused with his blood, or perhaps the needle used to inject him was used to inject someone else without being sterilized. *Perhaps*, a few weeks later, the virus was transferred to a third person through another injection or transfusion. This *might* have been enough to 'kick-start' the virus. It *might* have evolved through such 'passaging' to become able to grow vigorously in human cells. It *might* have been able to infect new people through means other than needles or blood transfusions. It *might* have become sexually transmitted, and it *might* have become deadly.[7] (Emphasis added).

The AIDS mainstream insists that changing sexual behavior is the key to stopping AIDS. My book scrutinizes those assumptions to show why African behavior modification projects have been spectacular failures. For instance, the Summertown HIV-Prevention Project was an initiative that lasted three years in an impoverished South African township. It was described as a 'mixed bag of disappointments and achievements…[as] many proposed activities [were] yet to be implemented, consistent and widespread condom use remains low… and the most damning lack of Project success over the three-year-research period is the lack of evidence for any reduction in STI [sexually transmitted infection] levels' (Campbell 2003). The tangled analysis by the project's director, Catherine Campbell, used such impenetrable prose that one is not surprised to learn that the project had no effect on sexual behavior, HIV rates, or AIDS cases. As Campbell concludes:

> In the interests of contributing to the development of a critical social psychology of sexuality, the research has illustrated the way in which sexual behavior, and the possibility of sexual behavior change, are determined by an interlocking series of multi-level processes, which are often not under the control of an individual person's rational conscious choice. Sexualities are constructed and reconstructed at the intersection of a kaleidoscopic array of interlocking multi-level processes, ranging from the intra-psychological to the macro-social.[8]

---

[6] An especially breezy account is Pisani (2008).

[7] Epstein (1999). Eight years later, Epstein (2007) barely altered her bizarre and circuitous reasoning in a book.

[8] *Ibid.*, p. 183. Despite the stunning failures of the Project, one reviewer, who happened to be the Series Editor for its publisher, called it "the best book yet written on the struggle to control HIV." De Waal (2004).

Like similar initiatives elsewhere in Africa, the researchers with the Summertown Project believed that sexual behavior changes would make Africans healthy and enable them to stay well. They did not imagine that their project failed because its core construct was erroneous and incapable of correction. They never considered that the production of HIV antibodies might be environmentally induced and had little to do with sexuality. Their well-meaning interventions and complex proposals were wholly inadequate for the task of sexual behavior modification. *The Plague That Wasn't* dissects the Summertown Project as an object lesson in how not to proceed with AIDS education and awareness.

A comparative study by anthropologist Robert Thornton of the University of Witwatersrand argues that merely accruing information about AIDS can make people anxious. According to Thornton, 'One of my students in Johannesburg, Zodwa Radebe, who has worked in AIDS research and prevention, once remarked to me, "The more I learn about HIV and the more people I work with who are HIV-positive, the less I seem to know; the more my understanding is shaken."' This led Thornton to muse that 'knowledge of AIDS is like knowledge of sex… it is anxious knowledge' (Thornton 2008).

Overall, the data used to create an HIV-is-everywhere in Africa imagery are either flawed or inaccurate, or involve small unrepresentative samples. I stress the unresolved scientific problems that bedevil the reliability of claims made about HIV and HIV tests within its critical review of mainstream African AIDS research.

17.4 Sex, Statistics, and Male Circumcision Assumptions

How do we account for historical changes in African mortality and morbidity? In tackling this question, I compare the state of African political economies in the first two decades of post-colonial independence (1957–1980) with what has happened to them since the early 1980s. In the 1960s, Africa was a net *exporter* of food. In 2008, the continent *imported* 24 % of its food as hunger and famine became recurrent phenomena with severe emergencies in southern and central Africa, the Sahel, and the Horn. The structural adjustment fiscal policies of the 1980s that coincided with the onset of the 'age of AIDS' were what caused decreased agrarian investments, rising unemployment, reduced social spending, diminished agricultural credits, and lower crop yields. Africa was at a crucial turning point in its post-colonial history precisely when westerners began investigating AIDS and sought its putative origins in Africa.

According to Oxfam, the number of sub-Saharan Africans living on less than $1 a day nearly doubled from 160 to 311 million between 1981 and 2001–2005. In Central Africa today, 55 % of its people are undernourished (Mayne 2006). As Paul Nugent writes:

> By the start of the 1980s, virtually every African country was manifesting signs of acute economic distress, reflected in a mounting and unsustainable debt burden, a permanent trade deficit and an acute fiscal crisis, which meant that the state was unable to maintain basic infrastructure or fund essential social services (Nugent 2004).

The effects of structural adjustment policies in deepening poverty are undeniable: human costs were grave, economic gains slow in coming, and the decline of quality of life in Africa was palpable. This is an equally plausible explanation for the level of ill-health across the continent today than HIV rates. But, I contend, recognizing such complex problems would demand complex social and economic solutions; whereas the focus on AIDS lends itself to a narrow preoccupation with individuals' behavior and the proposal of immediate, technical solutions that are easier to deliver and to measure.

The western obsession with African bodies, sexuality, and behavior patterns has led AIDS researchers to focus on how semen can kill, why the foreskin must be removed, or the dangers that lurk in mother's milk. They believe that the problems of hunger, poverty, and illness in Africa have technical solutions—wear condoms, practice abstinence, circumcise males, ingest pills, don't breastfeed. The AIDS orthodoxy resorts to a reactionary set of claims that harkens back to the Victorian era with its obsessions about sexual restraint.[9] These claims are cloaked in scientific language, which appear to add credibility: until the science is examined.

For example, the lead editorial from the October 3, 2009 issue of *The Lancet* stated:

> 'Breakthrough,' 'landmark,' 'an important day for the planet.' Such were some of the reactions to the news released on September 24th that, for the first time, an HIV vaccine has shown a modest degree of efficacy in a phase 3 clinical trial… [In 1984, Margaret Heckler declared that a vaccine would be available within 2 years.] A quarter of a century on, it seems as though the journey is only now just beginning. The development of an effective and practical HIV vaccine will take *more* basic research, *more* collaboration, *more* money, and *more* trust and goodwill from *more* volunteers. But the latest findings present a tantalizing hope that such efforts could one day pay off.[10]

What did this unprecedented trial actually find? Leaving aside the flaws, inconsistencies, and disclaimers about HIV tests, the results found that, in the intervention group of Thai volunteers, 8197 received vaccines over the three-year period, at the end of which 51 (six-tenths of one percent) were HIV+. In the control group, 8198 received placebos over the same period, at the end of which 74 (nine-tenths of one percent) were HIV+. This is an absolute difference of 0.3 % (three-tenths of one percent).

However, the relative reduction—the difference between 51 and 74—cynically became a 31 % reduction, widely touted by the media. Thus, on October 20, 2009, an Associated Press medical writer, Marilynn Marchione, claimed that 'researchers announced that a two-vaccine combination cut the risk of becoming infected with HIV by more than 31 % in a trial of more than 16,000 volunteers in Thailand' (Marchione 2009).

---

[9] A fine example is Adams and Pigg (2005).

[10] "A (Prime) Boost for HIV Vaccine Research?" *The Lancet* (vol. 374, October 3, 2009), p. 1119.

A similar distortion of statistics is present in investigations regarding male circumcision and alleged HIV protection in Africa. The first two randomized trials were based in Uganda and Kenya. The research results were reported in *The Lancet* in February 2007. According to the researchers, their studies showed that the circumcision of heterosexual men could reduce their risk of HIV infection by 50–60 % (Gray et al. 2007; Bailey et al. 2007). The results of the Ugandan and Kenyan trials were released to the media to coincide with World AIDS Day (December 1, 2006), two months *before* the studies were published in the journal. As one journalist wryly observed:

> This unusual move produced worldwide publicity that was heavy on eye-catching headlines and light on details, because–in the absence of the published studies themselves–few journalists took the time to dig beyond the press releases made available to them (Fauntleroy 2008).

It is necessary to look closely at the data to see how the HIV/AIDS researchers arrived at their conclusions. In Uganda, researchers started with 4,996 men and randomly divided them into two groups, medically circumcising one group (2,474 men) and leaving the other group intact (2,522 men). After 24 months, both groups were tested for HIV infection. Of the circumcised men, 22 tested positive, while 45 in the uncircumcised group tested positive. In other words, 67 out of 4996 (or 1.3 %) were HIV+ while the remaining 98.7 % remained HIV–. Yet researchers simply derived the 50 % 'risk prevention' figure from the difference in results between the two groups, i.e., the difference between 22 and 45. Hence, male circumcision was said to reduce heterosexual male acquisition of HIV from heterosexual women by 50 %.

The Kenyan trials began with 2,784 men and randomly divided them, with 1,391 undergoing circumcision and 1,391 left intact. Two years later, testing showed 22 new infections among the circumcised men and 47 among those left intact. Astonishingly, neither team of researchers ever attempted to determine the HIV status of any of the men's female partners, a glaring omission that effectively negated whatever statistical significance their findings were alleged to show.

The extremely small numbers of new infections in each group raise questions about extrapolating them to such larger populations as the African continent or the entire world. In the Ugandan trial, a mere 0.8 % of the circumcised men tested positive after two years, while 1.7 % of the uncircumcised men tested positive. Likewise, in Kenya, the claim of a 50–60 % rate of risk reduction was based on 1.5 % of circumcised men becoming infected, compared with 3.3 % of those left intact. In the Kenyan study, 2.4 % of all men tested HIV+, while 97.6 % remained HIV–. Furthermore, these were microscopically small studies.

Throughout the research history of AIDS in Africa, comparable figures typically became 'mutant statistics,' which took on a life of their own and enjoyed a remarkably long shelf life. The more they were repeated, the longer the shelf life. This is very important because policy decisions affecting millions of lives are based on sensational figures that did not reflect the realities on the ground. Any scientist who has respect for data and empirical verification should be well aware of this basic fact.

However, such is the power of the HIV/AIDS orthodoxy that even scientific studies that confound the original hypothesis are presented as supporting orthodox conclusions. A 2009 study from Uganda sought to determine any association between male circumcision and reduced risk of HIV infection among heterosexual female partners (Wawer et al. 2009). None was found. The investigators identified 922 uncircumcised HIV+ males, aged 15–49, who were asymptomatic for AIDS and had CD4 cell counts above 350. In the intervention group, 474 men were immediately circumcised. In the control group, 448 men were delayed circumcision for 24 months.

The researchers randomly selected 92 HIV− women who were sexual partners of men in the intervention group (92 couples). Of those 92 women, after 24 months, 17 (18 %) tested HIV+. The investigators randomly selected 67 HIV− women who were sexual partners of men in the control group (67 couples). Of those 67 women, only 8 (12 %) tested HIV+. In other words, a higher percentage of the female sexual partners of the circumcised males later tested HIV+.

The researchers conceded that 'the trial was stopped early because of futility [since] circumcision of HIV-infected men did not reduce transmission to female partners over 24 months.'[11] The research team found that consistent condom use was actually higher in the intervention group (50 %), where they found more seroconversions to HIV than in the uncircumcised control group (36 %).[12]

Yet, despite these findings, the investigators were so wedded to the orthodoxy that they reflexively concluded: 'condom use after male circumcision is essential for HIV prevention'.[13] They were concerned that 'circumcised HIV-uninfected men might use their circumcised status to negotiate unsafe sex'.[14] How would the Ugandan researchers reply if someone asked them to speculate on what the dialogue might sound like in the 'negotiations' for sex between the circumcised male and his unwitting female partner? This study is another example of how conventional HIV/AIDS researchers reduce African sexuality to lust and exoticism.[15]

17.5 AIDS and Medical History

As Charles Rosenberg writes in his study of the history of American medicine, in the modern era, the bureaucratic need 'for numbers that legitimate and trigger a sequence of additional diagnostic, therapeutic, and administrative actions [may]

[11] *Ibid.*, p. 229.

[12] *Ibid.*, p. 236.

[13] *Ibid.*, p. 229.

[14] *Ibid.*, p. 235.

[15] For a general overview, see Keim (1999); an important critique of the racism of conventional African AIDS research is Stillwaggon (2006).

obscure the very construction of those numbers.' He continues: 'The fact that such numbers are routinely generated by seemingly objective, highly technical tools and procedures works to endorse their plausibility and meaningfulness… [but] creates a reciprocal social rigidity as numbers become the measure and legitimation of presumed things' (Rosenberg 2007). This predicament describes what mainstream HIV/AIDS researchers assume they are counting when it comes to HIV or AIDS in Africa.[16]

The investigations discussed above are among the many examples of statistical manipulation and dubious claims that are reassessed in *The Plague That Wasn't*, as part of a broad-ranging critique of the entire African AIDS orthodoxy. Unless we are prepared to challenge some of the deep-seated assumptions about AIDS in Africa, we will remain blind to what scientific evidence and historical enquiry can tell us about what is really making Africans sick, and what interventions could possibly make things better.

References

Adams V, Pigg SL (eds) (2005) Sex in development: science, sexuality and morality in global perspective. Duke University Press, Durham

Altman L (2000) A new AIDS mystery: prostitutes who have remained immune. New York Times 2(3):A17 (3 Feb 2000)

Bailey RC et al (2007) Male circumcision for HIV prevention in young men in Kisumu, Kenya: a randomized controlled trial. The lancet (vol 369, Feb 24, 2007), pp 643–656

Bauer HH (2010) HIV tests are not HIV tests. J Am Physicians Surg 15(1):5–9

Benthall J (2010) Returning to religion: why a secular age is haunted by faith. Taurus, London

Campbell C (2003) Letting them die: why HIV/AIDS prevention programmes fail. James Currey, Oxford, p 185

De Waal A (2004) Sex in summertown. Times literary supplement, 6(5)

Epstein H (1999) Something happened. NY rev books 2:18

Epstein H (2007) The invisible cure: Africa, the West, and the fight against AIDS. Farrar Straus and Giroux, New York, pp 46–47

Fauntleroy G (2008) The truth about circumcision and HIV. Mothering magazine, US, p 45

Gray RH et al (2007) Male circumcision for HIV prevention in men in Rakai, Uganda: a randomized trial. Lancet 369:657–666

Hooper E (1999) The river: a journey to the source of HIV and AIDS. Little Brown Publishers, Boston

Keim C (1999) Mistaking Africa: curiosities and inventions of the American mind, Westview Press, Boulder

Marchione M (2009) New results show experimental AIDS vaccine only marginally effective. Enterprise-record, Chico (Calif.)

[16] The World Health Organization has defined health as "a stage of complete physical, social and mental well being and not merely the absence of disease or infirmity," a definition that psychiatrist Seamus Sweeney termed "a statement of awesome fatuity which renders health unattainable in this world." Seamus Sweeney, "Incredible Promises," *Times Literary Supplement* (June 20, 2008), p. 15.

Mayne R (2006) Causing hunger: an overview of the food crisis in Africa. Oxfam briefing paper 91:1
Nugent P (2004) Africa since independence: a comparative history. Palgrave Macmillan, New York, p 326
Oppong C, Oppong MYPA, Odotei IK (eds) (2006) Sex and gender in an era of AIDS: Ghana at the turn of the millennium. Sub-Saharan, Accra, p 304
Pisani E (2008) The wisdom of whores: bureaucrats brothels and the business of AIDS. W.W. Norton, New York
Rosenberg C (2007) Our present complaint: American medicine, then and now. Johns Hopkins University Press, Baltimore, p 26
Stillwaggon E (2006) Racial metaphors: interpreting sex and AIDS in Africa. In: Stillwaggon E (ed) AIDS and the ecology of poverty. Oxford University Press, New York
Taylor C (2004) Modern social imaginaries. Duke University Press, Durham
Thornton R (2008) Unimagined community sex, networks and AIDS in Uganda and South Africa. University of California Press, Berkeley, p 222
Wawer MJ et al (2009) Circumcision in HIV-infected men and its effect on HIV transmission to female partners in Rakai, Uganda: a randomized controlled trial. Lancet 374:229–237
Women's Health Interaction (1999) Uncommon questions: a feminist exploration of AIDS. Ottawa
World Health Organization (2010) Public health campaigns: getting the message across. WHO, Geneva

Author Biography

Charles Geshekter PhD, Professor Emeritus of African history at California State University, Chico, earned his PhD in History from UCLA and received numerous grants for his African field research. His writings examine modern Somali history, techniques of documentary film making, and reappraising AIDS in Africa. Geshekter established the Somali Studies International Association and coordinated its first conference in Mogadishu (1980). In 1985, he produced a PBS documentary, "The Parching Winds of Somalia" for WQED-TV. During the UN intervention in Somalia (1992–95), Geshekter was news analyst for CBS National Radio Network, KRON-TV/San Francisco, and PBS. Geshekter coordinated the program for the 1989 Meeting of the American Association for Advancement of Science/Pacific Division. From 1991–95, he chaired its History of Science Section and served on its Executive Council. In 1995–96, he was Chief Policy Advisor on Education Finance for the California State Assembly, he has served as a consultant and researcher on African immigration issues for the Department of Justice, and he was a member of the South African Presidential AIDS Advisory Panel (2000–03).
Chico, California, USA.

Chapter 18
Defying the Enlightenment: Jewish Ethnicity and Ethnic Circumcision

Leonard B. Glick

Abstract For much of their history, European Jews viewed religion and ethnic identity as inseparable; social behavior, not belief, mattered, and conformity was essential. The Enlightenment introduced rationalism, individualism, and modernity into Western Europe—all incompatible with an ethnically segregated lifestyle. Many European Jews adopted Enlightenment principles and became at least partly assimilated. But even those who abandoned most ritual practices continued circumcising male infants as an *ethnic* tradition. Two partly opposed doctrines became prominent in twentieth-century thought: *cultural relativism*, teaching that all cultural traditions merit equal acceptance and respect; and (an essentially contrary argument) that *human rights* apply to *individuals,* not to traditions. Some defenders of ethnic circumcision use doctrinaire cultural relativism to reject the human rights argument. With this as background, I discuss contemporary Jewish-American circumcision advocacy. A key question: Since few Jewish Americans now observe the more demanding ritual practices, why the insistence on retaining infant circumcision?

Keywords Jews • Religion • Ethnic identity • Individualism • Tradition • Cultural relativism • Human rights • Circumcision

18.1 Introduction: A Puzzling People

Among the many singular images of Jews in the public imagination is that they exemplify both sides of contrasting characteristics: wealthy capitalists and radical socialists, passive European victims and fierce Israeli warriors, dedicated liberals and resolute neoconservatives. Equally confusing, they seem to be among the most prominent representatives of the modern ("cosmopolitan") spirit, yet they still hold to premodern cultural practices: food taboos associated with kosher

L. B. Glick (✉)
Professor Emeritus of Anthropology, Hampshire College, Amherst, Massachusetts, USA
e-mail: quabbin@rcn.com

G. C. Denniston et al. (eds.), *Genital Cutting: Protecting Children from Medical, Cultural, and Religious Infringements*, DOI: 10.1007/978-94-007-6407-1_18,

regulations, special methods of animal slaughter, resistance to intermarriage (now admittedly fading)—and, most puzzling of all, circumcision of infants on the eighth day of life.[1]

18.2 Jewish Ethnicity Encounters the Enlightenment

Why do non-religious or fully secular Jews (the largest segment of the Jewish-American population) persist in preserving this anachronistic custom? Answering the question must begin with historical perspective on the European Jews who were ancestral to most contemporary Jewish Americans. Their way of life did more than is ordinarily recognized to shape the minds and social attitudes of their contemporary New World descendants. Above all, European Jews, particularly but not only in Eastern Europe, knew that they were a people apart: that they had been born into a world completely dominated by "Gentiles" who neither understood their way of life nor, for the most part, even thought of them as genuine neighbors. Most European Jews lived in collective, corporate communities that were essentially closed; local rabbis and other prominent men held political and legal authority, and meaningful social life took place solely within the local Jewish environment. Aside from a very few men who enjoyed privileged status in the Gentile world, for most Jews prospects for life outside the local group were minimal or nonexistent. They formed in every sense a separate and distinct social world, linked by unbreakable bonds of kinship, culture, and dependence on one another, and sustained by conviction that the Lord had designated them for a unique role and specific burdens and obligations. In that context, asking whether particular ritual practices were acceptable or not was out of the question; one was a Jew, and one acted accordingly.

Traditional Jewish society was rooted in what I shall call (without judgmental intent) *ethnic fundamentalism*—with emphasis on "ethnic" rather than "religious," because its definitive characteristics were social, political, and economic; its religious rituals symbolized the community's distinctive identity and difference from others. In Christian societies, religious identity was (and is) distinct from ethnicity or nationality; in fact, in medieval and early modern times most of Europe was described as *Christianitas*, the Christian world. The Jewish concept of personal identity differed completely. In the Jewish world *religion* and *ethnic identity* were one and the same; what mattered was not belief but *behavior* that conformed to community standards and expectations. The only alternative form of identity was to become a convert to Christianity (a rare and radical act that could sever a person forever from home and family).

[1] Although I'll refer specifically to Jewish Americans, all statements refer equally to Jewish Canadians.

The pivotal development in modern European history was the emergence in the eighteenth century of an intellectual transformation now known as the Enlightenment. As used (and debated) by historians, the term refers to a set of related ideas and principles, culminating in the American and French Revolutions, that heralded the onset of what we understand as "modernity." The term is associated with the pioneering publications of the seventeenth-century philosopher Benedict Spinoza and those of such widely recognized philosophers as Voltaire, Diderot, and Rousseau. The key principle of Enlightenment thought was *reason*, or rationalism; enlightenment meant accepting scientific knowledge over religious dogma, natural causation over supernaturalism. It meant also rejection of authority rooted in claims to elite status, and assertion of the *rights of individuals* as the foundation of a just society. What constituted those individual rights—how they were to be defined, whether they could be limited by the collective rights of culturally or ethnically defined groups—provided, and still provides, material for a seemingly endless debate that I'll epitomize here as *human rights* versus *cultural relativism*.

In accord with a key tenet of the Enlightenment, the foundational principle of the French Revolution was that henceforth all rights would adhere to *individuals*, not to members of particular socioeconomic classes, hereditary elites, religious orders, or any other social or cultural category. But we should note that despite the avowedly secular nature of its leaders, this truly revolutionary way of conceiving and organizing social relations was rooted in Christian beliefs about individual souls and their personal salvation—a way of thinking about the relation between individuals and their society fundamentally in contrast with the collective, communal emphasis of Judaism.[2]

For the designers of the new state, France's small Jewish communities stood out as uniquely problematic: Could they ever be fully assimilated into the new nation? Would they ever become truly French? In December 1789, the French National Assembly came around to debating the essential political issue: Could or should Jews be eligible for French citizenship, with the same rights and responsibilities as other citizens? That was no small consideration, since being a "citizen" meant that one belonged wholly to the nation, that one's sole identity was "French." Could Jews, notorious for their attachment to their alien ethnic identity, be accepted without substantial accommodation on their part? If not, how could they be citizens on equal footing with everyone else?

[2] A personal anecdote may help to emphasize this point. I once invited a group of young Christian missionaries to speak to my class on anthropology of religion. When the class ended, they dispersed among the students, trying to win converts on the spot. One young man came over to me and spoke earnestly about my salvation. When he sensed that the conversation was going in the wrong direction, he asked what I thought would happen when I died. Without really thinking, I replied, "There will be one more dead Jew." He was taken aback and abandoned the effort. I had responded, of course, with characteristic Jewish focus on community, while he was thinking of me as an individual needing personal salvation.

On December 23, the Count of Clermont-Tonnerre delivered a definitive conclusion to the debate. No compromise was possible: "The Jews should be denied everything as a nation," he declared, "but granted everything as individuals."

> They must be citizens.... There cannot be one nation within another nation.... It is intolerable that the Jews should become a separate political formation or class in the country. Every one of them must individually become a citizen; if they do not want this, they must inform us and we shall be compelled to expel them. The existence of a nation within a nation is unacceptable to our country.[3]

Leaders of the Jewish community, clearly understanding the significance of the challenge, opted firmly for complete integration, assuring the authorities that the Jews of France were prepared to accept all the duties and responsibilities of loyal citizens.

As I mentioned, the ideas and principles associated with the Enlightenment were the foundation for what we now call modernity—and if modernity can be said to have a single definitive feature, it is *individualism*. Individualism (not to be confused with selfishness or egocentrism) implies respect for the integrity and independence of individual persons, and recognition of each person's right to determine the course and direction of his or her life. In countries where public commitment to "enlightenment" and modernity took hold in the nineteenth-century—particularly France, Germany, England and other Anglophone nations, including the United States—Jewish society and social status were radically transformed. Like all other individuals in their countries of residence, Jews were now free to decide on their degree of personal Jewish identification, communal involvement, and ritual observance. For example, a Jewish man living in mid-nineteenth-century America would probably have been recognized as such (by name and occupation), but he was essentially free to ignore ritual requirements of traditional Judaism, to live apart from other Jews, even to intermarry. And over time many Jews came to be identified by others as the quintessential modern people: urbanized, cosmopolitan.[4]

Nonetheless, most Jews continued to practice infant circumcision as a sign of their ethnic "covenant" with the God of *Genesis*. The contradiction was obvious: Were they wholly committed citizens of their nation—modern, enlightened, liberated—or did they still believe in their divinely created special status? That contradiction was never truly resolved, either in France or in Germany, where it became even more of an issue during the nineteenth century. Many German Jews adopted a modernized form of Judaism, called "Reform," which modified or abandoned some of the more demanding (and self-segregating) ritual requirements, particularly food

[3] "The French National Assembly: Debate on the Eligibility of Jews for Citizenship," in Mendes-Flohr and Reiharz (1995); here, p 115.

[4] One recent author, claiming that the "Modern Age" is the "Jewish Age," defines "modernization" as "everyone becoming urban, mobile, literate, articulate, intellectually intricate, physically fastidious, and occupationally flexible." In other words, he concludes, modernization "is about everyone becoming Jewish." Slezkine (2004).

taboos, and emphasized unqualified loyalty to the German homeland. But even most Reform Jews, seemingly defying logic, maintained that the foreskins of their male infants had to be removed.[5]

To understand why so many European Jews insisted on preserving this one practice, we need to examine two ideas associated with modernity that are often cited to defend opposing positions on circumcision.

18.3 Responding to Cultural Difference: Relativism and Rights

Early twentieth-century anthropology—the anthropology of Franz Boas, Ruth Benedict, and Margaret Mead—was predicated on the principle of *cultural relativism*: that every society merits respect and acceptance as an autonomous way of life with its own culture and its own traditions. An influential textbook, published in 1948 by Melville Herskovits, explained the term and the argument: "With the possible exception of technological aspects of life," he declared, "the proposition that one way of thought or action is better than another is exceedingly difficult to establish on the grounds of any universally acceptable criteria.... The very core of cultural relativism is the social discipline that comes of respect for differences—of mutual respect. Emphasis on the worth of many ways of life, not one, is an affirmation of the values of each culture. Such emphasis seeks to understand, and to harmonize goals, not to judge and destroy those that do not dovetail with our own."[6]

But although on first consideration cultural relativism seems to be unexceptionable as an affirmation of respect for difference, it has generated an immense amount of controversy: How far can or should we go in condoning practices that appear unacceptable, even disgusting, and that seem to involve onerous restrictions or outright harm to individuals? I use the term *categorical cultural relativism* for those who unequivocally condone all alien cultural practices. Categorical cultural relativists maintain that whether or not we personally approve of the values and practices of culturally distant others, our role must be limited to objectively phrased description, explanation, and implicit acceptance. Often the watchword is "tolerance," but even that must never imply an attitude of superiority to other ways

[5] I discuss this history in some detail in *Marked in Your Flesh: Circumcision from Ancient Judea to Modern America.* New York: Oxford University Press, 2005, Chap. 5; and more concisely in "Jewish Circumcision: An Enigma in Historical Perspective," in Denniston et al. (2001). See also Judd (2007) Chaps. 1–3.

[6] Herskovits (1948). Both Boas and Herskovits were Jewish. On Boas's attitude to Jewish ethnicity see my article, "Types Distinct from Our Own: Franz Boas on Jewish Identity and Assimilation," *American Anthropologist,* Vol. 84, 1982, pp. 545–65; reprinted in Regna Darnell, ed., *American Anthropology, 1971–1995*. Lincoln and London: University of Nebraska Press, 2002, pp. 341–72. See also Herskovits (1960).

of life. Carrying this to its logical conclusion, categorical cultural relativists accept such practices as child labor (even to the point of virtual enslavement), enforced seclusion of women, denial of education to girls, widow burning, and honor killings. As this list shows, many such practices concern powerless members of society, particularly women and children. The persuasive character of arguments rooted in categorical cultural relativism offers some perspective on the mentality of those who support ritualized genital cutting of male and female children.[7]

Categorical cultural relativism is inherently supportive of ethnic fundamentalism—and the associated conviction that loyalty to an ethnically defined group and its collective rights overrides all other considerations. Many ethnic fundamentalists of various stripes will be the first to acknowledge that they reject the foundational principles of the social and political revolution that began with the eighteenth-century Enlightenment. They interpret individualism as a pernicious philosophy, antithetical to stability at every social level from family to national polity, maintaining instead that members of traditional ethnic groups must respect principles of belief and behavior that have been transmitted across time, even when adherence might require some sacrifice of personal freedom and independence.

In obvious opposition to categorical cultural relativists are those who believe that universal human rights transcend particular cultural traditions. People on this side of the divide believe that rights adhere not to individual cultures, ethnic groups, or religious communities but to *individual persons*. They insist that rights to personal autonomy and self-determination trump all considerations of what members of a particular society may consider desirable, or even essential, for promoting or preserving cultural traditions.

So one side we find cultural relativists, who focus on *communities,* arguing that individuals are always situated within social groups and inevitably find their identities within those groups; hence, that culturally constituted traditions, beliefs, and practices cannot be abandoned in the service of individual autonomy. And on the other we find those who insist that, while all cultures and religions do indeed deserve respect, in the final analysis they must take second place to the right of *individuals* to personal autonomy and freedom from oppression or exploitation, no matter how sacred or time-honored a traditional practice may be.

The conviction that rights belong exclusively to individual persons became a central tenet of the "human rights" movement of the twentieth century. Calls for

[7] Violations of male human rights usually involve atrocities (torture, slavery, massacre, etc.) that even the most confirmed relativists do not defend. But lest I seem to be misrepresenting categorical cultural relativism, see publications by the prominent University of Chicago anthropologist Richard A. Shweder, who finds nothing objectionable in male or female genital cutting, nor in rigorous seclusion of women in India enforced by beating of offenders. Commenting on human rights, he asks, "To whom shall 'rights' be granted? To male adults? To women? To children? To dogs? To the insane? To the elderly? To a fetus? To a sperm?" Shweder (1984). For his view of female genital cutting, see "What About Female Genital Mutilation? and Why Understanding Culture Matters in the First Place," in Shweder et al. (2002). I should acknowledge that many defenders of human rights are equally categorical.

human rights in particular situations always signified the rights of individuals to personal expression, freedom from coercion, release from exploitation, and so on.[8] Although modern societies vary somewhat in how they define human rights, it would probably be agreed that, in addition to obvious needs for adequate food, shelter, and medical care, basic rights include freedom from intentional harm or interference with one's physical and mental integrity. This means that a society cannot be called wholly modern unless it has legally encoded provisions and sanctions to protect its citizens from all forms of intentional harm, including torture, mutilation, rape, enslavement, political imprisonment, arbitrary discrimination, and other forms of oppression. It follows that modern societies are generally tolerant of diverse ethnic, religious, and cultural communities, *provided their actions do not threaten or diminish the individual rights of any persons.*

With this much as background, we are better prepared to think about why so many Jewish-American parents seem to cling to male infant circumcision as virtually their last remaining link to distinctive ethnic identity.

---

[8] The literature on human rights in relation to cultural relativism and collective rights is immense. Most publications focus on non-Western peoples, women, peasants, and indigenous ("tribal") groups. References to children's rights usually deal with child labor and/or female genital cutting. For some sense of the size and complexity of the literature on this subject, see Eva Brems, *Human Rights: Universality and Diversity*. The Hague and Boston: Martinus Nijhoff, 2001. Of the book's 574 pages (of rather turgid prose), 43 pages are devoted to bibliography (by no means complete). Although there is an index listing for "Female genital mutilation," I find not even a sentence on male circumcision. A few references most relevant for tensions between individual human rights and cultural relativism are the following: Howard (1992); Renteln (1988, 1994); Donnelly (1990); Adamantia Polis and Peter Schwab, "Human Rights: A Western Construct with Limited Applicability," in A. Polis and P. Schwab, eds., *Human Rights: Cultural and Ideological Perspectives*. New York: Praeger, 1980. It seems a safe generalization that male genital cutting is rarely if ever discussed by human rights scholars (most of whom are political scientists, lawyers, and anthropologists). Thus, despite the suggestive title, I found nothing on male circumcision in a book co-edited by an Israeli and including several articles on Israel: Gillian Douglas and Leslie Sebba, eds., *Children's Rights and Traditional Values*. Aldershot, Eng. and Brookfield, VT: Ashgate Publishing, 1998. The only references to male circumcision appear to be publications by scholars largely outside the mainstream of human rights discourse and concerned specifically with this topic. Notable in this small cohort are the following: Fox and Thomson (2005, 2009); Hodges et al. (2002); Svoboda et al. (2000); *Doctors Opposing Circumcision: Genital Integrity Policy Statement*, Chap. 9: "International Human Rights Law and the Circumcision of Children," available at www.doctorsopposingcircumcision.org. A widely publicized and debated defense of "parental discretion" in male circumcision is Benatar and Benatar (2003); multiple commentaries follow, pp. 49–66; and response by the authors is available at www.bioethics.net/journal/correspondence for the same issue of the journal. For a defense of parental rights by an Oxford University philosopher, see Viens (2004). A book on "ethical universals" by a bioethicist at Albert Einstein College of Medicine discusses female genital cutting (here called "female genital mutilation") extensively but never mentions male circumcision: Macklin (1999). Macklin says, "What I intend to show is that some things are relative, others are not. A convincing argument against ethical relativism need not conclude that nothing is relative, only that certain types of actions or practices—chiefly those that violate human rights—are not" (p. 24). She implicitly concludes that female genital cutting is a human rights violation but male circumcision is not. A summary of Macklin's published debate with Robert Baker is available in Svoboda and Darby (2008); here pp. 289–90.

18.4 Defying the Enlightenment: Jewish Americans and Ethnic Circumcision

Today few Jews in modern nations engage in much traditional ritual behavior. Some identify as "secular Jews," meaning that they accept Jewish ethnic identity but reject all elements of Jewish practice originating in biblical precepts or explained as divine commands. Nevertheless, as we know, the one practice that most Jews, secular and religious, *have* retained is male infant circumcision. Despite all evidence to the contrary, many Americans still think of circumcision as a peculiarly Jewish practice, and many, perhaps most, Jewish Americans share that misperception (which may reinforce their inclination to hold on to the practice). But whereas most Americans can ignore the circumcision controversy as irrelevant to their personal lives, Jewish Americans are forced to confront the issue, more often and more intimately, as parents and community members. The result has been that defensive literature on the subject, whether defending Jewish circumcision or *all* circumcision, has been disproportionately written (and probably read) by Jews. Sometimes the defense is phrased in explicitly religious terms harking back to ancient rabbinic times: circumcision is the inalienable possession of the Jewish people, the eternal sign of the covenant with Abraham, a tradition that must be preserved if the Jewish people are to survive. Other, more contemporary defenses offer a variety of pop-psychological, medical, or vaguely mystical explanations and rationalizations, nearly all avoiding or dismissing the unpleasant physical reality of the procedure in favor of claims for what it accomplishes socially—or, as it were, ethnically.

Thus it is that opposition to circumcision in America often runs up against strong Jewish objections, on the grounds that what's really at stake is the right of Jewish Americans to preserve their own ethnic heritage. This is an especially effective argument at a time when "multiculturalism" is fashionable (in public discourse if not in private behavior), and liberals of all kinds incline toward relativism as the proper attitude toward alien religious and cultural practices.

I use the term "ethnic circumcision" to emphasize the fact that most Jewish circumcisions, whether conducted ritually or performed non-religiously in hospitals, are motivated heavily or primarily by conviction that the practice must be continued if Jewish-American ethnic identity is to survive. Probably the most widely read expression of this argument appears in the closing pages of Philip Roth's novel, *The Counterlife*. Nathan Zuckerman (Roth's alter-ego) is a Jewish agnostic married to an upper-class Englishwoman who can no longer tolerate his seemingly endless preoccupation with his Jewish identity. Nathan intends to demand "that the child, if a boy, shall make his covenant with Yahweh through the ritual sacrifice of his foreskin." Circumcision may be a "barbaric mutilation," as his wife claims; he may be "irrationally Jewish," and the surgery may be the ultimate in "human irrationality." This he knows as well as she:

> Circumcision is startling, all right, particularly when performed by a garlicked old man upon the glory of a newborn body, but then maybe that's what the Jews had in mind and what makes the act seem quintessentially Jewish and the mark of their reality.

> Circumcision makes it clear as can be that you are here and not there, that you are out and not in–also that you're mine and not theirs. There is no way around it: you enter history through my history and me.[9]

Note Nathan's nod to the traditional religious argument (the "covenant" with Yahweh) followed by an obviously secular ethnic justification.

A far less distinguished writer on "Jewish uniqueness," Francine Klagsbrun, offered the same argument in even more explicit language.[10] In her one-page essay the term "primitive" appears twice: "[W]e need to admit that there is something primitive and, yes, frightening about the procedure.... Yet we, as a community, continue the practice despite a sense of the primitive because it represents our connectedness to God and to each other." The "connectedness" that really matters here is "to each other." Concluding with the quotation from Roth about "here and not there," and intent on making certain that no one equates mohels with wielders of knives in "primitive" (read African) societies, she hammers home her essential message: Jewish circumcision "may resemble the practices of other cultures, but it has a meaning of its own for our own uniqueness." Though the deity and his covenant retain their role in the shadowy world of biblical myth, the immediate concern is promotion and preservation of ethnic solidarity.

One final example in this mode should suffice—this time from a Reform rabbi and professor of rabbinics. The language of his article is remarkably similar to what we've just encountered. Why, he asks, do Reform Jews, who have "done away with a number of ritual observances that conflict with our contemporary cultural and aesthetic sensibilities," continue a practice that is so obviously "at odds with the views and habits of modern civilization"? The answer "lies largely in the words 'ancient tribal rite.' For that's what *berit milah* is. That's why we do it, and, really, it's the *only* reason we do it." Lest we miss the essential message (hardly likely!), he follows with an excursus in the anthropological mode (perhaps with the cultural relativism argument in mind):

> Every tribe in the world behaves in this way, proclaiming its sense of community through the performance of rituals that allow the tribe to tell its story and to recount its sense of self. And make no mistake: we Jews are a "tribe," a social grouping that has defined its existence and historical destiny as that of a family, an *ethnos*, a community that reproduces itself by giving birth to Jewish children.... To say that we are a "tribe" is simply another way of saying that we are the *people* of Israel, a community that asserts its ongoing historical existence.[11]

---

[9] Roth (1987). Roth does say, "out and not in," apparently meaning out of the social mainstream.

[10] Francine Klagsbrun, "Circumcision may resemble female genital mutilation, but it has meaning for Jewish uniqueness," *Moment*, April 1997, p. 22.

[11] Mark Washofsky, "Why Reform Never Abandoned Circumcision," *Reform Judaism*, Fall 2008; quotation from online publication, *Reform Judaism Online*; italics in original. Many older Jews know the term "M.O.T."—member of the tribe—as shorthand for saying that someone is Jewish.

Here, then, is a plain declaration (by a *Reform* rabbi) of "chosen people" ideology, and in effect a preemptive strike against those who argue that removing foreskins from infants has no place in contemporary Jewish-American life. Yes, he admits, circumcision does seem anachronistic, chauvinistic, perhaps even cruel; but it has a purpose that must not be abandoned. And that purpose cannot be explained in narrowly religious terms; it is *ethnic* survival.

18.5 Conclusion

Confronted by seemingly intractable Jewish opposition, activists working to end *all* infant and child genital cutting feel frustration and even resentment. They perceive the hostility they encounter as *religious* defense of *Judaism*, and indeed the most vociferous Jewish opponents often rely heavily on the "freedom of religion" argument. As I've tried to show, however, the principal underlying motive in Jewish defense of circumcision is dedication to ethnic survival. When Jewish defenders charge opponents of circumcision with covert "antisemitism" it is not primarily *Judaism* they have in mind but Jewish *ethnicity*.

Moreover, although the vast majority of infants circumcised in this country are Gentile, many, perhaps most, Jewish Americans have only the vaguest understanding of overall circumcision rates and prevalence. They (like their non-Jewish counterparts) still think of circumcision as a uniquely Jewish practice—and a uniquely Jewish sign of male identity. That's why (even though this may seem to defy logic) when they hear a call for an end to circumcision, they may instinctively understand it as a threat to Jewish ethnic continuity.

Opponents of circumcision routinely cite the principle closely associated with modernity and enlightenment: the right of every *individual* to freedom from unwanted physical alteration or harm. Of course, individual rights also pertain to infants, persons unable to speak for themselves but equally entitled to physical autonomy and integrity. Thus, the most recent major publication of the movement to end circumcision is titled *Circumcision and Human Rights* (Denniston et al. 2009). The logic of this "human rights" argument seems impeccable, unchallengeable. And yet it is challenged, effectively and paradoxically, by an argument grounded in the equally modern, equally reasonable, principle of "cultural relativism": that every social or cultural *community* has its own right to autonomy and integrity—and that includes the right to preserve rituals and ceremonies that symbolize the community's identity and assure its endurance.

Arguments in support of individual human rights over what is perceived as *religious* fundamentalism are likely to make little headway against the many Jewish Americans—even those most committed to modernity and secularism—who remain convinced that circumcision is part of the price that must be paid for Jewish *ethnic* survival. They are inclined to respond to assertions about human rights as just one more challenge to the inherent right of Jews to maintain their distinct identity.

A puzzling question remains: Why this particular practice and not others? Why not maintain kosher food requirements, for example, or regular synagogue attendance, rather than infant foreskin removal? I can only speculate here, but the answer may be that, while other Jewish ordinances (e.g., food taboos) require long-term behavioral commitment for adults, infant circumcision is a single experience (unpleasant primarily for the child!), rationalized as necessary and soon conveniently forgotten. For human rights advocates, responding effectively to this entrenched understanding of circumcision may require careful consideration of how to counter the cultural relativism argument for Jewish ethnic continuity.[12]

References

Benatar M, Benatar D (2003) Between prophylaxis and child abuse: the ethics of neonatal male circumcision. Am J Bioethics 3(2):35–48

Denniston GC, Hodges FM, Milos MF (eds) (2001) Understanding circumcision: a multi-disciplinary approach to a multi-dimensional problem. Kluwer Academic/Plenum, New York, pp 37–44

Denniston GC, Hodges FM, Milos MF (eds) (2009) Circumcision and human rights. Springer, Dordrecht

Donnelly J (1990) Human rights, individual rights, and collective rights. In: Berting J, Baehr PR et al (eds) Human rights in a pluralist world: individuals and collectivities, Westport, CT: Meckler, pp 39–62

Donnelly J (2003) Universal human rights in theory and practice, 2nd edn. Cornell University Press, Ithaca, p 102

Fox M, Thomson M (2005) Short changed? the law and ethics of male circumcision. Int J Children's Rights 13:161–181

Fox M, Thomson M (2009) Reconsidering best interests: male circumcision and the rights of the child. In: Denniston GC, Hodges FM, Milos MF (eds) Circumcision and human rights. Springer, Dordrecht, pp 15–31

Herskovits MJ (1948) Man and his works: the science of cultural anthropology. Alfred A. Knopf, New York, pp 70, 77

Herskovits MJ (1960) Who are the Jews? In: Finkelstein L (ed) The Jews: their history, culture, and religion, 3rd edn. Harper & Row, New York, pp 1498–1509

Hodges FM, Svoboda JS, Van Howe RS (2002) Prophylactic interventions on children: balancing human rights with public health. J Med Ethics 28:10–16

Howard RE (1992) Dignity, community, and human rights. In: An Na'im AA (ed) Human rights in cross-cultural perspectives: a quest for consensus, University of Pennsylvania Press, Philadelphia, pp 81–102

Judd R (2007) Contested rituals: circumcision, kosher butchering, and Jewish political life in germany, 1843–1933. Cornell University Press, London

Macklin R (1999) Against relativism: cultural diversity and the search for ethical universals in medicine. Oxford University Press, New York

Mendes-Flohr P, Reiharz J (eds) (1995) The Jew in the modern world: a documentary history, 2nd edn. Oxford University Press, New York, pp 114–116

[12] To end on a somewhat more positive note, we should keep in mind the contemporary understanding of "culture" as a dynamic process involving steady development in response to personal decisions by many individuals: "All forms of cultural relativism fundamentally fail to recognize culture as an ongoing historic and institutional process where *the existence of a given custom does not mean that the custom is either adaptive, optimal, or consented to by a majority of its adherents*" (my emphasis). Zechenter (1997). [Cited in Donnelly (2003). This book also includes a useful bibliography.] The same point and related matters are ably discussed in Preis (1996).

Preis ABS (1996) Human rights as cultural practice: an anthropological critique. Hum Rights Q 18:286–315
Renteln AD (1988) Relativism and the search for human rights. Am Anthropologist 90:56–72
Renteln AD (1994) Is the cultural defense detrimental to the health of children? Law and Anthropology 7:27–106
Roth P (1987) The counterlife. Farrar, Straus and Giroux, New York, pp 314–15, 323
Shweder RA (1984) Anthropology's romantic rebellion against the enlightenment, or there's more to thinking than reason and evidence. In: Shweder RA, LeVine RA (eds) Culture theory: essays on mind, self, and emotion, Cambridge University Press, New York, p 47
Shweder RA, Minow M, Markus H (eds) (2002) Engaging cultural differences: the multicultural challenge to liberal democracies. Russell Sage Foundation Press, New York, pp 216–251
Slezkine Y (2004) The Jewish century. Princeton University Press, Princeton, p 1
Svoboda JS, Darby R (2008) A rose by any other name? symmetry and asymmetry in male and female genital cutting. In: Zabus C (ed) Fearful symmetries: essays and testimonies around excision and circumcision. Rodopi, Amsterdam, pp 252–297
Svoboda JS, Van Howe RS, Dwyer JG (2000) Informed consent for neonatal circumcision: an ethical and legal conundrum. J Contemporary Health Law and Policy 17:61–133
Viens AM (2004) Value judgment, harm, and religious liberty. J Med Ethics 30(3):241–247
Zechenter EM (1997) In the name of cultural relativism and the abuse of the individual. J Anthropol Res 53:319–347

Author Biography

Leonard B. Glick MD, PhD, received his medical degree from the University of Maryland and his doctorate from the University of Pennsylvania. He is Professor Emeritus of Anthropology, Hampshire College, Amherst, Massachusetts, and the author of *Abraham's Heirs: Jews and Christians in Medieval Europe* (1999), "Religion and Genocide," in I.A. Chaney (ed.), *The Widening Circle of Genocide* (1994), and *Marked in Your Flesh: Circumcision from Ancient Judea to Modern America* (2005). New Salem, Massachusetts, USA.

Chapter 19
Circumcision: Gender and Power

Miriam Pollack

Abstract When people hear the term "circumcision," many associations pop up, depending upon cultural, religious and educational backgrounds. For many Americans, Jews, and Muslims, circumcision is an unquestioned rite of passage, be it secular or religious. For secular Americans, it is an assumed medical "improvement." For religious Jews, and Muslims, it is a sacred mark of belonging, and for secular Jews, the tribal connection is often paramount. For non-circumcising cultures, circumcision is a confounding, primitive rite with no imaginable redemptive value. When viewed without the heavily laden trappings of tradition and pseudoscience, circumcision is most basically about the removal of functional sexual tissue from an unconsenting, forcibly restrained human being. Both in origin as well as in its effects, circumcision is neither about medical benefits, nor that which is holy. Indeed, circumcision, most fundamentally is a cruel distortion and reconfiguring of the most primary attributes of gender and power. This is its true purpose, and this is what we must understand if we are to make the world safe for our baby boys.

Keywords Jews • Muslims • Circumcision • Ritual • Sacred • Mitzvah • Commandment • Sacrifice • Patriarchal fears • Empowerment of women • Brit b'lee milah

I am a Jew, a proud and somewhat literate Jew. Yet, I do not simply question the practice of ritual or routine infant circumcision, I condemn it. I understand that this places me in an awkward position, at best, vis-a-vis many Jews. Unlike my Muslim sisters, such as Soraya Mire and Ayaan Hersi Ali, who publicly campaign against genital mutilation in spite of ongoing threats to their very lives, I am not forced to summon such breathtaking courage. I need not fear that something akin to a fatwah will be issued against me. Fortunately, Judaism has a long history of dissent; and intolerance is usually confined to verbal incriminations and shaming. Unpleasant as that may be, that is not what concerns me as I undertake this very public critique of one of Judaism's most central tenets. What does give me pause

M. Pollack (✉)
Educator in private practice, Boulder, CO, USA
e-mail: m3pollack@comcast.net

G. C. Denniston et al. (eds.), *Genital Cutting: Protecting Children from Medical, Cultural, and Religious Infringements*, DOI: 10.1007/978-94-007-6407-1_19,

is the fear that I may unwittingly be giving ammunition to those who are invested in seeing Judaism in simplistic, reductionist terms and who may choose to use my argument to further their own anti-Jewish agenda. Today, at a time of intensifying anti-Semitism, I take this risk very seriously. And yet, that is not sufficient reason for me to avoid an honest and critical examination of this ancient rite of genital alteration. With deep love and respect for my tradition, for the Jewish people, and the land of Israel, I am here to challenge the rite of circumcision on behalf of all male babies, yet to be born.

Let me begin by saying this: Judaism is central to my core identity, spiritually and culturally, ethically and linguistically, to say nothing of my peculiar culinary preferences and sense of humor. The questions I ask, as well as my sense of entitlement to question anything, are firmly rooted in my Jewish upbringing. Judaism has formed and informed my understanding of the sacred, and how we are to conduct ourselves as ethical and compassionate human beings. It has taught me that my purpose in this life is to repair the broken places, and part of that process often requires the ability to embrace paradox: the necessity of finding truth by allowing and holding opposing views. Love and justice must be intertwined and always sought after for, when they are out of balance, suffering results. Indeed, reverence for life is the guiding principle that must inform all of our actions. Ultimately, spirituality must be in alignment with ethics in order to be valid. It is in this spirit, that I undertake this radical analysis of circumcision.

Circumcision is seen as the central mitzvah (or commandment) of Judaism. Even for non religious Jews, circumcision continues to be perceived as the sine qua non of Jewish identity. And, yet, unlike any other controversial topic that we Jews address, the subject of circumcision is not to be challenged. We can calmly discuss whether there is a G d or no G d, if G d is masculine, feminine, or neuter, or whether homosexuals should become rabbis (hardly debatable outside of orthodoxy). Yet, questioning circumcision has been out of bounds. This taboo, in and of itself, is indicative of how strong are the feelings that surround this ancient rite, and how much lies below the surface, in the dark silence where powerful forces have coalesced for thousands of years.

In order to attempt to understand the role of circumcision in Judaism, we need to explore not simply the biblical injunction found in Genesis 17 (Genesis 17:10–12, 1955). We are also obliged to focus on the functions that male genital cutting serves–socially, politically, psychologically and individually–in order to see what and whose invisible needs are being fulfilled. Some of this information comes to us from scholarship; some, can only be derived by examining the more subtle ramifications, which result from the permanent alteration of male sexual organs.

Circumcision is hardly unique to Judaism. However, two elements distinguish the Jewish version of male genital cutting. First, in Judaism circumcision is expressed as the divine mandate, which seals and perpetuates the covenant, G d's contractual and eternal relationship with the Jewish people. Second, it is commanded to occur on the 8th day of the baby boy's life. Other than these unique identifiers, circumcision in Judaism shares much with rites of circumcision in other societies.

What I intend to do here is to show that cutting out a portion of a child's genitalia, fundamentally, is about gender and power. This is true whether the mandate is divine, tribal, secular, or pseudo-medical and pertains to little girls as well as little boys.

For those of us who have grown up with the normalcy of newborn male circumcision, this may seem like a bold, perhaps, even outrageous statement. As Paige and Paige state in their book, *The Politics of Reproductive Ritual*, according to the many theories advanced that attempt to explain the function of reproductive ritual, all agree that "the purposes of ritual are seldom if ever the object of conscious knowledge."(Paige and Paige 1981)

In each and every circumcising society, circumcision functions to fulfill multiple unspoken social, political-tribal, and sexual needs. Paige and Paige claim that male circumcision originally functioned as a vehicle for attempting to achieve, by means of ritual, what could not be accomplished by means of political arrangement: that is, the defusing of possible competitive claims by male progeny for the same limited resources.[1] In pre-industrial societies, where clan and tribal loyalties formed the basis of economic and military security, the father's willingness to expose, sacrifice, and risk the tender organ of his son's procreative potential and the promise of his own male progeny to the knife was a dramatic demonstration to the elders (read that as male elders) of the father's allegiance to his tribe (Glick 2005; Paige and Paige 1981, p. 151). For this reason, circumcision is rarely a private surgical event. Rather, it is most commonly a communal ceremony accompanied by feast and celebration. Circumcision, typically, is public declaration of alignment and thus not simply a social event, but a political statement as well. Without a whisper of the true hierarchical intentions of this ceremony, the outcome was always, and continues to be, a re-assertion and institutionalization of a power structure based on gender.

The timing of male circumcision furthers the political/social relationships in less obvious ways. Even though the age for circumcision ranges widely across all circumcising societies, what is most universally constant is the requirement that circumcision occur before marriage.[2] This rule not only establishes the father's status in the male dominant community, but it also works to achieve another salient objective: marriageable girls are entrained to view any uncircumcised man as undesirable, thereby ensuring the ethnic stability of the tribe. Girls know from an early age that they would risk social ostracism by mating with an uncircumcised male. By enculturating all group members to the necessity, normalcy, and moral superiority of circumcision, circumcising children not only re-affirms the political and social structure of the tribe, but also deepens the identity formation of the group. In this way, circumcision functions as a primary and potent entrainment for group bonding.

1 Ibid., 166.

2 Ibid., 150.

At an even more muted level, circumcision does more than restructure identity based on contemporary and historical alliances of gender and power. On a meta-historical and biological level, circumcision acts to rename, remap, and invert our fundamental and primal relationship to the feminine. It is not coincidental that this ritual of tribal belonging necessitates the cutting, blood letting, and altering–in a public ceremony–of the male child's sexual organ. As Leonard Glick points out in his landmark book, *Marked in Your Flesh*, "...Female blood contaminates, male blood sanctifies." Thus, he explains, "the shedding of male blood is an act of consecration."[3] By creating historical and social linkage through this sacrificial ritual, circumcision functions to supersede and transcend our most primary maternal and biological system of relationship making patrilineal and patriarchal hierarchy appear "natural and inevitable,"(Jay 1992) as Nancy Jay noted in her brilliant book, *Throughout Your Generations Forever.* Karen E. Fields, in the Forward to this same book, commented as follows:

> In no other major religious institution is gender dichotomy more consistently important, across unrelated traditions, than it is in sacrifice. This is true not only of ancient and so-called primitive religions. Even among contemporary Christians, the more vividly the Eucharist is understood to be itself a real sacrifice, the greater the opposition to ordaining women....Consequently, a study of sacrifices focusing on gender leads to a new understanding: sacrifice as remedy for having been born of woman.[4]

Thus, in both the Hebrew Scriptures[5] and the New Testament (Matthew 1:1–16, Luke 3:23–38, 1964), legitimacy is established by citing and repeating the lineage of male progenitors. The names of the mothers are usually unmentioned, irrelevant in a male dominant culture.

Circumcision subverts the community's relationship to the life-giving principle of the feminine, not only by obliterating the woman's rightful identity in structuring the historical social network of her tribe, but also by trivializing and implicitly forbidding her to acknowledge, much less act upon, her deepest mammalian instincts to protect her newly birthed child. She knows, long before she has even conceived, that in order for her child to be bonded to the male community, past, present, and future, and to a male-imaged god, she must surrender him to the men with a knife to cut, wound, and cause great pain to this newly birthed life on his most vulnerable sexual organ. Typically, a mother's feelings are dismissed or ridiculed. Her voice is silenced, even to herself. Can it be a coincidence that we have language for the primary disempowerment for men, but not for women? When men are wounded in their primal potency of manhood, we say they have been "emasculated." When women are wounded in their primary potency of womanhood, we rarely notice. We have no language, no conceptual structure, no word to claim, much less attempt to heal, the experience of core female disempowerment.

---

[3] Glick LB, 21.

[4] Ibid., 37, Forward Fields KE, University of Rochester, 1991.

[5] I Samuel 1:1 The Holy Scriptures.

The wounding of circumcision irreversibly alters both mother and child: the mother, fractured at the base of her deepest womb-wisdom, that knows she must protect her child no matter what; and the baby, shocked and traumatized, fractured in his ability to absolutely trust the protective arms of the mother he has biologically and innately trusted as his primordial place of safety. From the beginning, masculinity is now defined as that which must be cut off from the mother and all that is female, nurturing, and essential for human survival. In this way, women are made complicit in this masculine-defined model of motherhood. Nancy Jay states, "Gender is therefore unequalled as a cornerstone of domination."[6] Circumcision is the weapon that not only destroys a boy's foreskin, but it also deftly excises maternal authority over the ultimate wellbeing of her child. For, if a woman cannot allow herself to feel not only entitled, but also honoured for her instinctive need to protect her newborn child, what feelings of her own can she ever trust?

In all circumcising societies, the sacrifice endured by the child is considered incidental to the social, political, and/or religious forces that require it. Typically, the extremity of the baby's pain is denied, ignored, or made the object of countless jokes. Because we Jews circumcise at eight days of age, when a child is easily overpowered and, we believe, may not consciously recall this event, we deem those who circumcise children at later ages barbaric. Many of us Jews are capable of witnessing a bris, a ritual circumcision, looking into the eyes of the shocked, terrified, and shrieking baby, his head flailing and chin quivering, as his foreskin is severed from the delicate surface of the glans, cut, and crushed, and concluding that this is no different than a routine infant protest of having a wet diaper changed. We ignore or choose to be ignorant of not only what our hearts and wombs are telling us, but of the plethora of scientific data, replicated numerous times in the past several decades, which leave little question about the reality of the baby's experience. Heart and respiratory rates, as well as cortisol levels of babies undergoing circumcision point to the unambiguous conclusion that circumcision is not only excruciatingly painful to any baby but, as is the case in other severe trauma at the neonatal level of development, the implications of lasting sequelae in the nervous system are serious (Van Howe 1999). Science has not yet turned its attention to identifying what these sequelae may be. Nevertheless, a modicum of psychological awareness is sufficient to suggest that issues of trust, fear, comfort with intimacy, sexuality, and gender relationships would be reasonable places for scholarly investigation. While traumatizing an infant is neither the stated nor conscious intention of circumcision, it is an inevitable corollary of cutting off a child's genital organs with possibly unspecified but hardly neutral alterations in the nervous system.

Although vigorously denied by the proponents of circumcision, the forcible removal of the foreskin also has profound and long-lasting effects for a male's sexual experience. Even during ancient times, when circumcision was less radical

[6] Jay, 148.

than it is today, the unique quality of the foreskin was understood. In Biblical Judaism, circumcision consisted of cutting the foreskin that extended beyond the glans, leaving most of it intact. The full reaming and ablating of the entire foreskin, known as *periah,* was only innovated by rabbinic decree during Hellenic times in response to the practice of some Jewish men who were attempting to avoid ridicule by their fellow Greek athletes by tying and stretching their foreskins so as not to look circumcised (Kohler 1964).

Both the Hellenic Jewish Philo[7] in the first century C.E. and Moses Maimonides, also known in the Jewish tradition as the Great Rambam, in the twelth century wrote of the consequences of violently removing the most sensuous part of a man's sexual organ before he is old enough to understand or consent to this loss. Many centuries later, Cold and Taylor would confirm their understanding when they discovered that, indeed, there are over 20,000 specialized, fine touch receptive cells in the human foreskin, which allow for far greater nuanced sensation and control than any other penile tissue (Cold and Taylor 1999). Removing the foreskin creates a secondary loss of sensitivity, as well. Not only has the most erogenous tissue of the male sexual organ been removed but, as the man ages, the glans loses its mucosal covering, becomes dried out, and keratinizes over time. Typically by middle age, the glans of the circumcised penis has lost much sensitivity and the man requires more abrasive stimulation to achieve orgasm. Often this is just as a woman is becoming peri-menopausal and experiencing decreasing vaginal lubrication. The problem is usually identified as the woman's entry into menopause, but the contribution of the circumcised partner is rarely acknowledged. In subtle, but profound ways, circumcision functions to diminish a man's pleasure potential, allowing his bond to his partner to be subordinated to his bond to his tribal male peers. Both Philo and Maimonides, knew beyond a doubt that, as in all other aspects of biology, altering form alters function. Here is what Maimonides, the great philosopher, physician, and Talmudist, had to say in his famous book, *The Guide of the Perplexed,* written in 1160:

> The fact that circumcision weakens the faculty of sexual excitement and sometimes perhaps diminishes the pleasure is indubitable. For if at birth this member has been made to bleed and has had its covering taken away from it, it must indubitably be weakened. The Sages, may their memory be blessed, have explicitly stated: It is hard for a woman with whom an uncircumcised man has had sexual intercourse to separate from him (Genesis Rabbah LXXX). In my opinion this is the strongest of reasons for circumcision (Maimonides 1190/1963).

There they are, the twin patriarchal fears: the fear of woman and the fear of pleasure. Circumcision is both the vehicle and the product, the menace and the antidote, which simultaneously assuages and perpetuates these ancient terrors. This is the achievement and true function of circumcision. Circumcision achieves this by violently breaching the maternal-infant bond shortly after birth, by amputating and marking the baby's sexual organ before he knows what he has lost,

[7] Glick LB, 33.

by disempowering, "taming," the mother at the height of her instinctual need to protect her infant, by bonding the baby to the community of men past, present, and future and to a male-imaged G d, by restructuring the family and the society in terms of male dominance and by psycho-sexually wounding the manhood still asleep in the unsuspecting baby boy. In all of these ways, socially, politically, religiously, ethnically, sexually, tribally, and interpersonally, the cutting of our baby boys' sexual organs is the fulcrum around which patriarchy exerts its power. Circumcision is a rite of male domination–domination and the entitlement of domination over other men, women, and children, both institutionally and personally. It is the essence of patriarchy.

Nevertheless, it would be grossly oversimplifying to characterize Judaism as a purely patriarchal religion, nor would it be accurate to view Judaism as the source of patriarchy in Western religions. The emphatic and elaborate emphasis on this life, on the sanctity of all life as a primary organizing value throughout both Biblical and Talmudic texts is in complete contradiction to the practice of circumcision. Removing functional sexual tissue is harmful: it is harmful to the infant, to the pleasure potential and sexual bonding of the mature man, and to the mother who is entrained to surrender her sacred bond with her infant in order for his masculinity to be redefined in terms of his community. The rabbis explain that, because women are closer to the divine due to our ability to give birth and sustain life, men are in need of other ways to access spirituality–circumcision being the primary one. However, the notion that trauma can be a bonafide path, much less an ethical avenue to greater spiritual awareness would be vociferously challenged by contemporary neonatologists as well as epigeneticists. What is unethical cannot be spiritual. The dichotomy and hierarchy assumed and taught for millennia in multiple religions between sexual aliveness and spirituality is false and has led to ages of human suffering. Spiritual sexism is still sexism and needs to be discarded.

I remember when I first learned about the phenomenon of female genital cutting. I was appalled. How could they? How could anyone? It took years before I could hear them say, "It's who we are, who we've been for thousands of years. No one will marry us if we're not cut. Intact genitalia are ugly. They are unhygienic." Then, I realized, we say the same things. Yes, there are significant differences between female and male cutting, but it is not honest to claim that one is physically and sexually insignificant and the other barbaric; that one is enlightened, the other primitive. Holding a child down and forcibly removing genitalia is sexual abuse. We would not hesitate to use that label for an individual or culture that countenanced sexual fondling of children. Why do we think slicing off genitals is acceptable? Circumcision is not holy, it does not transmit the Jewish spiritual heritage, nor does it secure Jewish continuity.

For religious as well as tribal and secular reasons, many Jews believe that "circumcision ensures our survival." Without circumcision, we tell each other, the Jewish people will disappear, a very frightening prediction to a people for whom annihilation is a perpetual possibility. Again, the transparent sexism of such a contention is only too apparent. Are males the only ones who count as

Jews? Is the contribution of Jewish women irrelevant, invisible, insignificant? More fundamentally, why can Jewish women carry on our spiritual legacy and remain whole, but Jewish men cannot? How, indeed, did circumcision further our survival needs during the desperate epochs of Jewish purges when the enemy only had to pull down pants in order to eliminate Jewish males? In the US, when most men over 30 have been circumcised, or in the Middle East, where circumcision is normative for Muslims, are naked Jewish men distinguishable from their non-Jewish counterparts? And, if circumcision is the quintessential protector of Jewish identity, why do we have tens of thousands of Jewish men in the US who have had their genitalia radically and permanently altered who are Judaically ignorant and completely Jewishly unaffiliated? The question of how we are to secure and sustain Jewish survival is extremely serious, but the answer is not circumcision.

An orthodox rabbi, interviewed by Eliyahu Unger-Sargon in his brilliant movie, *Cut: Slicing through the Myths of Circumcision*, stated unequivocally that circumcision was tantamount to sexual abuse. Yet, this thoughtful man went on to justify the practice of circumcision for religious reasons, saying that this is where "the rubber hits the road" if you are a Jew. It is a commandment. We have no choice.

Indeed, we do have a choice. What is sacred is our obligation to protect the integrity and privacy of all of our children's genitals. They are not the province of family, community, or anyone else. Spiritualizing the wounding of circumcision does not change the damage, nor make it ethical. As Deuteronomy 30:6 teaches, what is truly required of us in order to contact the divine has to do with the architecture of the heart, not the alteration of male genitals (Deuteronomy 30:6, The Holy Scriptures). Creating a joyful and loving Jewish home and providing our children with meaningful and in-depth Jewish education are the only authentic means we have to ensure our survival. Cutting our babies' penises will not do it.

We do have a choice. Circumcision may be an ancient rite, but it is wrong. Over the ages, Judaism has demonstrated a remarkable ability to mutate in practice and retain the integrity of its spiritual legacy. Judaism was not vanquished when the first temple was destroyed nor when the second temple was razed. The discarding of animal sacrifice as the primary mode of worship did not result in an unravelling of Jewish spirituality or continuity. Legally, Jewish identity is defined both by halachah, Jewish law, as well as the Israeli Supreme court, by the status of the child's mother: if the mother is Jewish, the child is Jewish. Circumcision does not trump maternal lineage.

Without compromising our children's identity or the survival of our people, we can invite all of our Jewish children, our baby girls and our baby boys, into a brit b'lee milah, a covenant without circumcision, school them in the wisdom, love, and beauty of the Jewish tradition. Unlike Christianity, which teaches that a child is born into original sin and must be redeemed, Judaism teaches that the soul is pure…only the penis needs "redemption." The truth is that the whole baby is pure, body and soul, including his tender genitals, and it is both a mitzvah and our most sacred duty to protect him.

References

Cold CJ, Taylor JR (1999) The Prepuce. Br J Urology 83(Suppl 1):34–44
Genesis 17:10–12 (1955) The holy scriptures. Jewish Publication Society, Philadelphia
Glick LB (2005) Marked in your flesh: circumcision from ancient judea to modern America. Oxford University Press, Oxford, p 18
Jay N (1992) Throughout your generations forever. University of Chicago Press, Chicago, p 148
Kohler K (1964) Circumcision. The jewish encyclopedia. KTAV Publishing House, Inc., New York, p 93
Maimonides M (1190/1963) The guide of the perplexed, trans. Pines S, vol 2, part 3, chap 49. University of Chicago Press, Chicago, p 609
Matthew 1:1–16, Luke 3:23 38 (1964) The holy bible: revised standard version. World Publishing Company, Cleveland
Paige KE, Paige JM (1981) The politics of reproductive ritual. University of California Press, Berkeley, p 3
Van Howe RS (1999) Anesthesia for circumcision: a review of the literature. In: Denniston GC, Hodges FM, Milos MF (eds.) Male and female circumcision: medical, legal and ethical considerations in pediatric practice. Kluwer Academic/Plenum Press, New York, pp 63–97

Author Biography

Miriam Pollack an educator in private practice, has been advocating for genital integrity for Jewish as well as non-Jewish baby boys for the past 19 years by writing, speaking, counselling Jewish parents, and providing alternative brit b'lee milah ceremonies for interested parents. Her article, "Circumcision: A Jewish Feminist Perspective," was published in *Jewish Women Speak Out: Expanding the Boundaries of Psychotherapy* (Seattle: Canopy Press, 1995) her paper, "Circumcision: Redefining the Sacred," was published in *Sexual Mutilations: A Human Tragedy* (New York and London: Plenum Press, 1997), and her paper "Circumcision: If It Isn't Ethical, Can It Be Spiritual?, was published in *Circumcision and Human Rights* (New York and The Netherlands, 2009). She appeared in the documentary, *Whose Body, Whose Rights?,* and has spoken at international symposia at the University of Maryland, University of Lausanne, Switzerland, University of Washington, and University of Keele, Staffordshire, England. Miriam lives in Boulder, Colorado, USA.

Chapter 20
Reclaiming Circumcision: Armenian Stories

Astrik N. Vardanyan

Abstract A significant number of Armenian Americans are adopting the practice of circumcision, a procedure that historically has not been a custom among Christian Armenians. Currently, the reasons given by Armenian Americans mimic the American rationale of "health" and "hygiene," however, historic evidence shows long-standing resistance to circumcision imposed by Islamic dominators. Circumcision was perceived by Armenians as the bodily mark that stigmatized them as forcibly Islamized. Circumcision denoted assimilation; resistance to it ensured Armenian survival. However, an unexpected shift in cultural attitudes took place among Armenians. Circumcision was rapidly embraced after genocide and the strict line between the circumcised and uncircumcised was crossed. Centuries-old denigration and rooted historical anxieties were reconciled and conveniently resolved in the "medical" justification of the practice. Armenians reclaimed the practice anew. This presentation explores the latent motives of such a cumulative ethnic response through anthropological and psychological analyses.

Keywords Armenian Americans • Christians • Jews • Muslims • Islam • Anthropology • Psychology • Circumcision • Genocide

20.1 Introduction

A significant number of Armenian Americans have adopted the practice of circumcision, a procedure that historically has not been a custom among Christian Armenians. The practice of circumcision among Armenians serves no religious purpose and is mainly performed for "hygienic" reasons mimicking the American rationale of hospital circumcision. Some parents have been victims of negligent doctors, who circumcise children without the parents' informed consent. Others have been aggressively solicited by hospital staff, which promotes the procedure for financial incentives. Still others in the Armenian community seem to be inclined to it in order to

A. N. Vardanyan (✉)
Independent Anthropologist, California State University, Northridge, California, USA
e-mail: astrikvardanyan@yahoo.com

G. C. Denniston et al. (eds.), *Genital Cutting: Protecting Children from Medical, Cultural, and Religious Infringements*, DOI: 10.1007/978-94-007-6407-1_20,

assimilate into the dominant American cultural norm, alleged medical justification, and perceived sexual benefits. Some even circumcise in admiration of Jewish and Muslim wisdom. While circumcision of male infants has been a much-debated issue in the US, nonetheless, it remains an especially uncomfortable topic of discussion among most Armenians. The uneasiness surrounding circumcision goes beyond the social embarrassment of touching upon a personal issue; it has historic roots.

20.2 The Circumcision Issue in the Lives of Armenians: Symbolic Mark of Islam

For centuries, being geographically surrounded by Islamic dominating nations, Armenians struggled to keep their ethnic identity by leaving boys intact as a crucial differentiating factor. As known from history, the Muslim rulers led systematic and coercive policies to convert Armenians to Islam (Daranaghtsi 1965; Papazian 1971) part and parcel of which was ritual circumcision (Davrizetsi 1988; Dadrian 2003). Under the Ottoman Empire, from the fifteenth to nineteenth centuries, every three to seven years, all healthy male children were forcibly taken as "child levy," a system called Devshirme, and made into slaves of the Sultan to serve as Jenissaries (Daranaghtsi 1965). These boys were forced to take a ceremonial oath to convert to Islam, got Turkish names, and were then ritually circumcised. As the Sultan's standing army, Janissaries were instrumental in the Empire: trained by the Ottoman Turkish officials, these Christian children were brainwashed to kill their own people (Papazian 1971; Erdem 1996).

20.3 Circumcision in Arakel Davrizetsi's "History"

Given the historical apprehension about forcible Islamization, Armenians associated circumcision as a threat to their Christian identity. The seventeenth-century historian Arakel Davrizetsi [of Tabriz] in his *History* writes about the martyrdoms of Christian Armenian youth who resisted conversion to Islam and circumcision and chose death instead (Davrizetsi 1988). These martyrs were venerated as saints among Armenians. There is ample evidence of coercive circumcisions referenced by Davrizetsi. In one passage, Davrizetsi describes how Persian king Shah-Abas sends a group of circumcisers to carry out massive circumcisions and convert Armenians to Islam. Out of fear of the circumcisers, many Armenians run away to the mountains, change their names and appearance. In gut-wrenching detail, Davrizetsi writes:

> Thus, they forcefully hung them upside down, circumcised them and made them recite benedictions according to their religion.[1]

[1] Davrizetsi . 1988:131. [My translation].

Davrizetsi's stories often end with martyrdoms, which are an unequivocal assertion of cumulative ethnic response; it is better to die and see their young die as "saints" than be subject to forceful Islamization and circumcision. In Davrizetsi's *History*, traitors circumcise.

20.4 Genocide and Circumcision

Circumcision as a cultural marker of ethnic cleansing continued in the twentieth century. During the Armenian Genocide of 1915 architected by the Ottoman Turkey, thousands of Armenian children were murdered by a variety of brutal methods, (Balakian 2003) such as "serial rapes," (Künzler 1921) "burning alive," "mass poisoning" and "en masse drowning" (Dadrian 2003). Despite the appalling torture of the Armenian children, Turks had also another *modus operandi*: massive assimilation of Armenians through coercive conversion to Islam, which entailed name change and, for boys, circumcision. In other words—the making of Turk (Dadrian 2003). The following is a personal account of a genocide survivor:

> ...Now I was supposed to be a Muslim... and Muslims had a practice of circumcision. When the man came to circumcise me I ran away to the hills (Jamgojian 1991).

Thus, for many centuries, circumcision was perceived by Armenians as forcibly Islamized.

20.5 Adopting Circumcision: Embracing Modernization

However, circumcision's cultural meaning of survival and resistance was soon destined to be erased with the medicalization of the procedure. Rapidly, circumcision made its way into Armenian communities of the Middle East with the same rationale and through the same sources as they emerged in the English-speaking countries. The circumcision that Armenians were adopting was not the Muslim rite, it was the new, the "medical," the "scientific" one introduced from the Western countries. Repeating the scenario of the West, where the Jewish rite was normalized and incorporated into the routine hospital practices, Armenians with higher social class and standing came to associate circumcision with medical sophistication.[2] Inconspicuously, circumcision lost the cultural/religious stigma attached to it. As the Middle Eastern Armenian communities immigrated to the US, the practice was further reinforced in the American milieu, where circumcision was a norm. It is fascinating that those,

[2] Data collected from numerous interviews taken from Middle Eastern/Diaspora Armenians 2004.

who once escaped circumcision, later circumcised their sons and grandsons as a health measure.[3]

20.6 A Multi-Group Analysis of Circumcision Practice

There appears an intriguing statistical discrepancy between different groups of Armenians. While there are no accurate statistics the incidence of circumcision varies dramatically from 3–5 % among Eastern Armenians, whether in homeland or as recent immigrants from Armenia in the US, to 70 % among Armenians in the Middle East or among American Diaspora. Beyond some data that I collected from a day-care center,[4] a medical practitioner,[5] and ethnographic interviews,[6] I attempted to find out the underlying attitudes associated with the two different groups by designing a questionnaire to test the automatic response to the word "circumcised" that was carefully hidden in other culturally obvious expressions. The survey was designed to test the various attitudes of the two groups. The Eastern group surveys are carried out in Armenia and the US, and the Middle Eastern group surveys are carried out in the US Diaspora exclusively[7] Table 20.1.

The following data has emerged from 31 respondents, college students in California identified as Middle-Eastern or descendants of Middle-Eastern Armenians Table 20.2.

Quite different responses came from 17 respondents of Yerevan State University students in Armenia (Eastern Armenians) and 13 respondents of Glendale College students in California, identified as Eastern Armenians, or descendants of Eastern Armenians Table 20.3.

The majority of Eastern Armenian respondents associated "circumcised" with Turkishness and Muslims. Judging from the value-laden language of Eastern Armenians ("dog," "worthless") one can see that circumcision is not a medical issue for them. Circumcision is perceived as a cultural taboo, even though they did not suffer the threat of coercive circumcision directly in the Eastern part of Armenia. By contrast, among Middle-Eastern/Diaspora Armenians, circumcision has become so ubiquitous that some state that it's a "family tradition." The old identity of the "traditional" Armenian male, Christian, not-circumcised, ready to die for the preservation of this identity, and repeatedly victimized, has vanished right after the Genocide, giving way to a

[3] Grigor Alagagian. Unpublished memoir, *Four Years in Der-Zor*.

[4] Data collected from daycare center (Artek Child Educational Center, information provided by the Principal 2004).

[5] Data collected from a Glendale pediatrician, Dr. Vigen Zargarian 2004.

[6] Comparable statistics are extrapolated from my ethnographic interviews taken from Middle Eastern/Diaspora Armenians 2004.

[7] Surveys in Armenia in the US are done on May 2006 and September 2007, respectively.

Table 20.1 Questionnaire

Please fill out the blanks without too much thinking:
Place of birth________________
Sex________________________
Santa ______________________
North and ___________________
Paris _______________________
Armed ______________________
Shaved ______________________
Circumcised __________________
Wicked ______________________

Table 20.2 Glendale respondents

Circumcised	Number of responses
Penis/dick	19
Baby	1
People	2
Clean	2
Jews	2
Ouch/Uhh!	2
No	1
Circle	2

Table 20.3 Yerevan (Armenia) respondents

Circumcised	Number of responses
Turk	9
Mohammedans/Islamic	7
Dog	3
Worthless Turk/person	2
Non-Armenian/Muslim	1
Suffered	1
Persian	2
Jews	2
Unprotected-Muslim, Jew	1
Baby	1
No	1

new construction of Armenian—"modern," "scientifically inclined," and "not-so-ready-to-fight" for his identity with respect to circumcision status. While most cultural features have been strongly preserved in the Middle Eastern Armenian communities—language, inter-group marriage, religion, customs of everyday life—the strict line between the circumcised and uncircumcised has been crossed. Thus, the two groups of Armenians are deeply committed to two different "traditions," one to the centuries-old (which is now too old), and one freshly invented.

20.7 Reclamation

The challenge is to comprehend why Middle-Eastern/Diaspora Armenians, on whom circumcision has been inflicted, have adopted the practice and not the Eastern Armenians? Why has something forced on them, that marked them as religiously and culturally robbed, later become a body mark of "medical sophistication" and "modernism?" The answer could be explored in anthropology, in a phenomenon described as *reclamation:*

> Reclamation happens when subjugated groups reclaim or re-appropriate, for the purposes of identity creation and maintenance, (re)presentations of them created by the dominant culture (Magliocco 2001).

A typical example of reclamation is branding practice reclaimed by African American college students within fraternities and sororities. Brands, once used by plantation owners for identification of slaves, are generally third-degree burns that burn the skin open and heal as a scab. The practice was revived by Black Greek-letter organizations as a permanent signifier of allegiance and brotherhood, as well as a way of identifying those blacks able to gain higher education (Brown et al. 2005). The practice emerged anew not as a sign of subjugation but as a sign of "dominance," "honor," and "success." While extremely painful and often times dangerous, submitting to an act of violence inflicted on the flesh in a context of brotherhood and on one's own terms has shifted the meaning radically (Magliocco 2001). Branding is reclamation of the body not enslaved but empowered.

Jewish circumcision is another prime analogue of reclamation. Circumcision among Jews was prevalent long before the formation of formal Judeo-Christian religion and subsequently, the covenant. Moreover, some theorists propose that it was a mark of subjugation and slavery (DeMeo 1997; Eilberg-Schwartz 1992; Goldman 1997). If this is so, then Jews reclaimed the practice by ascribing a divine commandment to it and, thus, shifted the meaning fundamentally—what was a mark of suppression became an honor badge, a sacred law upon which the Jewish identity was constructed.

Reclamation of circumcision by Middle-Eastern Armenians may be viewed as another such example. They embraced the "medical" argument en masse to rationalize what was imposed on them for centuries by the dominating Turks and Persians. They resolved their rooted anxieties in reclaiming circumcision not as victimized converts but as "progressive" and "scientifically" inclined citizens in line with the dominant strata of their communities back in the Middle East, as well as in American society. "Medical recommendation" became culturally appropriate justification. Circumcision no more victimized but rather empowered Armenians. Asked about circumcision as an ethnic and cultural issue, most go into extremes to debunk such a connection by presenting circumcision as a "purely medical" issue without any connection in history or identity. Interestingly, the most ardent denial comes from those, who are indeed familiar with historic context, but who show defensive, aggressive, or avoiding reactions to circumcision discussion, indeed attesting deep conflict with it, whether conscious of it or not. Here are some vignettes from my ethnography to illustrate my point.

Historian: (May, 2004, truncated telephone conversation, which was meant to be a telephone interview)

- ...You mention circumcision accompanying forceful conversion by Turks. Do you know other historical sources that engage the theme of such forceful circumcisions by Turks?
- What circumcision? I never wrote about circumcision! And I'm not interested in the topic at all!
- But you *did* write about it in your... (I mention the article).
- Why are you pursuing this? (hung up the phone)

Documentary filmmaker: (September, 2004 at a cultural event)

- I'm researching the circumcision issue and I'd like to talk to you about it.
- Well I'm not a doctor.
- I know, but you've worked with genocide survivors.
- Yes!
- Did you come across personal accounts of forceful circumcisions?
- Circumcision is a medical issue; I don't know anything about it.

(This filmmaker indeed had used a survivor's account on circumcision in his documentary).

Middle-ranked clergy: (June, 2007, at a wedding party, sitting next to me. All guests have pocket bibles on the table as a wedding gift. The clergy starts the conversation.)

- What are you reading?
- I'm reading Paul's preaching on circumcision.
- Paul said neither circumcision nor *uncircumcision* matters to Christ!
- Paul said many things about circumcision, not just that.
- Why are you interested on the subject though?
- I have a professional interest; my thesis is on circumcision...
- How interesting is that! I know that it's medically beneficial.
- Not necessarily. I think Armenians were wise to reject it.
- What exactly is your purpose?
- Well, I want to bring more awareness about this issue in our community.
- You're wasting your time.
- Why?
- It's a futile pursuit!
- Why is it futile?
- Don't waste your time!

There are a wide range of defense mechanisms used in the above situations, the most obvious ones—denial and repression—so shockingly evident that one would be negligent not to see them. In my experience, those Armenians, who are earnestly unfamiliar with the historic repressions, are quite forthcoming to talk about it and can even fast-change their position if provided with adequate medical information. Armenians, thus, employ double-layered defense mechanisms when discussing circumcision—one on the individual, and one on the level of cultural identity.

To conclude, while the prepuce is a natural fact present in all mammals and primates for millions of years, societies have created their own socially constructed phallus. Foreskin has been the prime site where cultural meanings have been ascribed. Warriors, religious authorities, and medicine men have carved the male genitalia with an aim of domination, blessing, or hygiene. The history of circumcision reveals a chronicle, wherein meanings attached to the practice have been continuously changing and metamorphosing from a mark of slavery to divine power, from coercive conversion to disease prevention. The practice has been fought and reclaimed anew, denigrated and sanctified. However, in recent decades, throughout the world and especially in the US a new form of reclamation has increasingly been manifest; *reclamation of the whole body and genitalia.* The American cultural trends are moving towards the acceptance of the foreskin as an integral body part and an irreducible ontological reality; a reality that is not subject to cultural meanings. That is the reclamation par excellence!

References

Balakian P (2003) The burning Tigris: the Armenian genocide and America's response. Perennial, New York

Brown T, Parks G, Phillips C (2005) African American fraternities and sororities: the legacy and the vision. University Press of Kentucky, Kentucky

Dadrian V (2003) Children as victims of genocide: the Armenian case. Journal of Genocide Research, vol 5(3), pp 421–427. http://myweb.tiscali.co.uk/cragsite/Children.htm last retrieved 2 Nov 2003

Daranaghtsi G (1965) Zhamanakagriutiun [Chronology]. Jerusalem Press, Jerusalem

Davrizetsi A (1988) History. Yerevan Press, Yerevan

DeMeo J (1997) The geography of genital mutilations. (Presented at the fourth international symposium on sexual mutilations, University of Lausanne, Lausanne, Switzerland, 9–11 Aug 1996). In: Denniston GC, Milos MF (eds) Sexual mutilations, a human tragedy. Plenum Press, New York link to www.nocirc.org

Eilberg-Schwartz H (1992) Why not the Earlobe? Moment, pp 28–33, February

Erdem HY (1996) Slavery in the Ottoman empire and its demise. St. Martin's Press (Davrizetsi 1988:131). [My translation]

Goldman R (1997) Questioning circumcision: a Jewish perspective. Vanguard, Boston, pp 11–12

Jamgojian H (1991) From the documentary: the Armenian genocide, Atlantis production

Künzler J (1921) Im Lande des Blutes und der Tränen. Erlebnisse in Mesopotamien Während des Weltkrieges (In the Land of Blood and Tears. Experiences in Mesopotamia during the World War). Berlin-Potsdam, pp 77, 87

Magliocco S (2001–2002) Coordinates of power and performance festivals as sites of (Re) Presentation and reclamation in Sardinia, Ethnologies, vol 23(1), pp 167–189; 168

Papazian A (1971) Turkish documents about Armenia and Armenians from 16–19th Century. Yerevan Press, Yerevan

Author Biography

Astrik Vardanyan BA, received her BA in English Linguistics and Literature from the Institute of Foreign Languages, Yerevan, Armenia, in 1996, and her Masters degree in Anthropology at California State University, Northridge. She is a recipient of McArthur scholarship in journalism, a fellowship at the Bulletin of the Atomic Scientists in Chicago, Illinois, where she published articles on social and environmental issues. Her recent interests are cross-cultural child-rearing practices. She is an advocate of genital integrity for boys and girls, prolonged breastfeeding, co-sleeping, and natural birth. Vardanyan is inclined toward action or advocacy anthropology and employs her research to outreach the general public through media, seminars, and small group and individual talks. Northridge, California, USA.

Chapter 21
Self-Made Intactivism in the Middle East

Hatem Kamal Saied

Abstract Throughout the past decades, there has been little progress in the Arab world for promoting the end of the long-held practice of MGM. It is taken for granted that males should be circumcised, under several pretexts, where the strongest one is the absence of true information. With the emergence of a new means of communication, promoting anti-MGM thought has become easier. As a group of online activists, we created a Facebook group in Arabic, to be the strongest movement in the region so far promoting the end of MGM.

Keywords Islam • Koran Middle East • Circumcision • Facebook • MGM • UNICEF • WHO

I will mention a little bit about my experience as an example of how a person, even in the most highly circumcising region in the world, without prior knowledge or help, reached alone the realization that circumcision is wrong, and then did intensive work with others who joined in a campaign to stop circumcision in the Middle East. I was pleasantly surprised to find that there was an international campaign for the same cause. I will also address the issue of Islam and circumcision.

21.1 Introduction

Around 12 years ago, I read an article by Nawal El Saadawi stating that male circumcision is as wrong as female circumcision (Saadawi 1998). This was the first time I had heard such an opinion. At this time, there were no organizations in the Middle East dedicated to ending male genital mutilation (MGM). In fact, there are no such organizations even today. Scientific facts about circumcision

H. K. Saied (✉)
Founder of the first Arabic online society opposing MGM, Alexandria, Egypt
e-mail: htm_kml@yahoo.com

G. C. Denniston et al. (eds.), *Genital Cutting: Protecting Children from Medical, Cultural, and Religious Infringements*, DOI: 10.1007/978-94-007-6407-1_21,

are unknown there. This article opened my mind to the disaster that is circumcision. Fifteen months ago, when I learned about Facebook, I noticed it is widely used in campaigns of all kinds. I also noticed that there are many groups addressing female genital mutilation (FGM) in our region but no one is talking about MGM. I tried to convince these groups to incorporate both genders, but they were not interested. I discovered that MGM is a neglected subject, and reasoned that someone has to do it. I was so confident of my beliefs that I started a campaign.

21.2 Protecting Human Beings

I was armed by the logic that God did not create two separate types of human beings—man and woman—but only one type of human being, which comes in either one of two shapes, the male and the female. Therefore, the same organs or same tissues in one will certainly exist in the other—but just maybe different in size or shifted a little in place.

- Exist, yes.
- Perform the same function, yes.
- Give the same feeling, yes.

So protecting the genitals of one sex and cutting the other does not make sense and is not acceptable.

I was completely confident of that without even being a medical physician. I was convinced that, although this society worships medical physicians, what the medical community is doing is wrong.

Soon many people responded and some supporters became activists with me. We needed support at the beginning so we began by targeting people and organizations that were more secular and open-minded. We then broadened our campaign and attempted to raise public awareness for all people.

I do not know why at that time I could not find one organization like NOCIRC or one website like Doctors Opposing Circumcision. But we were always ready to enter discussions and debates armed by the amount of knowledge that we had, and we did just fine because it is a fact of nature and we are right, while circumcision supporters are wrong.

Most of the people we spoke to had never before heard anyone telling them to stop circumcising their boys. When the word circumcision is said without defining male or female, people think immediately about FGM but then are shocked when they realize that you are asking them to stop MGM.

After this shock, however, when they give themselves a chance to research and to read our literature, many agree with us. So there are potentially a large number of supporters, but many people are just waiting to hear the message.

21.3 Scientific Education Needed

Regarding scientific education about circumcision, for about 300 million Arabic speakers, there isn't any scientific book elaborating the functions of the foreskin and the harm of circumcision. There is not even one single scientific or medical book opposing circumcision written in the language (Arabic) spoken by people in nearly 20 countries. I hope that an author of such a book would consider issuing an Arabic version. The need is great, and I think the market is ready.

While the media in general does not publish positively about our activity, they do immediately publish reports about circumcision and HIV from such agencies as the CDC, AAP, or WHO, as if they were the ultimate truth.

I want to tell everyone who works for genital integrity that, by your organizations' work, you save children not only in your own countries, but you also save children far away from you in places you do not know. We in the Middle East use your information, research, and news of your activities to confront the news favoring circumcision. For example, if the MGM bill had passed in Massachusetts, the news would have travelled to shores thousands of miles away.

21.4 UNICEF

Another point to say is that one of the earliest arguments we faced from our opponents is the call of World Health Organization (WHO) to circumcise Africa for the supposed purpose of controlling the HIV epidemic. Our opponents frequently used that against us. We thought about UNICEF, the United Nations organization responsible for children, as the possible solution. Why don't we go and talk to them, and tell them something which it seems they do not know?

We thought we should tell them, "We are trying to protect our children from circumcision, and you are responsible for children, but another UN organization (WHO) is annoying us. WHO keeps issuing statements recommending circumcision to control HIV. WHO neglects to include a warning not to circumcise minors. In fact, they even monitored a circumcision of a 5-year-old boy." We imagined that if we told UNICEF that the child circumcisers in our country depend on WHO, that UNICEF would step in and help us. To our shock, we found that UNICEF knows all about it already. Moreover, UNICEF is itself involved in recommending, teaching, and advising (and possibly funding) for circumcision, although they are not directly involved in a program for clinically performing the surgery.

On page 8 of their document, *Children and AIDS: Third Stocktaking Report* (Children and AIDS: third stocktaking report 2008), UNICEF calls for infant male circumcision as a means of AIDS prevention, although infants and children do not perform sex. So, there is no justification to fear that they may contract STDs.

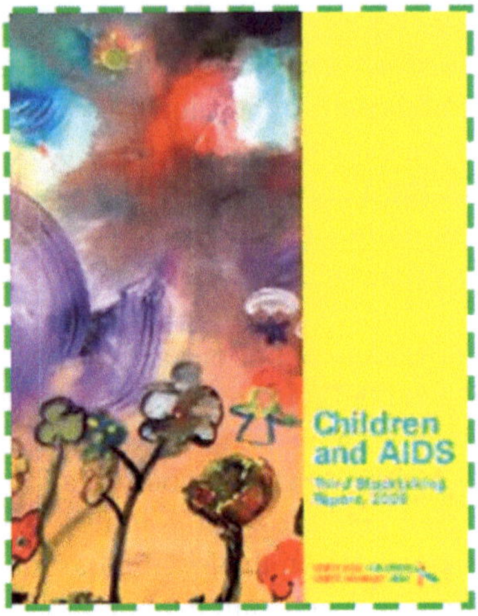

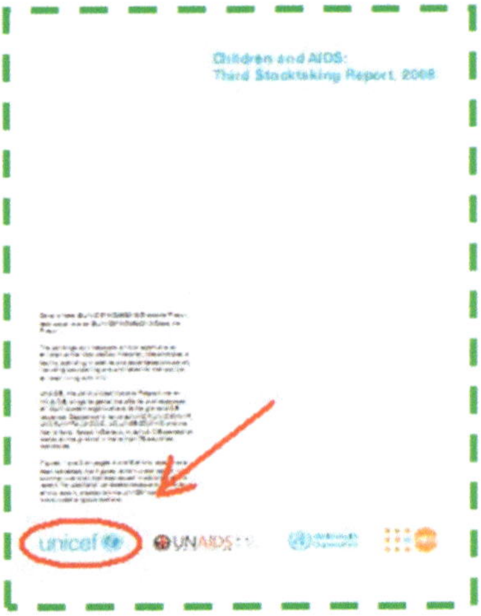

> Maternal and child health services, including PMTCT services, can be linked with male circumcision, including neonatal male circumcision and circumcision of HIV-negative male partners. These services can be delivered using a family-centred approach as part of an integrated programme of HIV prevention for mothers (both HIV-negative and HIV-positive) and, more broadly, for women of childbearing age, including adolescent girls. Implementation will need to be contextualized to the country situation and take into account the fact that investing in neonatal male circumcision will not result in tangible impacts for many years.

On page 20 of the same document, UNICEF suggests that adolescents be told positive information about circumcision at school and in their communities, and by advocates giving this same information to their fathers. They also suggest providing such surgical procedures during school vacation, training the circumcisers to speak friendly with the youth in order to involve them in trapping others into circumcision, involving the children as participants in making policies and strategies to attract their peers to circumcision, and recommending adoption of adolescent circumcision as part of countries' health strategies.

Male circumcision

Male circumcision, with full attention to safety, needs to be introduced as an additional strategy in a comprehensive package of prevention measures that includes condom use, reduction in number and concurrency of partners, and delaying the onset of sexual activity. In Swaziland, strategies are emerging on how best to reach adolescents through their schools and communities with accurate and relevant information about male circumcision. Activities include awareness raising among parents, making male circumcision available during school holidays, training staff to be 'youth-friendly' and reducing the cost of the procedure. Male circumcision can provide an important entry point for promoting safer sex practices, improving sexual and reproductive health and contributing to positive gender attitudes and behaviours.[66]

A September 2008 consultation on male circumcision in the Eastern and Southern Africa region, organized by the UN Inter-Agency Working Group on Prevention with the participation of youth organizations, recommended young people's involvement in the review and development of policies and strategies, in national mobilization efforts to increase demand for male circumcision and in the development of information materials. The consultation also recommended that male circumcision become part of countries' adolescent sexual and reproductive health strategies, thus having the potential to 're-energize' adolescent-friendly health services, among several other recommendations. Following the consultation, young people participated in the preparation of a question-and-answer document on male circumcision for use with other young people.[67]

In another document, Botswana Summary Results Matrix (2010–2014), on page 3, UNICEF states explicitly that one of its key tasks in Botswana is to increase male circumcision. Clearly, UNICEF is not addressing adults in this document because it is not an organization for adult affairs, so, who is UNICEF's discourse meant to address? Undoubtedly, it targets male infants, boys, and adolescents. An infant, child, or adolescent cannot even sign to open a bank account of his own, let alone to make a decision about an irreversible alteration of his body by cutting a healthy functional body part.

Summary Results Matrix: Government of	
MTSP Focus Area	**UNICEF Key Results Expected in this Focus Area/ Baseline Estimates for these Results**
	increase safe male circumcision, and correct and consistent condom use among adolescents
	3. 5 The proportion of vulnerable children whose households received external care and support from non family sources that supplement existing family-based activities, reaching at least 60%.

While the facts are against the procedures taken by UNICEF, WHO, and the UN Program to combat AIDS, those organizations, in a joint press release, say "Access to HIV therapy grew significantly in 2006"(http://www.unicef.org/media/media_39392.html. http://amcirc0.blogspot.com/. http://www.facebook.com/groups/37736989287/.)

> Recognize male circumcision as an important additional HIV prevention intervention. Recent clinical trial data demonstrate a significant reduction in the risk of heterosexually acquired HIV infection among circumcised men. Male circumcision could have a major public health impact in countries where HIV prevalence is high, transmission is predominantly through heterosexual contact, and rates of male circumcision are low. Such countries should urgently consider scaling up access to safe male circumcision services. Key issues in implementation include the quality and safety of services, cultural considerations, and adherence to human rights principles in the provision of male circumcision, including informed consent, confidentiality, and absence of coercion.

This document talks mentions "adherence to human rights principles in the provision of male circumcision, including informed consent, confidentiality, and absence of coercion." "Informed consent" cannot, of course, apply to male infants or minor boys.

There is even more evidence regarding UNICEF, but I will not elaborate as that research is available for you, if you wish to look at it.

We tried to approach the UNICEF Cairo office for discussion. The secretary, who supposedly is an educated person working in an international organization, didn't believe what she was hearing and asked me to repeat the phrase "male circumcision" five times to make sure she heard correctly. Finally, we were declined and treated impolitely.

The bad news is I learned that, at the AIDS Conference in Vienna 2010, UNICEF announced it is going to promote more or adopt a program for neonatal circumcision. I really wish they had heard us in Cairo.

21.5 Connecting with Others

After a while of working on our campaign, we received a contact from one Egyptian intactivist, Dr. Seham Abd el Salam, and a greeting from someone named Marilyn Milos. I thought, "Who is she?" Gradually, I came to know a lot of activists and organizations and saw their videos, read their papers, learned from them, and followed their activities.

I was inspired so much by what I saw, and we were able to convert the group to an information center (KNMG 2010). I filled it with selected videos, translating the content inside most of the videos and introducing activists to people in our region. I also introduced circumcision proponents under a special category (called "Know your enemy")—people like Brian Morris and Edgar Schoen. I told people to beware of their websites and to compare their messages with what is provided on other web sites. We provided summaries and answers suitable for replying to every claim. Because of what others have done, we can provide more powerful answers to each claim and alleged reason for circumcision. And we can provide many studies showing how harmful circumcision is, and we can state with much more detail the other side of the story. Our campaign crossed the borders of Egypt to other Arabian countries and some from these countries became activists with us. We never planned to do it, and never imagined we would do it, but here we are—an Arabic coalition, coming from different backgrounds and religions, Muslims, Christians, and Agnostics from many countries. We believe that, by now, many individuals have heard about our activity and we have managed to save some children from mutilation.

21.6 Islam and Circumcision

We often hear the counter-argument that male circumcision has not been completely prohibited in any European country. That is why, in our letters to the AAP and the CDC, we appealed to them not to recommend circumcision. But before

Western countries and organizations pass a law that completely prohibits neonatal non-therapeutic circumcision, they may need to communicate with the religious communities in their territory. That is what KNMG in Holland (KNMG 2010) tried to do and we sent a letter to support them.

It seems that the governments do not wish to prohibit circumcision as long as religions still practice it. And, religions do not renounce it because the government is still allowing it. It is a vicious circle and a Catch-22. Religions and governments each cannot stop circumcision until the other does.

Dr. Sami Aldeeb Abu-Salieh has written a very valuable book that addresses circumcision in Judaism, Christianity, and Islam (Abu-Salieh 2001). However, it is quite a lengthy tome (more than 1,000 pages). Honestly, the majority of the people in our nations do not have the energy to read. In addition, activists in foreign organizations would have difficulty in dealing with this research, due to its use of difficult ancient theological jargon and expressions. It is not accessible for general study or as a ready source of arguments against circumcision enthusiasts.

Now, we have experience in Muslim dialogue when it comes to this highly controversial debate. About ten of our members have engaged in heated debates over the past fifteen months with pro-circumcision enthusiasts. We have heard all the arguments, provided the counter arguments and also come up with new ideas and discoveries. That is why we thought about collecting the best of what we have read, written, or discovered and the most successful answers from the debates we have had, into a 4-page guide, our *Quick Guide to Dealing with Muslim Communities about Genital Integrity.*

According to Islam, when God had commanded Abraham to slaughter his own son, the father asked the son and the latter made the decision himself and told his father to carry out the order. This is an important point that no one paid attention to before; the Islamic story tells us that Abraham did not force his son to do something, even though it is a divine order. But, the decision was the son's and he accepted the slaughter. Therefore, we used this argument to respond to our opponents, calling on them to follow the manner of Abraham, if they really love to follow him, and leave the resolution to the son. Nobody could make a valuable counter argument to this point. It is also evident that, in the Koran, it is forbidden to cut or wound anybody, even an animal, and the Koran describes those who do this as followers of Satan.

Also, the Koran describes the human as "created in the best shape." The exception to that is when people do not believe in the perfection of the human body and engage in body modification, which actually degrades the body.

The Koran never mentions circumcision either explicitly or implicitly. All the "short statements" that are alleged to be Muhammad's and promote circumcision are contradictory, confusing, and false, as is proven brilliantly in Dr. Aldeeb's book and in our arguments with male circumcision enthusiasts.

We have emphasized that children do not have religious obligations and it is necessary that, when they do, they should perform such obligations out of free will and a mature mind.

Also, we have attempted to draw pro-circumcision enthusiasts' attention to an interesting analogy. The ritual of "confirmation" in Catholicism consists of an individual announcing his religious belief out of free will. We see this as similar to asking Muslims to wait until their children are old enough to use their own free will to decide whether or not to be circumcised. This gives children a chance to grow up and research circumcision themselves instead of it being forced upon them at birth.

Islam, for most of its adherents, relies not only on one book, the Koran, but also several extra books. These extra books contain the snapshots and short stories from the life of the Prophet and also short statements claimed to be said by the Prophet, and ideas and thoughts of ancient people and scholars. But in my opinion, true Islam is the holy book only, not these extra books. Every day, many more people come to this same belief.

One friend told me that he has read the Koran but, what he means is that he had read a translation of the Koran. What he read is erroneous because, when translators come to an expression in the Koran, they go to the extra books to get the meaning from them, and use it, giving the reader the erroneous translation, too. For example, there is no slavery in the Koran, but slavery is very prevalent in the extra books, so translators give you this meaning in the translation. As another example, you are aware that women wear head scarves, but there is nothing about scarves in the Koran. And, in the Koran, you can find a verse where God asks the women when they sit not to open their legs. That suggests that women at that time, the time of the Prophet, were wearing short skirts. Circumcision is just one more thing like that. It is not in Koran but in the extra books, and the clergy lead people to think it is part of the religion.

Parents, regardless of religion, sect, or belief, should be responsible for the safety of their children's bodies until they are grown up enough to make the decision to be circumcised or not for themselves.

We believe that all medical and children's rights organizations all over the world should pass strict laws that prohibit non-therapeutic genital modifications of children and leave no place for manipulation of the law.

Acknowledgments I want to thank Marilyn Milos and NOCIRC for the invitation to speak, Seham Abd El Salam for her support and for offering for me to go to the symposium in her place, Nihal Nour for her help in editing, Aya Sami and Saied Abd El Moaty for their brilliant ideas, and Amy Rosenberg for her endless unconditional heart and support.

References

Abu-Salieh SAA Dr (2001) Male and female circumcision among Jews, Christians and Muslims: religious, medical, social and legal debate, Warren Center, Shangri-La Publications, PA, p 400

Botswana Summary Results Matrix (2010–2014) http://www.unicef.org/about/execboard/files/Botswana_Summary_Results_Matrix_2010-2014__8_March_.pdf

Children and AIDS: third stocktaking report, 2008 http://www.unicef.org/StocktakingReport08_Full_FINAL_18_Nov_08.pdf.

KNMG (2010) http://knmg.artsennet.nl/Publicaties/KNMGpublicatie/Nontherapeutic-circumcision-of-male-minors-2010.htm

Saadawi NEL (1998) Stop male circumcision. Rose Alyousef Magazine, 21 Dec 1998

Author Biography

Hatem Kamal Saied BSc, Graduate Diploma, MSc, physics and IT, Alexandria University, is the founder of the first Arabic online society opposing MGM. Alexandria, Egypt.

Chapter 22
Genital Autonomy: A New Approach

David Smith

Abstract This chapter addresses the fundamental legal and medical issues involved with the phenomenon of genital cutting. The activities of existing international organizations dedicated to the eradication of harmful practices are highlighted, and a call is made for the formation of a new international and broad-ranging council that will harmonize the efforts of the existing organizations that address male and female circumcision as well as intersex issues.

Keywords Circumcision • Human rights • Genital integrity • Genital autonomy • Intersex • International child for genital autonomy

22.1 Introduction

The term "genital autonomy" came about at the 10th International Symposium on Circumcision, Genital Integrity, and Human Rights at Keele University in 2008. The international child was brought into focus when the concept for a truly universal, all-embracing organization for female, male, and intersex developed in discussion.

The International Child logo was created by Ofra Pleban, a Jewish woman, for the International Symposia on Circumcision, Genital Integrity, and Human Rights, a special project of the National Organization of Circumcision Information Resource Centers. The child not only embraces the subject matter but more importantly has worldwide appeal because the color is the perfect mix of every race, creed, and color. This instantly appealing symbol is not only evocative of the human form but also provides the initial letter of the word "Autonomy." With the International Child as its logo, Genital Autonomy (GA) was born.

D. Smith (✉)
General Manager, NORM-UK, Stone, Staffordshire, UK
e-mail: info@norm-uk.org

G. C. Denniston et al. (eds.), *Genital Cutting: Protecting Children from Medical, Cultural, and Religious Infringements*, DOI: 10.1007/978-94-007-6407-1_22,

22.2 What is Autonomy?

According to Wikipedia, autonomy refers to the capacity of a rational individual to make an informed, non-coerced decision. In moral and political philosophy, autonomy is often used as the basis for determining moral responsibility for one's actions. One of the best known philosophical theories of autonomy was developed by Kant. In medicine, respect for the autonomy of patients is an important goal, though it can conflict with a competing ethical principle, namely beneficence. Politically, it is also used to refer to the self-government of the people.

Distilling that concept down, Paul Mason gave the perfect definition when he said,

> This is the symbol for the right of all children—girls, boys, and intersex babies—to choose the form of their own genitals when they are old enough to decide.

Unnecessary genital surgery on babies is said to be cheaper and easier than on adults. All abuse of babies is easier. They are powerless and history will judge us by how we protect the powerless.

Let the children decide for themselves—all in good time—Paul Mason

22.3 Genital Autonomy

Having understood the concept and the worldwide need, it was a logical step to form Genital Autonomy into a charity. On June 2, 2010, the first meeting of the embryo organization was held in London, following which it has been registered as a UK charity with an initially small board of trustees headed by Richard Duncker, Margaret Green is the treasurer, Professor Michael Thomson, from Keele University School of Law is the Secretary, and the other trustee is Mary Cronk, MBE, who is a well-respected midwife. GA will be based in the small market town of Stone in Staffordshire, where it will initially share office premises with NORM-UK.

Although GA will be based in the UK, it is enhanced, in this age of instant technology and global communications, by having an international board, currently encompassing Paul Mason for Australasia, Seham Abd el Salam for Egypt, Michelle O'Brien for New Zealand, and, of course, when it came to covering the USA, there was nobody better nor more fitting than Marilyn Milos. You will be pleased to know that she has accepted.

22.4 Genital Cutting

Globally, most people have pre-conceptions as to not only why the procedures are done but, in most civilized nations, the belief that these barbaric practices are a thing of the past. When the dark satanic mills were the norm and showing a female ankle was considered racy, male circumcision was started in a vain attempt to stop or lessen masturbation, which was blamed, at that time, for dozens of diseases with unknown origins. What is not commonly known is that tens of thousands of girls were also circumcised for the same "reason." This was also recommended and found in US medical journals as late as 1959. Patricia Robinett gives a good account of this in her book, *The Rape of Innocence*. Interestingly, France has no special law against female genital cutting but the UK has prosecuted some 30 people already. We have a beautifully designed piece of FGM legislation that gathers dust on a shelf.

22.5 Intersex

Worldwide, even today, many babies are born intersex where doctors play god. With regard to intersex variations and genital autonomy, I can do no better than quote the words of Michelle O'Brien from OII:

> Intersex refers to atypical internal and/or external anatomical sexual characteristics, where features usually regarded as male or female may be mixed to some degree. This is a naturally occurring variation in humans. From the late 1950s onward, starting in the USA, intersex infants and children were increasingly subject to cosmetic surgeries intended to ensure that their genital appearance and internal gonads conformed to that usually expected for their assigned gender. This also tended to entail hormone treatments aimed at conforming them to those associated with being "male" or "female."

From the early 1990s to the present day, hundreds of intersex adults have come forward to say they regard these medical practices as being extremely harmful, both physically and psychologically. Despite this high level of dissatisfaction, there has been little follow-up of adults who were treated this way as children, so without any clear understanding of outcomes, there is no real evidence upon which to justify this approach. On the contrary, the little evidence there is suggests that physiologically, functional outcome is poor. A study conducted in England of intersex individuals who electively chose to undergo such surgery as adults revealed that the large majority were dissatisfied; treatments resulted in physical pain and diminished sexual response, and were not able to provide them with the sense of normalcy for which they had hoped.

There is no evidence that intersex variations alone will negatively impact the quality of life of the individuals who have them, nor that "normalizing" medical treatments are a solution. What evidence there is suggests the opposite—intersex adults who have not received unnecessary medical intervention have said they feel lucky to have "escaped" such treatments. They lack the psychological trauma from treatments imposed on others, and report satisfaction with their sexual response and their unique physical attributes.

Such treatment is often justified from the assumption that intersex children and/or adults will be subjected to discriminatory behavior because of their bodily differences; however, this is not necessarily correct, because their differences are sometimes only evident when naked, or not evident visually at all. Where differences are visible, this is no different than the situation of people from other minority groups. The solution to such challenges is not to alter the characteristics themselves, but to combat the prejudicial attitudes that stigmatize.

Cosmetic surgery on intersex genitals appears to harm intersex infants, children, and even adults, yet, it still persists. As with male circumcision, it is often driven by parental desire to provide their children with bodies that conform to certain beliefs about how genitals should be. Also, the presumption that atypical sex anatomy will result in atypical sexual orientation and/or gender identity, homophobia and a fear of atypical gender presentation are seen by some intersex as the motivation driving these surgeries. In many societies today, gender expression and sexual orientation are seen as a human right, and this is recognized by the UN. Performing unnecessary surgeries on infants and children in order to influence adult sexual orientation and/or gender identity outcomes should be seen as a human rights abuse. There is no evidence that sexual orientation or gender identity are affected by genital surgery one way or the other.

22.6 Treatments

We seek recognition that all humans have the right to autonomy over their own bodies, including their genitals. Because infants and children are too young to assert their autonomy, they should not be subjected to unnecessary surgeries that may irrevocably harm them, and that they may not have chosen as adults. We recognize that cases requiring medical treatment for the maintenance of health or preservation of life should be managed as with any other situation where a child needs treatment. Intersex infants and children should be raised without cosmetic surgery and/or steroidal hormones until they are old enough to decide for themselves whether they wish to undergo these procedures and treatments or not.

We recommend avoidance of genital cutting, where possible, until a child can fully participate in decision-making. This would be worked towards through communication between parents of intersex children, the children themselves, intersex adults, support groups, and clinicians who are sensitive to the needs of the child. Counselling should be available for those affected by the situation to ensure they are fully informed and equipped to make the best decisions. Wider education about intersex as a human variation is also necessary; the cultural anxiety and social pressure that encourage surgery, hormone therapy, and physical conformity need to be addressed. Through a process that includes education, communication, and counselling, public shame will decrease, along with a reduction of cultural anxiety and social pressure, ultimately allowing people the liberty to maintain autonomy over their own bodies.

22.7 Male Circumcision

In the UK, circumcision is not routine but is a recognized medical treatment, and we want to see the use of the excision of the foreskin restricted to the appropriate medical situations, which should make male genital cutting very rare.

Suzanne Jenkins, who is part of the Keele University Law Team headed by Professor Marie Fox and Professor Michael Thomson, is currently looking at NORM-UK's enquiries of interest. These reveal that, in the UK, those adults who have their foreskins excised for a medical problem, usually Type 2 phimosis, have few complaints. Type 2 is the grade given by Dr. Peter Ball to those men who cannot retract their foreskins either flaccid or erect. For such men, sex has been a painful and sometimes bloody process and the removal of the foreskin results in a more comfortable sex life. Better education for boys might well cure this problem. I personally favor the method pioneered by Dr. Michel Beaugé, that an effective masturbation technique was a fun way for teenagers to cure phimosis. The other group Suzanne looked at, those cut as children, had many complaints: feelings of inadequacy, rage, and a range of psychological problems (for example, depression, suicidal). MIND, a leading UK mental health charity, recognizes MGM as leading to this problem of psychological damage.

All non-therapeutic surgery, by definition, is harmful and there are many casualties and no proven benefits. Even if there are benefits, the boy in question cannot benefit until he becomes sexually active, at which time he can make up his own mind and decide how he wants to manage his own sex life. Circumcision is a risky surgery on a small and developing structure. It is easier and has the possibility of effective anesthesia when performed on an adult.

22.8 Joining Forces

The three separate strands—female, male, and intersex—have been plowing lonely furrows over the years, making heavy weather of the constantly slammed doors, non-returned phone calls, and lack of publicity. Together, by highlighting the basic foundations of human rights as well as shared problems, they become a much more powerful force with which to be reckoned. Cooperation should provide a significant support network of ideas, answers, and solutions, where one of the three strands has forged ahead in a particular area.

Harmful traditional or non-therapeutic genital cutting practices must not only be stopped but, initially, global publicity about the definite harm being caused by those practices needs its champions and exponents, the advocacy of whom will be the bedrock of the constitution of GA.

22.9 Objectives of Genital Autonomy

1. To promote, preserve, and protect the health and wellbeing of female, male, and intersex children by protecting them from non-therapeutic genital surgery or modification.

2. To promote human rights of children in relation to genital surgery or modification (as set out in the United Nations Convention on the Rights of the Child) throughout the world by all or any of the following means:
   (a) Relieving need among victims of human rights abuse;
   (b) Raising awareness of human rights issues;
   (c) Researching human rights issues that recognize the autonomy of diverse individuals;
   (d) Contributing to the sound administration of law, policy, and practice consistent with human rights.

Genital Autonomy will not replace or subsume organizations such as NORM-UK, NOCIRC, Intact America, FORWARD, or OII but, because it will be working with them, it will make a much more powerful voice in the world media and, hopefully, will gather greater momentum to influence government policy and ultimately change the relevant laws safeguarding children worldwide, once and for all.

A good example of this could be the huge publicity drive of Intact America and the lessons learned from the media coverage, where this evaluation can be shared and provide a valuable basis for GA. Similarly, the pioneering work of NOCIRC and NORM-UK, under the leadership of Marilyn Milos and John Warren, will provide the catalyst for moving the male issue of GA upwards and outwards and many of the lessons we have learned through these organizations will be equally appropriate to the other two strands within GA.

This is going to be a mountain to climb. We are not averse to working with any organization or individual that can provide contacts to move GA forward because, without your individual support and enthusiasm, as we all know from our experiences, tackling this complicated and complex subject matter, is never high on the agenda of those in medical fraternities. GA needs to break down the barriers so that, like the change in HIV/AIDS, it becomes a universally acceptable topic discussed without embarrassment or censure.

In popular literature, the plight of Somali women has been used as a sub plot by the author, Ruth Rendell, in her novel, *Not in the Flesh.* The review of this book says: The second social aspect that runs like a red thread through the book is genital mutilation and cultural tolerance. Chief Inspector Wexford and his wife are friends with a Somali family. This family came to Great Britain so that their daughters would be protected from genital mutilation. Other families, however, still practice this ritual. Chief Inspector Wexford is drawn into the debate through several avenues, one of them his daughter's activist stance against female genital mutilation. Another one is his officers' action when they have a chance to prevent a case, at least for the time being.

Chief Inspector Wexford thinks about genital mutilation from various perspectives, but like in real life, he does not come to a conclusion. The question is where cultural tolerance ends and becomes a feminist or human rights issue. Although female genital mutilation is illegal in Great Britain and in the United States, enforcing this law is difficult. And what are the results? In "Not in the Flesh," the girl eventually ends up in state custody because of the fear of genital mutilation.

Now, is that a better solution than being in a loving family? This and related questions have no easy answers as *Not in the Flesh* makes very clear.

The plight of the intersex has also been featured by Jeffrey Eugenides in Middlesex, which is partly set in San Francisco but to date nobody has been brave enough to cover the male aspect of our subject. The story of David Reimer did not focus on circumcision as the cause of his problem. Hopefully, one day an author will be brave enough to tackle male circumcision as the main plot rather than the sub-plot and write what would become a national best seller.

Combining all three strands of the Genital Integrity Movement will help each to become more widely appreciated. Universally discussed as the sum of the three parts is a more powerful and meaningful message than individual aspects battling alone and facing the inevitable political comment.

Worldwide, the plight of the child is beginning to be more widely examined. In the UK, NORM-UK has been working closely with both the London and Manchester Metropolitan Police who now recognize that male circumcision has the same horrific consequences as FGM. Pioneering research is being carried out by Marie Fox and Michael Thomson at Keele University. In Holland, the Royal Dutch Medical Association (the KNMG) has published a ground-breaking position paper on non therapeutic male child circumcision, which calls for a "powerful policy of deterrence," if not an outright ban. This can only strengthen our case.

In the world media, the advocacy of intersex is now openly discussed, thanks to the controversy surrounding the gender of South African runner, Caster Semenya. In a statement to the press, Semenya stated that "God made me the way I am and I accept myself."

In the wake of the Semenya publicity, nothing is more powerful than having Sarah Graham on national radio in the UK eloquently describe how the medical profession treated her, disguising the truth that she was born intersex by telling her parents, when she was nine, that her ovaries—when in fact they were testicles—could become cancerous and needed to be removed. The truth was only told when Sarah was in her twenties, causing untold psychological damage in the process.

She, through her courage, has opened a tiny crack in the door of knowledge and understanding, which GA needs to open wider and broadcast to the population, not only in the numbers of children born intersex even today but about leaving them alone. The matter can be rectified at a later stage, without an ill-informed surgeon deciding for and on behalf of the child, especially where they have a minimum 50 % chance of inaccuracy.

The medical procedures undertaken at the neonatal stage for the intersex can be equally channelled to the movement of the anti male and female circumcision cause, which has been the ultimate taboo subject in cultured civilizations. Activists need to help break down the barriers about the whole subject matter.

We need GA to receive the same recognition internationally as Amnesty International and Greenpeace have, but this will only happen by everybody supporting the embryo organization and assisting GA to be like the proverbial pebble rolling downhill, not gathering moss but, instead and more importantly, gathering momentum so that the symbol is recognized worldwide and the topic the subject of polite conversation in every family group.

Author Biography

David Smith Was educated at St. Joseph's College, Market Drayton, and he qualified in business studies at Underwood College. He worked for Re-Solv, a solvent abuse charity, and is currently General Manager of NORM-UK, a charity dedicated to giving men a choice and the General Manager of Genital Autonomy, a charity dedicated to protecting the genital autonomy rights of male, female, and intersex infants and children. He created and now edits *NORM NEWS,* the organization's magazine for members and concerned individuals. Stone, Staffordshire, UK.

Index

G. C. Denniston et al. (eds.), *Genital Cutting: Protecting Children from Medical, Cultural, and Religious Infringements*, DOI: 10.1007/978-94-007-6407-1,

MIX
Papier aus verantwortungsvollen Quellen
Paper from responsible sources
FSC® C105338

If you have any concerns about our products,
you can contact us on
ProductSafety@springernature.com

In case Publisher is established outside the EU,
the EU authorized representative is:
Springer Nature Customer Service Center GmbH
Europaplatz 3, 69115 Heidelberg, Germany

Printed by Libri Plureos GmbH
in Hamburg, Germany